STONEWALL INN EDITIONS
Keith Kahla, General Editor

By Larry Kramer

Reports from the holocaust:

the story of an AIDS activist

Larry Kramer

St. Martin's Press
New York

REPORTS FROM THE HOLOCAUST: THE STORY OF AN AIDS ACTIVIST. Copyright © 1981, 1982, 1983, 1984, 1985, 1986, 1987, 1988, 1989, 1990, 1991, 1992, 1993, 1994 by Larry Kramer.

Foreword copyright © 1994 by Simon Watney

Design by Robin Malkin

Library of Congress Cataloging-in-Publication Data

Kramer, Larry.
    Reports from the holocaust / Larry Kramer.
      p. cm.
    ISBN 0-312-11419-2 (paperback)
    1. AIDS (Disease)—Social aspects—United States.
2. Homosexuality. Male—United States. 3. AIDS activists—United States. I. Title.
RC607.A26K73   1994
362.1'969792'00973—dc20   94-21883
                                          CIP

For Rodger McFarlane

They have spoken against you everywhere,
But weigh this song with the great and their pride;
I made it out of a mouthful of air,
Their children's children shall say they have lied.

—"He Thinks of Those Who Have
Spoken Evil of His Beloved"
by W. B. Yeats

Contents

Part Four

Acknowledgments

M any people, some unknowingly, conspire to help one become an "activist." Particularly when, as in my case, I never wanted to be one. If the playwright Robert Chesley had not attacked me one day in 1981, long ago when we were young, in the columns of the gay newspaper the *New York Native,* and if I had not at that time been in therapy with the prescient Dr. Norman Levy, who encouraged me to stop kvetching and respond, I often wonder if I should have been so caught up in what at first was only to be a slight and momentary adjunct to my "other" writing. So, ironically, I must first thank Bob Chesley (and, of course, as always, Norman), and it is to him that my friends and foes can give their gratitude; certainly he has mine.

I thank Chuck Ortleb, the editor-in-chief and publisher of the *Native,* for allowing me the many pages of his newspaper my prose has gobbled up, even when our opinions differed, and his two impeccable editors, first Brett Averill and then Patrick Merla. For those gaffes they caught and I refused to budge on, I take full blame.

Michael Denneny has been all that any writer could ask for in an editor. That he suggested this book puts me in his debt for a start, but the energy and enthusiasm he has lavished on an enterprise that is as far from being a remunerative best-seller as can be imagined have been extremely moving to me. His help on the long essay that is Part Two of this book is particularly acknowledged.

Because I'm convinced everything I've ever written always falls on deaf ears, it is to those who have been kind enough to write or call me, or stop me on the street to offer encouraging words for my efforts, that I also owe appreciation. It's helped keep me going, particularly when I've been roundly criticized, as well as got me back after my periodic burnouts when I vowed Never Again.

No one involved in fighting AIDS does so without the constantly insistent, haunting, painful memories of many too many friends who aren't here in body anymore. They, more than anyone or anything else, have provided all the necessary fuel my energy requires.

My dear loving and loved Rodger McFarlane has lived through all of this with me, and has read, critiqued, and contributed no small input into most of these pieces. He is one of the noblest human beings ever to grace this currently crummy world. This world, and this writer, is lucky to have him, and it is with great admiration, respect, and devotion that I dedicate this book to him.

May he, and I, and everyone still with us, remain among the living.

Foreword

THE PERSISTENCE OF MEMORY

*Ever since the Mayflower Compact was drafted and signed
under a different kind of emergency, voluntary associations
have been the specifically American remedy for the
failure of institutions, the unreliability of men,
and the uncertain nature of the future.*

Hannah Arendt*

L arry Kramer is probably best known in Europe as the Oscar-nominated screenwriter of Ken Russell's *Women in Love* and the author of the best-selling satirical novel *Faggots*. Yet he spent most of the 1980s working relentlessly to communicate the grim realities of AIDS against the grain of the massive sensationalism, trivialization, and flagrant misreporting of the American mass media. Nobody has written with greater passion of the American AIDS epidemic, and nobody has done more to help gay men take the threat of HIV infection seriously, especially in the long years before the discovery of the virus. Nor has anyone done more to draw public attention to the continuing scandal of official U.S. government neglect and the mismanagement of a health crisis that has already claimed more than a hundred thousand lives in the United States alone.

Reports from the holocaust contains a chronological selection from the steady torrent of articles and speeches that Kramer has produced since the very beginning of the epidemic. In this respect it should be noted that activists such as Kramer have now

---

**Hannah Arendt, "Civil Disobedience," in *Crises of the Republic* (New York: Harvest/ HBJ, 1971), p. 102.

been campaigning about AIDS for longer than the duration of
the first and second world wars *combined*. This work has been
immensely complex and exhausting. As he explains: "Everything
was uncharted territory for all of us. Events were happening too
quickly to bear. Issues were constantly shifting in importance.
And becoming hugely complicated. Quickly we had to master
these complications, understand new scientific, medical, pharmaceutical vocabularies, and juggle them adeptly so we could
defend ourselves. . . ."* Indeed, one of the most important aspects of the book is the direct way in which it provides a sense
of the constantly changing debates that have characterized the
course of the epidemic, and the extreme difficulties facing community leaders and organizations dealing with institutions that
refuse to accept their validity and show no interest in, or understanding of, the actual lives and values of the social groups most
drastically affected by the results of widespread HIV infection
in the years before the existence of HIV was even suspected.

Yet Kramer's work has not only been defensive. He has also
been centrally involved in establishing organizations that have
been able to represent and campaign on behalf of the needs of
people living with HIV and AIDS, and their communities. His
own involvement in the AIDS crisis stemmed from only too real
and immediate experience. Friends and acquaintances were sick-
ening and dying all around, yet there seemed to be no great sense
of urgency to provide care and social service support, or medical
research, or preventative health education, from either Washington or New York's City Hall. It was not until Thanksgiving
1987, with a known total of 25,644 dead from AIDS in the United
States, that President Reagan was able even to so much as mention the word AIDS in public, and then only to state that he was
asking the Department of Health and Human Services "to determine as soon as possible the extent to which the AIDS virus
has penetrated our society."** This is the shocking context in
which we can begin to appreciate Kramer's fury at the scale of
indifference to the lives of those most directly threatened by

---

*See Kramer's introduction to this volume, page xxxi.
**Cited in Douglas Crimp, "AIDS: Cultural Analysis/Cultural Activism," in D. Crimp
(ed.), *AIDS: Cultural Analysis, Cultural Activism* (Cambridge, Mass.: MIT Press, 1988),
p. 11.

HIV. As he notes: "One of the saddest lessons I have learned from this epidemic is that the true heterosexual liberal, for some unaccountable reason, is not necessarily the gay person's friend. He or she will fight for blacks, women, Hispanics, abortion, nuclear disarmament, keeping the Jefferson Library open all week. But when it comes to homosexuality, they get queasy."*

Since 1981 Kramer has been writing and giving interviews in a huge variety of American publications, from *The New York Times* to the *New York Native*, which was at the time the most important weekly gay newspaper in the USA. He has also been instrumental in the establishment of two of the most important AIDS organizations in America. Thus it was that Kramer, together with a small group of friends, began to raise funds in the summer of 1982 in order to found Gay Men's Health Crisis (GMHC) in New York, which is now the largest nongovernment AIDS service organization in the world. However, as he points out: "Most of GMHC's efforts are devoted to providing services the *city* should be providing. . . ."** His analysis of the situation facing New York in 1982 makes both inspiring and depressing reading, since so much of what he had to say was extraordinarily perceptive, while few of the urgent needs that he accurately recognized have been subsequently met. For example, he identified six initial areas of concern: first, the need for medical research; second, the dismal track record of American journalism; third, the ignorance about gay men among professional care providers; fourth, the need for local and national planning; fifth, the failure of local government in New York; and, last, the scale of initial denial among gay men.

It was in response to this last factor that Kramer launched his most celebrated invective, "1,112 and Counting," in the spring of 1983, which must be counted as one of the most important public statements in the entire history of the U.S. epidemic. Addressed to gay men, it began: "If this article doesn't scare the shit out of you, we're in real trouble. If this doesn't rouse you to anger, fury, rage and action, gay men may have no future on this earth. Our continued existence depends on just how angry you

---

*See "Second-Rate Voice," pages 98–99 of this volume.
**See "An Open Letter to Richard Dunne and Gay Men's Health Crisis," page 103 of this volume.

can get."* His outspoken evangelical tone has offended some, but
it is important to think about whom he was trying to reach and
what other forms of rhetoric might have been more successful
in communicating his message. Here, as in so much else, he
proved himself a brilliant strategist, able to stimulate debate and
action in all the many tribes that make up American gay male
society. He assumed the onerous mantle of the gay community's
punitive father-figure; and, as he is well aware, this could not be
guaranteed to endear him to all gay men. However, the dismis-
sive accusations that he is "hysterical" and overstates his case
should always be measured against the truly frightening official
understating of the gravity of the AIDS crisis throughout the
entire history of the epidemic. It also ignores Kramer's deeper
aim, which is to bond gay men together in the shared awareness
that they have been systematically denied their rights—to
potentially life-saving health education and potentially helpful
treatment drugs.

Throughout the AIDS crisis Kramer's work has been distinguished by his refusal to prioritize health education or treatment
issues and by his assertion that both are vitally important. As
he has constantly insisted: "THERE IS NOTHING IN THIS
WHOLE AIDS MESS THAT IS NOT POLITICAL!"** Read-
ing *Reports from the holocaust,* one realizes the full extent of his
prescience. As early as March 1983 he was remarking on the
probable need for civil disobedience to obtain adequate funding
and other resources: "I hope we don't have to conduct sit-ins or
tie up traffic or get arrested. I hope our city and our country will
start to do something to help start saving us. But it is time for
us to be perceived for what we truly are: an angry community
and a strong community, and therefore *a threat.*"† By early 1983
he was also already criticizing GMHC, which he had helped to
set up, for opposing the extension of their efforts from providing
services to an active advocacy role, which the organization refused to assume. By now he already had something of the reputation of a "crazy man" in some circles, though his supposed

---

*See "1,112 and Counting," page 33 of this volume.
**See "An Open Letter to Richard Dunne and Gay Men's Health Crisis," page 110 of
this volume.
†See "1,112 and Counting," page 48 of this volume.

craziness consisted of no more than the repeated insistence that gay men might have to take direct action in order to obtain their rights: "It doesn't cost any money to have a troop of volunteers picket City Hall . . . [or] flood switchboards with complaints when *The New York Times* runs something ignorant and hateful."* In 1987 he sadly described how "for the past five years I have painfully watched as GMHC has attempted to be all things to all people, in so doing losing complete sight of the larger picture, of what is happening. . . . The bigger you get, the more cowardly you become; the more money you receive, the more self-satisfied you are. No longer do you fight for the living; you have become a funeral home."**

However, in one of the several retrospective "asides" with which the book is punctuated, Kramer describes how he persuaded GMHC to employ Dr. Barry Gingell as the head of a new Office of Medical Information. This in itself was a major achievement, for Barry Gingell, who sadly died in the summer of 1989, was soon to become the first editor of *Treatment Issues*, a newsletter of experimental AIDS therapies that has proved to be one of the most useful publications in the entire AIDS field. It continues to provide reliable, up-to-date scientific information to people living with HIV and AIDS and to the wider AIDS community, nationally and internationally.

Nonetheless, although GMHC took up the challenge of addressing medical issues, including the scandalous delays in testing new drugs, and making such trials open to as many people as possible, the organization was not willing to take on the direct advocacy role that Kramer had wanted. So in 1987 he called an open meeting at the New York Lesbian and Gay Community Center, from which the AIDS Coalition to Unleash Power (ACT UP) was born. It is no exaggeration to state that ACT UP became the most significant direct-action campaign in the United States since the anti–Vietnam war movement in the 1960s.† As he has described: "ACT UP became strong and healthy very

---

*See "We Can Be Together," page 81 of this volume.
**See "An Open Letter to Richard Dunne and Gay Men's Health Crisis," pages 101–2 of this volume.
†See Simon Watney, Introduction, in E. Carter and S. Watney (eds.), *Taking Liberties: AIDS and Cultural Politics* (London: Serpent's Tail, 1989).

quickly. The group is, for me, infinitely moving to witness, because it is composed mostly of such young people. These are men and women, some barely in their twenties, who have a comfort with their homosexuality that I never had at that age, and a desire to be politically active that, at such a young age, for such large numbers, is actually historically new and important in the ongoing struggle for gay rights."*

This gives the lie to critics who have accused Kramer of losing sight of the wider objective of gay rights and of becoming obsessive about AIDS. For, as historian Jeffrey Escoffier points out: "Not only has the AIDS epidemic mobilized more gay men than any other issue in the history of the gay movement, but it has led to a greatly increased appreciation of gay rights."** In both these respects Kramer has played a central and indispensable role. Moreover, attempts to brand him as a ranting extremist ignore the extent to which he has successfully drawn attention to the iniquitous condition of American private medicine and the conflict of interests between the financial priorities of the multinational pharmaceutical industry and people's health. Furthermore, he has consistently helped translate medical opinion into the terms of community awareness. He has deliberately set out to transform people's personal anger, and their sense of loss, into a genuine popular movement, into collective *action*. More than anybody else it was Larry Kramer who recognized the political implications of the stark observation by Dr. Mathilde Krim, founding co-chair of the American Foundation for AIDS Research (AmFAR), that "everything about this epidemic has been utterly predictable, utterly, utterly and completely predictable, from the very beginning, from the very first day. But no one would listen. There are many people who knew exactly what was happening, what would happen and has happened, but no one of importance would listen."†

Eventually it did prove necessary to conduct sit-ins, to tie up traffic, and for large numbers of people to get arrested. But the effects of such direct action have been spectacular, both in terms of media coverage and in forcing the testing and release of po-

---

*See "The Beginning of ACTing UP," page 139 of this volume.
**Jeffrey Escoffier, letter in the *Nation*, March 20, 1989, p. 377.
†Cited by Kramer in "The Plague Years," page 150 of this volume.

tential treatment drugs after years of official recalcitrance and red tape. Kramer concludes without apology: "If I use gross language—go ahead, be offended—I don't know how else to reach you, how to reach everybody."* This book is but one further means to that end. It is also a major contribution to the testimonial literature that the epidemic is now beginning to accumulate. Yet it is far more than just a personal account of what one man did in the AIDS crisis. In his essay "Report from the holocaust," Kramer provides an overview of the epidemic, trying to make sense of the levels of bigotry and neglect that have played such a crucial part in delaying effective community-based health education, services, and medical research. He also locates his work in the moving personal context of his relations with his own Jewish family. He explains how and why he has reluctantly come to believe "that genocide is occurring: that we are witnessing—or *not* witnessing—the systematic, planned annihilation of some by others with the avowed purpose of eradicating an undesirable portion of the population. I know that straight Jews, and other heterosexuals, find this comparison of holocausts repugnant. . . . I am not unfamiliar with charges of hysteria and hyperbole. To read Primo Levi is to know that our suffering, as of this moment, is still small in comparison. But Primo Levi also writes, 'A certain dose of rhetoric is perhaps indispensable for memory to persist.' One inadvertent fall-out from *the* Holocaust is the growing inability to view any other similar tragedies as awful . . . the insistence on its primogeniture frustrates efforts to arouse equal public concern when the newest children on the block arrive, demanding immediate succor."**

At this point, British readers might care to contemplate the full significance of the fact that every penny of the £40.5 million that the Medical Research Council has received for medical research has gone to the development of a vaccine for the uninfected, while none has gone to the development of clinical trials for potential treatment drugs. People living with HIV and AIDS have simply been written off in their entirety. This is hardly surprising, given the belief stated by a leading British professor of microbiology, whose work is supported by the Medical Re-

---

*See "I Can't Believe You Want to Die," page 171 of this volume.
**See "Report from the holocaust," page 263 of this volume.

search Council, that treatment research raises a "moral dilemma" since it would "run the risk" of "prolonging the lives of people who would remain infectious in the community."* One wonders of what other social group afflicted by an incurable sexually transmitted virus might it be said that treatment research raises a "moral dilemma." Nor can such sentiments be dismissed as aberrant, since the same eloquently murderous homophobia was recently restated on the editorial page of the widely read and respected science magazine *Nature*, which pointed to the "bizarre possibility that, by prolonging the period of normalcy of the infection, general use of AZT might increase the potential for spreading infection."** Hence the urgent need to reconcile the currently conflicting interests of bio-medical research and clinical medicine. It is no surprise that Kramer should choose to quote from the 1988 Presidential Commission on AIDS, which concluded: "The Administration's response to AIDS has from the start been torpid, fitful, fragmented and riven with prejudice against those infected with the virus."† The Commission's report has, of course, been entirely neglected.

"Report from the holocaust" is also taken up with the widespread political passivity of many gay men, in spite of the AIDS crisis. Looking back over the 1970s, Kramer has remarked of himself that "the kind of person I was then would infuriate me now."‡ Yet he is also well aware that "there is no way in the world that there is ever going to be 'unity' in any population as large as ours. It's a waste of breath even wishing for it. It's totally unrealistic. There are too many constituencies, which is as it should be."§ In this context it is surely significant that none of the organizations that have successfully emerged to meet the many changing challenges of AIDS has derived from traditional mainstream politics. They have all been community responses, inspired above all by the concept of civil rights, and they have been beset by similar problems throughout the West. For ex-

---

*Cited in Simon Watney, "Tasks in AIDS Research," *Gay Times*, No. 128, London, May 1989, pp. 18–19.
**Anon., "AIDS Now a Tractable Disease?" *Nature*, Vol. 340, August 31, 1989, p. 663.
†See "Report from the holocaust," page 267 of this volume.
‡Personal communication.
§Larry Kramer, "A Word from Larry Kramer," *New York Native*, July 4, 1989, p. 8.

ample, the conflict between effective service provision and political advocacy is as pronounced in London and Paris and Berlin as it is in New York or Chicago. Nongovernment AIDS service organizations invariably face the impossible situation in which they are simultaneously expected to educate and support "everyone," thereby ignoring the special needs of injecting drug users and gay men, and to provide special services for the worst-affected communities that governments refuse to acknowledge for fear that they will be accused of "promoting" either drug use or homosexuality. There can be no more brutal index of the depths of anti-gay prejudice than the direct governmental interference and censorship of effective safer sex education for gay men in Britain and the USA at the height of an epidemic for which preventative medicine currently holds the only solution.* Indeed, the British and American governments appear to be enthusiastically willing to intervene in the AIDS crisis only in order to hinder and impair effective community-based AIDS education and awareness. As the American critic Cindy Patton has concluded: "It is a mark of the intransigence of homophobia that few look to the urban gay communities for advice, communities which have an infrastructure and a track record of highly successful behaviour change."** Such attention would run the grave risk of acknowledging that gay men are much like everybody else, except in the seriousness of their response to HIV, and that their experience might prove to be of vital importance for the rest of the population. Hence the significance of Kramer's description of how he wrote his internationally successful play *The Normal Heart:* "to make people cry: AIDS is the saddest thing I'll ever have to know. I also wrote it to be a love story, in honor of a man I loved who died. I wanted people to see on a stage two men who loved each other. I wanted people to see them kiss. I wanted people to see that gay men in love and gay men suffering and gay men dying are just like everyone else."† Research strongly supports the belief that countering anti-gay prejudice

---

*See Simon Watney, Introduction, *Taking Liberties.*
**Cindy Patton, "Resistance and the Erotic," in P. Aggleton et al. (eds.), *AIDS: Social Representations, Social Practices* (Lewes: Falmer Press, 1989), p. 238.
†See "We Can Be Together," page 94 of this volume.

should be a central theme in effective AIDS education for heterosexuals, who will continue to ignore the epidemic for just as long as they continue to regard it as only a gay issue.*

Larry Kramer is a man who found his voice in a crisis. While it is still too early for extensive histories of the epidemic, we may be sure that the material contained within *Reports from the holocaust* will eventually be recognized as an unparalleled record of personal achievement. As the crisis deepens, more and more people will come to agree with his own verdict that he is "blessed with hard-nosed, cold sanity, which becomes more objective and realistic day by day."** He alerted an entire generation of gay men, and many others, to the unthinkable realities of HIV and AIDS. Nor has he ceased to chide and cajole. Although he has often referred to the sheer number of his friends and acquaintances who have died of AIDS, it is important to note that the safer-sex revolution among gay men was, in the great majority of cases, motivated not by direct personal loss but by the establishment of community values, for which Larry Kramer is as responsible as anyone. Since October 1988 he has known that he also has HIV. The last time I saw him was at the third national Lesbian and Gay Studies Conference at Yale in September 1989, modestly selling ACT UP T-shirts to incoming delegates opposite the registration desk. In the meantime, as he points out, "Each day things get worse and worse." When I recently asked him what sustains him, it seemed entirely in keeping with the man that he replied it was the knowledge that he is HIV antibody positive. He is also inspired by the example of his favorite writers—Waugh, Zola, Dostoyevsky, and, above all, Charles Dickens, of whom he says: "He saw a society he didn't like and a lot of injustices and he dramatized them, and I feel that's what writing should be for me. . . . In this country, the writer as moralist or the writer as a presence in the work is considered as very bad taste and bad form: the writer should somehow mysteriously disappear. God

---

*See Simon Watney, "Safer Sex as Community Practice," in P. Aggleton et al. (eds.), *AIDS: Individual, Cultural and Political Dimensions* (Lewes: Falmer Press), 1990.
**See "An Open Letter to Richard Dunne and Gay Men's Health Crisis," page 103 of this volume.

forbid that he should have an opinion that's reflected in the work. I think that's all bullshit!"*

In November 1989 he distributed an article entitled "We Must Make Tomorrow Happen Today" at a regular ACT UP meeting in New York.** After summarizing an increasingly difficult situation in the United States, and explaining why he believes that the AIDS community is in more trouble than for some time, he concludes inspirationally: "Personally, ACT UP gives me my greatest energy and my greatest reason for being alive. We have already proved so much to the world and to our fellow gay men and lesbians. Mark Harrington is fond of saying the world's revolutions did not happen when there was no hope. They happen when there *is* hope, and when the system can't keep up with the rising expectations of the maligned and the downtrodden. We have discovered that there is hope that this epidemic, as Dr. Broder says, can be cured. We must clutch this hope every day to our hearts and use what we are entitled to— what is just out there, over there, is being denied to us and we demand it, that it be ours. It's there, still out of reach, but coming closer. We can't stop now. We've started the revolution. We can't quit until we finish it."

In the course of the relatively few years that I have known Larry it has frequently struck me that he embodies a certain American tradition of rugged faith in the possibility of community values that is intimately connected to the notion of *consent* that is the cornerstone of American jurisprudence. As Hannah Arendt has argued: "Consent and the right to dissent became the inspiring and organizing principles of action that taught the inhabitants of this continent the 'art of associating together,' from which sprang those voluntary associations whose role Tocqueville was the first to notice, with amazement, admiration, and some misgiving; he thought them the peculiar strength of the American political system."† The creation of such vitally important organizations as GMHC and ACT UP has been en-

---

*Personal communication.
**See "We Must Make Tomorrow Happen Today," page 294 of this volume.
†Hannah Arendt, "Civil Disobedience," p. 94.

tirely consistent with the spirit that has for centuries informed
the construction of essentially ad hoc voluntary associations with
specific, concrete goals. To this should be added the powerful
American sense of *citizenship* and the aspiration of lesbians and
gay men to enjoy the same rights as all other American citizens.
The absence of an equally powerful sense of civil rights in the
United Kingdom makes *Reports from the holocaust* all the more
important for British readers. Larry has sown dragons' teeth,
and they have grown up fast to become the most confident, organized, and articulate generation of lesbian and gay activists on
earth. For this reason alone it remains possible to agree with
Hannah Arendt's conclusion some twenty years ago concerning
the United States, that "as distinguished from other countries,
this republic, despite the great turmoil of change and of failure
through which it is going at present, may still be in possession
of its traditional instruments for facing the future with some
degree of confidence."* As for Larry Kramer, he will only state
that he doesn't consider himself an artist: "I consider myself a
very opinionated man who uses words as fighting tools. I perceive certain wrongs that make me very angry, and somehow I
hope that if I string my words together with enough skill, people
will hear them and respond. I am under no delusion that this will
necessarily be the case, but I seem to have no choice but to
try."**

Meanwhile, the AIDS crisis continues, and the question of
why so little has been done becomes more pressing than ever;
hence the significance of Kramer's emphasis on the most murderous, and even genocidal, aspects of the social policies that
have determined the course of the epidemics in both Britain and
the United States. For it would be invidious indeed if we were
to abandon any attempt to learn, in the midst of one catastrophe, from another and earlier tragedy. If there are lessons to
be learned from all of this, they seem not dissimilar to those
suggested by Zygmunt Bauman's book *Modernity and the
Holocaust:* "The lesson of the Holocaust is the facility with
which most people, put into a situation that does not contain a
good choice . . . argue themselves away from the issue of moral

---

*Ibid., p. 102.
**See "Message Queen," page 145 of this volume.

duty . . . adopting instead the precepts of rational interest and self-preservation. *In a system where rationality and ethics point in opposite directions, humanity is the main loser. . . .* And there is another lesson of the Holocaust, of no lesser importance. . . . The second lesson tells us that putting self-preservation above moral duty is in no way predetermined, inevitable and inescapable. One can be pressed to do it, but one cannot be forced to do it, and thus one cannot really shift the responsibility for doing it on to those who exerted the pressure. *It does not matter how many people choose moral duty over the rationality of self-preservation—what does matter is that some did."*

Simon Watney
January 1990

Postscript

And so things stood in 1990. Rereading *Reports from the holocaust* four years later, together with the subsequent material now included in this updated second edition, only serves to reinforce my previous sense of the enduring, powerful significance of the original text. The U.S. Public Health Service currently projects that by the end of 1994 in the United States, "the cumulative number of diagnosed AIDS cases will be in the range 415,000–535,000, with 320,000–385,000 cumulative deaths. In 1994 alone there are expected to be 43,000–93,000 newly diagnosed cases of AIDS, and 45,000–76,000 deaths—primarily among persons diagnosed in previous years."** As of November 1993, 201,775 Americans had already died from AIDS, with between 1 and 1.5 million infected by HIV. Meanwhile, in the United Kingdom by the end of 1993, of the 5,653 deaths from AIDS since the beginning of the epidemic, no fewer than 4,291 had been of gay or bisexual men—a staggering 76 percent of the total.†

---

*Cited in Istvan Deak, "The Incomprehensible Holocaust," *New York Review of Books* Vol. XXXVL, No. 14, September 28, 1989, p. 72.

**Centers for Disease Control and Prevention, Atlanta, Georgia, Document No. 320210 January 1993.

†Center for Disease Surveillance and Control (UK), June 2, 1994.

At the same time no modern catastrophe has been more consistently badly reported throughout the length and breadth of the Anglo-American mass media than HIV/AIDS. Nor is there any single area in which governments of all known political persuasions have intervened (or failed to intervene) with more immediately disastrous consequences for contemporary society than in relation to the epidemic. As I have written elsewhere:

> This epidemic is unique in so far as its prevention has been prevented, rather than transmission. Resources and education campaigns have been relentlessly targeted at those at least risk of contracting HIV, as if the priority of preventing an epidemic amongst heterosexuals had been established at the expence of halting the epidemics that are actually raging throughout the developed world.*

For example, recent statistics reveal that while 67 percent of AIDS cases in Glasgow, Scotland, have been among gay men, only 3.5 percent of the local budget for HIV education and prevention has gone toward work for gay men. At a recent two-day conference on the Scottish AIDS epidemic, only fifteen minutes were allocated to "the epidemic in homosexual/bisexual men."**

Over the course of the past few years I have had a few differences of opinion with Larry on some issues. For example, I think he tends to exaggerate the size of the "gay community" in the United States, and that this exaggeration may sometimes have led him to be overly critical of the response of lesbians and gay men to the AIDS crisis. He can be very hard on his friends and allies. But these are not issues concerning which we should, as it were, go to the Cross. Far more important is his continued exemplary courage, and his refusal to compromise with those who actively collude with the systematic neglect of those in demonstrably greatest need. As Larry recently pointed out:

---

*Simon Watney, "Powers of Observation: AIDS and the Writing of History," *Practices of Freedom: Selected Writings on HIV/AIDS* (London: Rivers Oram Press; Duke University, Durham, N.C., 1994), p. 277.

**Ross Wright, "AIDS Scandal in Glasgow," *The Pink Paper*, London, February 11, 1994, p. 4. For the most comprehensive and devastating survey of the "de-gaying" of AIDS in Britain and the United States, see Edward King, *Safety in Numbers: Safer Sex and Gay Men* (London: Cassell, 1993; New York: Routledge, 1994).

"There's no community in the world in which everyone gets along with everyone else. Or approves of every action everywhere."* And we forget this at our peril.

It is surely far more important to recognize that in relation to the vast majority of the many topics on which he has written over time he has been consistently right on target, and only too correct. Witness his majestically searing indictments in these pages of *The New York Times*. How easy it is to criticize "discrimination" in the abstract, or to talk in impressively general terms about the "tragedy" of "the global epidemic." In truth, however, the epidemic is invariably experienced at national and local levels, where concrete institutions and individuals are only too immediately responsible for otherwise avoidable specific forms of suffering, pain, harm, and deaths. It is precisely at this level that Larry Kramer remains most consistently and fearlessly accurate. In his 1985 play, *The Normal Heart*, Kramer's surrogate character, Ned Weeks, screams at the indifferent, incompetent mayor of New York City, who has refused to meet with community-based gay AIDS workers: "Fourteen months is a long time to be out to lunch!"** As Larry more than anyone is doubtless agonizingly aware, today one would have to write: "Fourteen *years*". . . .

Simon Watney
London, August 1994

---

*Larry Kramer, *Some Thoughts About Evil*, page 433 of this volume.
**Larry Kramer, *The Normal Heart* (1985) (London: Nick Hearn Books, 1993; New York: Plume Books, 1985), p. 45. For an interesting analysis of Larry Kramer's influence in the field of HIV/AIDS research, treatment, and care in the United States, see Robert M. Wachter, "AIDS Activism and the Politics of Health," *The New England Journal of Medicine*, January 9, 1992, pp. 128–132. Sadly, even this perceptive article dismisses unsafe sex among gay men as "recidivism," as if fucking without a condom were some kind of criminal or pathological act. If this were indeed the case, most heterosexual sex could equally casually be dismissed as a form of criminal pathology. Such are the double standards we continue to face.

Introduction

Fresh from Yale and the army, I started out, at the beginning of 1958, to do something in the theater—probaby become a producer or an actor; I didn't know yet that I could write. The theater, then as now, offered precious little opportunity, so, by chance, I found myself working for a movie company. The theater was forgotten as I attempted to focus my energy and ambition on becoming a film producer. I only half-jokingly wagered with my fellow members of Columbia Pictures' "Executive Training Program" (I ran the teletype machine) that I'd produce my first movie by the time I was thirty. (I almost made it; I was an associate producer at thirty and produced my first film on my own when I was thirty-three.)

I knew I was gay, and there were other homosexuals in the film business with me, but, trying not to think too much about it, we all lived double lives. I duly brought a young woman with me for Monday-night executive screenings when I was assistant to Columbia's head of production in London, and later, when I was assistant to the president of United Artists in New York. I was more interested in learning what my professional talents might be and how to get to the next step on the ladder of success.

I certainly wasn't interested in gay politics. Like many others, when Gay Pride marches started down Fifth Avenue at the end of June, I was on Fire Island. Gay politics had an awful image. Loudmouths, the unkempt, the dirty and unwashed, men in leather or dresses, fat women with greasy, slicked-back ducktail hairdos. Another world. Certainly not a world that connected to mine. Nor did I want it to. On Fire Island, we laughed, in those long-ago days of health, when we watched the evening news on Sunday night flash brief seconds of those straggling, pitiful marches.

There are a lot of us who felt like that, then and now. For me, the change was a slow one. First it took coming to terms with being gay in the first place. That wasn't so easy, and it took many years of psychoanalysis and therapy and many fights with and estrangements from my family. But that's another story. Eventually I not only came to terms with being a gay man, but I came to recognize that I love being one, and want to be no other. That's been, and continues to be, a miraculously wonderful coming of age.

Its onset coincided with a coming of age in my career. I'd produced my movie, and also learned I could write. I wanted to make movies that I could identify with personally. This meant, if not actually dealing entirely with homosexuality, at least including it. I soon discovered this was impossible. The movie industry wasn't interested in any of my concerns. And yet, like all writers discovering themselves, I desperately wanted to write about what I thought and felt. There was no other choice but to try another medium. I wrote a play. It was a resounding failure. I panicked. I quickly wrote a "heterosexual" screenplay and tried to reenter Hollywood. Hollywood again rejected me. When I found most of my daylight hours spent jogging around the complete perimeter of the UCLA campus in Westwood in useless attempts to outrun my anxiety attacks, I came home to New York to write a novel. I was writing my second one when what was to become known as AIDS came along.

It's obviously been sad for me to reread these words of mine, written during the years of AIDS. Depression overcomes me as I count the dead who need not have died. James Baldwin went to his grave filled with anger for the blind hatred against his people, but also with compassion for the frailty of individual man. My anger is still with me, but compassion hasn't arrived yet. And I don't think dying will bring it.

I've always slightly bristled when I'm described as an "activist." It's a word I'm uncomfortable with. I think it's usually meant pejoratively. It's used as a categorizer—to set one apart. I don't think I'm doing anything especially different. I'm a writer writing. I guess the tradition of writers being vociferous political animals is more European than American. Here, this territory comes along with being considered radical, bearded, and unwashed—all the things I had myself disliked in the breed before. I confess to the beard, but I think everything I write and say is eminently sensible, not radical at all. And if one is an "activist," does that mean those who aren't sensible are "passivists" or "pacifists?"

I remember years go, when my novel, *Faggots*, came out, not wanting to be labeled a "gay novelist." I'm a novelist, pure and simple, I huffily defended myself, at the same time demeaningly pushing aside the notion that this novel was in any way a "political act." Well, gay writers have come a long way since 1978. I certainly have. I'm proud to be called a gay novelist, and I certainly realize that almost everything I say and do now falls under the heading "political." Hell—at this period in the history of gay men, just staying alive is a political act.

I guess what I'm trying to say is that I didn't start out to write anything I eventually wrote, but I'm mighty glad I was able to do so. Even if I have to be called an "activist." (I've also been accused of being a "moralist"—my accusers not realizing that nothing they could say would please me more.)

And—if I was a writer writing—I didn't know it then, but I was also a gay man learning as I went along, learning much I had to learn and much I didn't want to learn. Everything was uncharted territory for all of us. Events were happening too quickly to bear. Issues were constantly shifting in importance. And becoming hugely complicated. Quickly we had to master these complications, understand new scientific, medical, pharmaceutical vocabularies, and juggle them adeptly so we could defend ourselves against those who tried to use their presumed "greater" knowledge to lord it over us.

And the cast caught up in playing this morbid drama was coming and, all too frequently, going. And we were all making mistakes faster than we were achieving certain modest wins. We all had hope, then, that if we only worked fast enough . . .

The one question I'm asked more than any other is how I can take all the criticism, attacks, denunciations, slurs, and scorn that have been hurled at me over these years. I don't mean to be simplistic when I say that after a while you get used to it. (And most gay people have had many years of practice.) But as I said, through writing, I've been fortunate to learn many valuable lessons. For starters, I discovered that no matter what you say, x number of people are going to agree with you and x number aren't. So you might as well say what you want to say.

So, to reread these writings from my past—such agonizingly long years, but how did they pass so quickly?—has not only been sad but rather educational. I again realized that not only am I grateful to be alive still (there have been a few days here and there when I wasn't so sure) but that I, along with many others, have grown up.

If being an activist has made both of these possible, I guess there's value in it. But—along with all the others—I know the cost has been too great.

■ ■ ■

To give a sense of the historical context I've appended notes to most of the pieces, detailing the occasion that led me to write or other relevant facts.

Reports from the holocaust:

the story of an AIDS activist

Part One

Gay "Power" Here

Harvey Milk was shot and killed in San Francisco on November 27th by Dan White. Mr. White also shot and killed Mayor George Moscone. Mr. Moscone wasn't homosexual. Harvey Milk was. He was the first openly acknowledged homosexual ever to be elected to the San Francisco Board of Supervisors, in a city with a homosexual population that is large but not so large as New York's.

I am not a crying man but I had tears in my eyes, as well as shivers of pride, while I was in San Francisco that week, all for a man I had never known and only vaguely heard about.

Thirty thousand people gathered outside City Hall, carrying lit candles in memory of Mayor Moscone and Mr. Milk. Five thousand gathered inside and outside of Temple Emanu-El, and six thousand did the same at the Opera House, with Governor Edumund Brown, Jr., in the front row center, for memorial services for Mr. Milk. There Anne Kronenberg, a lesbian and Mr. Milk's administrative assistant, spoke of his constituents, who loved him. "Harvey understood the necessity of us all working together," she said. The Reverend William H. Barcus

* The Op-Ed page of *The New York Times,* December 13, 1978.

of the Church of St. Mary the Virgin, who had recently disclosed his own homosexuality to his congregation, expecting the worst but receiving warm support instead, asked, "If you were shot down tomorrow, would the people you love know you as well as you knew Harvey?" Then Dr. David R. Kessler, a psychiatrist on the staff of the University of California Medical School and the Langley-Porter Psychiatric Clinic, and president of the Bay Area Physicians for Human Rights, a group of more than 250 homosexual doctors and psychiatrists, spoke: "Harvey asked us all to come out to our families and friends, to the people we work with and to those we shop from . . . so that we can shatter the myth, once and for all, that we were freaks, weirdos, or sickies . . . Harvey Milk fought for us. Now it is our turn to fight for him." Inside the Opera House, four thousand people rose as one to shout.

The new Mayor, Dianne Feinstein, had said, outside City Hall, "The fact of his homosexuality gave Harvey an insight into the scars which all oppressed people wear. . . . He believed that no sacrifice was too great a price to pay for the cause of human rights."

I returned to New York to discover that our City Council, on November 29th, had again, for the eighth year, rejected homosexual human rights. Councilwoman Ruth Messinger said that the homosexual civil rights bill, which the council refused to release from committee for full council consideration, involved the rights of "an estimated 10 percent of the population; on this basis there is a homosexual in one of every three families in every state in the country." She said there were an estimated one million homosexuals in the city.

I am back in New York, missing, very much, the sense of community I felt in San Francisco. I call several of my friends, but no one is home. I know that most of my friends are at the bars or the baths or the discos, tripping out on trivia.

We haven't had an acknowledged homosexual member of the City Council representing our constituency. But, gruesomely, I wonder if what happened there should happen here, would Governor High Carey be in the front row? He has refused even to meet with the New York Political Action Council, a homosexual professional group organized to interview all candidates on homosexual issues. Would City Councilwoman

Aileen Ryan make a laudatory speech of tribute? On November 29th, she had said that adequate consideration had been given to the legislation, and urged defeat of the motion.

What temple here would open its doors? The gay rights legislation was actively opposed by Jewish organizations.

Would our one million homosexuals march with lit candles? Will we join with San Francisco's 100,000 homosexuals on July 4th, 1979, in the march on Washington that Harvey Milk was planning at his death?

Where *are* our one million homosexuals?

Several months ago, I listened to Lieutenant Governor-elect Mario Cuomo speak to the homosexual Greater Gotham Business Council. He said that until homosexuals organized, until we prepared accurate demographics on our numbers and our purchasing power, we would get nowhere, that political power—and therefore rights—is based on numbers and money.

I heard Percy Sutton say essentially the same thing two years ago at a very sparsely attended anti–Anita Bryant rally. Mr. Sutton said, in effect: You don't know how many of you there are; until you do, you'll get nowhere.

The City Council was right. We are not ready for our rights in New York. We have not earned them. We have not fought for them. California homosexuals mobilized an entire state to defeat the Briggs Amendment, which would have banned the hiring of homosexual teachers in public schools. New York City's one million homosexuals cannot mobilize a city.

Harvey Milk, William, Barcus, Anne Kronenberg, Dr. David Kessler—we have no one like you here.

When my novel, *Faggots,* was published, the Random House publicity department suggested I write a piece for the Op-Ed page of the *Times.* I'd just returned from promoting the book in, among other cities, San Francisco, and my experiences there formed my debut with what I now see was a purely political statement.

I received a number of phone calls and letters, all saying, more or less, "Who the fuck are you and what right do you have publicly mouthing off?" Indeed, I was criticizing an entire community and its leadership that I hardly knew and that certainly didn't know me. "Where have you been all these years, while we've been working our asses off fighting for the gay rights bill?" was screamed at me by not a few.

I particularly aroused the wrath of some Jewish members of the gay synagogue Beth Simchat Torah, who were offended by my criticism of "Jewish organizations"—by which, of course, I meant heterosexual Jewish organizations, and particularly Orthodox and Hasidic Jewish organizations. When I was invited to speak at Beth Simchat Torah, I was barely allowed to do so, so persistent was the heckling. It was an early and, at the time, very frightening experience. But a valuable one. I learned that if one is going to speak one's mind, best be prepared to get as good as you give. This was a lesson—violent, vocal, vociferous—I was to learn a thousand times over with the appearance of *Faggots*.

I thought I'd written a satirical novel about the gay life I and most of my friends were living. I'd meant it to be funny. I loved Evelyn Waugh. I would use him as my model and guide. Everybody would laugh and learn. It never occured to me that *Faggots* would be *controversial.*

I was completely unprepared for its hostile reception in certain political quarters. I didn't know then (and I must confess to not knowing now) what the words "politically correct" or, in relation to *Faggots*, "politically incorrect" meant. But from these very first appearances I was to learn that, whatever they meant, I wasn't, to gay leaders, the former, and I most certainly *was* the latter.

Even though the book was a best-seller, at the time I was wounded and frightened by the criticism. I found myself actually shunned by friends. My best friend stopped speaking to me, even to this day. People would cross the street to avoid me, or ignore me at parties, to a fewer number of which I suddenly found myself invited. On a visit to Fire Island Pines, the summer retreat for many from New York's, and the world's, gay population, and the setting of my novel's concluding section, it was made pointedly clear to me that I was no longer welcome.

For the next three years, until the appearance of what was to become known as AIDS, I kept a pretty low profile. I didn't know it then but I was learning—not originally by choice—that necessary lesson for anyone who insists on speaking his mind: how to become a loner.

A Personal Appeal

It's difficult to write this without sounding alarmist or too emotional or just plain scared.

If I had written this a month ago, I would have used the figure "40." If I had written this last week, I would have needed "80." Today I must tell you that 120 gay men in the United States—most of them here in New York—are suffering from an often lethal form of cancer called Kaposi's sarcoma or from a virulent form of pneumonia that may be associated with it. More than thirty have died.

By the time you read this, the necessary figures may be much higher.

The men who have been stricken don't appear to have done anything that many New York gay men haven't done at one time or another. We're appalled that this is happening to them and terrified that it could happen to us. It's easy to become frightened that one of the many things we've done or taken over the past years may be all that it takes for a cancer to grow from a tiny something-or-other that got in there who knows when from doing who knows what.

* *New York Native,* Issue 19, August 24–September 6, 1981.

In four months, the number has risen to 120 of us stricken and 30 of us dead.

The majority of Kaposi cases are being tended to at New York University Medical Center. The doctor who is most on top of this situation is there, Dr. Alvin Friedman-Kien. He and his associates are passionately determined to help take care of us and to find out what's going on here.

Money is desperately needed, both for their research, which is going on around the clock, and for the treatment and chemotherapy of many of the patients who have no money or medical insurance.

I hope you will write a check and get your friends to write one, too. This is our disease and we must take care of each other and ourselves. In the past we have often been a divided community; I hope we can all get together on this emergency, undivided, cohesively, and with all the numbers we in so many ways possess.

A few friends had died mysteriously. Several others were sick with unrecognized symptoms. An old friend, Dr. Lawrence Mass, was writing in the *Native* of puzzling appearances of rare cancers and pneumonias in the gay community. And then, on July 3rd, 1981, *The New York Times* ran, buried on an inside page, its first (and for a tragically long nineteen months only one of seven) article, "Rare Cancer Seen in 41 Homosexuals."

I don't know why, but I was scared. I'd had many of the sexually transmitted diseases that the article said I shared with these forty-one homosexuals. I called Larry Mass and he suggested I visit Dr. Alvin Friedman-Kien, at New York University Medical Center, who reported the New York cases. I did so.

The genesis of the above appeal is discussed in the following article.

The First Defense

"**R**ead anything by Kramer closely," Robert Chesley has written to your publication recently [Letters, *Native* 22]. "I think you'll find the subtext is always: the wages of gay sin are death."

I am not interested in sin. I am interested in the difficulties people have in loving each other; I am also interested in how we use sex as a weapon, and I think anyone will find that all of my writing, including my film adaptation of *Women in Love*, concerns itself with explorations of these subjects, which have nothing to do with "the wages of gay sin are death."

Since Bob also suggests—among many other things—that I am self-righteously thrilled by the death of my gay friends from Kaposi's sarcoma (even as I appeal for funds to fight it), I think I must respond beyond the above, even though I have been told it's improper for an author to defend his point of view, his artistic endeavors, or his philosophy in any place other than this artistic work itself. Please excuse me if this response encompasses a rather strange-bedfellowed assortment of topics: death, cancer, my writings, particularly my novel, *Faggots*, and

* *New York Native*, Issue 27, December 21, 1981–January 3, 1982.

10

my own rather low opinion of our New York gay community as a community. And since it was Bob Chesley who lumped all these subjects together, forgive as well a first-person narrative that might otherwise appear self-serving.

■ ■ ■

I do not understand, and never shall, why criticism of ourselves and some of our actions constitutes "gay homophobia." The literary critic Leslie Fiedler has made the point that only when a minority is mature can it respond to self-criticism in art; and its horrified response to its depiction in anything less than the most "positive" terms is an indication of its immaturity.

■ ■ ■

Bob has not been completely honest with either *Native* readers or his political constituency. We had been friends, and I find it curious that his attacks upon me in print commenced with the cessation of this relationship. From the reporter who arrived at my apartment as a "fan," quoting to me his favorite lines from *Faggots*, effusive in his admiration for it, he turned, rather too suddenly I thought, into someone who has been attacking me in print ever since. His list of my malfeasances is endless. He has already trotted out homophobia, anti-eroticism, self-loath-ing, sex-as-evil, Anita Bryantism, brainwashed-by-psychoanaly-sis, fascism.

It has not been necessary for him to drag Kaposi's sarcoma into this and, with the unwitting complicity of the *Native*, to put a symbolic but not less effective damper on our fund-raising campaign. This is outright savagery.

■ ■ ■

I initially involved myself with fund-raising for Kaposi's sar-coma for the simple, uncomplicated reason that three of my friends had died from it. (Now there have been five.) Donald Krintzman, the one among these who was my closest friend, was still alive when he, his good friend and former lover Paul Rapoport, Dr. Lawrence Mass, and I joined together to try to collect funds for the research and treatment being conducted at New York University Medical Center by Donald's doctors, Alvin Friedman-Kien and Linda Laubenstein. Anyone who has read Larry Mass's interview with the "unnamed Kaposi victim" in *Native* issue 19 will understand how a friendship with this extraordinary, courageous man could be so inspirational.

I first learned that Donald had KS last July 29th [1981], when I went to New York University Hospital for information and tests myself. We ran into each other in the waiting room of the laboratory. As we waited for our blood to be drawn, we talked about almost anything else, inanities, rather than confront the coincidence that had brought us together in such a location. Each of us was terrified to ask if the worst was true for his friend. Finally he said, in the firm and confronting way that was to be typical of his death, "Yes, I've got Kaposi's sarcoma."

I had just come from Dr. Friedman-Kien's office upstairs. There I'd seen a young man I recognized. Everything in his expression and posture told me what he'd just been told. He sat down next to me in the waiting room and we nodded to each other and I shook my head softly from side to side in what I hoped would pass for sympathy and understanding. "I don't have anyone I can tell," he finally said to me. "I'm afraid to tell my friends, because they won't understand, and I can't tell my boss or I'll lose my job. There isn't anyone I can talk to." This young man, who is still alive, was the first of the many KS victims whom Donald took under his wing and supplied with his own special tonic of honesty and courage.

Dr. Friedman-Kien had asked me, as someone known in the gay community, to organize a solicitation of funds. He cited several patients who had no medical insurance, and he spoke of his own research. He felt something important was happening with KS: a cancer was occurring in a specific and controlled community; perhaps studying this cancer might reveal something about cancers in general. He also felt it was vital to educate the gay community about the cancer's very existence, and its symptomatology.

He also said he thought what was happening was only the tip of the iceberg. He didn't think what was happening would go away. This was very frightening to me, and still is. He said the numbers would continue to increase. This has unfortunately proved to be correct. There were forty KS-related cases (Kaposi's sarcoma, *Pneumocystis* pneumonia, certain lymphomas) on that day we met, and there are more than 180 cases five months later. Clear-headed friends have pointed out to me that this is not so many, in the scheme of things. Perhaps not. But I still have five friends who have died.

On August 11th, our committee of four held a fund-raiser in my apartment. We called all the friends we could think of who had money for charitable contributions or were well known in the gay community and could help get the word around. Hundreds were invited, including every doctor with a gay practice. Eighty men came.

Donald had prepared contribution circulars, and Dr. Friedman-Kien addressed the gathering and answered questions. He said he thought an epidemic was occurring (it was officially declared such in October by the government) [subsequently to be back-dated to June 5th by the Centers for Disease Control], that the causes were unknown, that there were a number of possible "culprits," none of which could be discounted.

We raised $6,635 as a result of this first night.

Two committees were formed to carry forward the endeavors: one to organize a solicitation of Fire Island, chaired by Philip Gefter, and another to plan a benefit dance, chaired by Edmund White. Each committee had over a dozen members. We all felt we were off to a good start.

■ ■ ■

Bob Chesley is very critical of the appeal I then wrote for the *Native.* This is an appeal the wording of which was approved by Dr. Friedman-Kien and Dr. Mass. I wanted it to be stirring and emotional and thought-provoking and scary. I didn't, and don't, think that anything less than scary was, and is, occurring. Neither does anyone else who has had anything to do with KS. Perhaps if Bob Chesley has had nothing to do with this cancer, it's hard for him to believe it exists. It is hard for me to believe that on August 11th Donald Krintzman was alive and energetically passing out his pledges for contributions in my living room and that on November 12th he was dead from *Pneumocystis* pneumonia and I was attending a memorial service for him at Frank Campbell's, filled with hundreds of men stunned and crying for his loss.

The sentence that has caused Bob, and several other *Native* correspondents, so much difficulty, is medically accurate: "It's easy to become frightened that one of the many things we've done or taken over the past years may be all that it takes for a cancer to grow from a tiny something-or-other that got in there who knows when from doing who knows what." But *something* we are doing *is* ticking off the time bomb that is causing the breakdown of immunity in certain bodies, and while it is true that we don't know what it is specifically, isn't it better to be cautious until various suspected causes have been discounted, rather than be reckless? An individual can choose to continue or cease smoking, where the same warnings have been presented, pointed out to us, and questioned by many. But isn't it stupid to rail against the very presentation of these warnings?

■ ■ ■

Over Labor Day weekend we canvassed Fire Island. Philip Gefter had photocopied several thousand copies of Larry Mass's ground-breaking *Native* article, "Cancer in the Gay Community," which, together with two of Donald's contribution circulars, made a six-page brochure. George Wilson saw to it that one brochure was placed in front of every door in both the Pines and the Grove. Enno Poersch, whose lover Nick Rock was one of the first to die, made posters for our tables, which we manned in the harbors of both communities throughout Saturday and Sunday, and where money could be donated and further information and additional brochures obtained. Jack Fitzsimmons provided cash boxes. Of the original committee formed at my apartment several weeks earlier, only a handful came to the island to help. I cite the following who did help us, and apologize if I have inadvertently overlooked someone: Paul Popham, Enno Poersch, Dr. Jeffrey Marmor, Dr. John Raftis, David Margolis, Joey Hernandez, Mark Rosenberg, Bill Touw.

These people manned the tables with Philip Gefter over the two days. Additionally, Paul Popham (who has in one year lost his lover, Jack Nau, to lymphoblastic lymphoma, and a best friend, Rick Willikoff, to KS) and Rick Fialla and I stood at the door of the Ice Palace on Saturday night with cash boxes. From midnight until 8:00 A.M., from thousands of dancers, we collected $126. The Pines Pavilion would not let us solicit on its premises, despite several appeals.

The entire Labor Day weekend in both communities on Fire Island brought us $769.55. Joey Hernandez went out with a cash box the following weekend and collected a further eighty dollars.

However, checks started coming in through the mail. We comforted ourselves that even if contributions were small at the Island, at least we were educating our community about KS, something few had known anything about before.

■ ■ ■

In four months we have raised $11,806.55. Over half of this money came in from our first fund-raiser in my apartment on August 11th. Five people gave $1,000 each and two people gave $500 each, which means that the rest of the entire gay community in the city of New York has contributed to this cause the sum of $5,806.55

■ ■ ■

Ed White's benefit dance committee was unsuccessful in making any sort of reasonable arrangements with our leading discotheque. Its owner's demands were too greedy. (The benefit has now been set for a Tea Dance on Sunday, January 17th, 1982, at the Paradise Garage.) Appeals to famous gay rock and disco stars, who would not be famous were it not for gay dancers, to appear at this benefit have been turned down.

■ ■ ■

Special solicitations were made to two of the richest homosexuals in the world, without success.

■ ■ ■

The mayor's office was completely unresponsive to our request for any kind of help. Herbert Rickman, who is Mayor Koch's liaison with the gay community, said to me on the phone: "This is something we definitely want to get involved with. I'll get back to you tomorrow." We wanted help in getting non-gay press attention for this disease. *The New York Times* had refused to run special articles prepared and delivered to them by hand. Even the *Village Voice* has yet to run an article with any comprehensive information. Rickman has yet to call.

■ ■ ■

I quote now from more of Bob Chesley's letter in the *Native:*

> I think the concealed meaning in Kramer's emotionalism is the triumph of guilt: that gay men *deserve* to die for their promiscuity. In his novel, *Faggots,* Kramer told us that sex is dirty and that we ought not to be doing what we're doing. Now, with Kaposi's sarcoma attacking gay men, Kramer assumes he knows the cause (maybe it's on page 37 of *Faggots?* Or page 237?), and—let's say that it's easy to become frightened that Kramer's *real* emotion is a sense of having been vindicated, though tragically: he told us so, but we didn't listen to him; nooo—we had to learn the hard way, and now we're dying.
>
> Read anything by Kramer closely. I think you'll find that the subtext is always: the wages of gay sin are death. I ask you to look closely at Kramer's writing because I think it's important for gay people to know whether or not they agree with him. I am not downplaying the seriousness of Kaposi's sarcoma. But something else is happening here, which is also serious: gay homophobia and anti-eroticism.

In *Faggots,* I set out to try to understand one main issue: Why did I see so little love between two homosexual men? Love is what I wanted and want, and what most of the friends I have say they want, too. Whatever reasons I came up with in my novel, they, and it, seem to have touched a most responsive chord in the gay community. The book has sold exceedingly well and I have received letters from all over the world thanking me for it. Not one of these letters has been negative. I did not receive one angry or "hate" letter from the entire American gay community. The only hate letters I have received have been from the American gay "political" press.

Can it be, I have begun to wonder, that the gay "political"

press and critics are out of touch with the realities of their audience and their lives? Can it be that these critics are writing for a very small group, quite possibly only each other?

Can it be possible that, as the feminist Vivian Gornick suggests, this reaction from one's own is predictable, that the people with whom one has shared the experience are incapable of seeing their version portrayed in a different way? "No one forgives an interpretation that is at variance with one's own," Gornick has said. "Nobody forgives you for growing up in their presence."

■ ■ ■

Of the sheer floodtide of gay literature which has been appearing over the past three years in America, perhaps nothing has stirred up so much controversy as *Faggots;* perhaps no other title has been so reviled by the gay media; perhaps no title has been so grotesquely misunderstood. . . .

It is one of the macabre ironies of fate that the world's moralists—not to mention gay activists—have branded (and no doubt will continue to brand) *Faggots* as obscene and self-oppressive . . . though they will almost certainly miss the deeper implications of the book. For Larry Kramer . . . has written a deeply moral . . . book.

. . . It is . . . Larry Kramer's sense of . . . unease with the world of instant sex which appears to have annoyed so many of the American activists—those who seem to equate sex with sexual liberation. . . .

—Peter Burton, *Gay News*, London, June 26, 1980

Mr. Kramer's "sin" is that he has accurately put down (in both senses of the expression) the heartless promiscuity of homosexual New York.

Mr. Kramer's view is a personal one—and it must be remembered that anyone's perceptions are distorted through the prism of their beliefs, ideals, desires. . . . Those who read *Faggots* with due care and attention will discover a novel of deep and abiding morality (and morality can never be out of place); bitter, harshly humorous, grotesque, frightening, comic, and as honest as one individual's perceptions can make it.

—Peter Burton, *Gay News*, London, July 10, 1980

Kramer . . . is asking pointed questions about the nature of urban gay lives which most gay men don't want asked . . . the book lays the blame for "our" rotten image at our own doorstep. Kramer accuses his fellow gays of misusing their freedom and shirking their responsibilities to each other as people. "Yes," says Laverne, one of a trio of male characters completed by Patti and Maxine, "we're all out of the closet but we're still in the ghetto and all I see is guys hurting each other and themselves . . . and yes, the world is giving us a bad name and we're giving us a bad name and one of us has to stop and it's not going to be the world."

—Vito Russo, *Gay News*, London, July 10, 1980

The extraordinary moral invective that attends discussion of books . . . in the wake of the Gay Liberation Movement . . . savaged [*Faggots*]. . . . This insistence on optimism in the face of oppression occludes discussion of actual contradictions within our lives, and relegates cultural production to the realm of facile propagandism.

. . . the point is missed both that *Faggots* is a best-seller, an important fact for any Marxist looking at a cultural product, and that *Faggots* might illuminate the material conditions that made it possible and expose the ideological forms through which those conditions are seen.

. . . the move from literary representation of homosexuality . . . to one in which gay men are plural, engaged with each other, creating, choosing, changing partners, are *social*, seems to me to be of emphatic importance. . . . It marks the entry of homosexuality into society, and thereby creates the possibility of deprivatising the experience of homosexuals.

—Philip Derbyshire, *Gay Left 9*, London

What can become of passion when the beloved wallows in the same pleasure-spots, when each dim corner

of the baths reveals him given up to anonymous ca-
resses, when hour after hour his aura fades because the
same carnal evidences cause him to grow pale? This is
the heart of the narrative, the de-mythification of physical love. . . .

Fags [the title in France] . . . dares to dismantle the
mechanism of feelings, it mocks the alibi of "forbidden
sex" in order to underline all the more heavily that the only
question is our identity and, beyond that, the question of
human identity.

. . . We cannot deny that it lays bare the reality of a
universe temporarily without tenderness. This novel has
the merit of shifting its scrutiny, and its analysis from
within is a revolution.

. . . A revolutionary book, *Fags* is one of the rare novels
in which the gay man carves out for himself the hero's
role—entirely for himself. Still a victim? Perhaps, but of
himself, and no longer of the fragile gods whom the
straights have mummified in order to glorify the anguish
of their loins.

—Hugo Marsan, *Le Gai Pied,* Paris, September 1981
(Translated for me by Richard Howard.)

Why has the reception of *Faggots* by the gay press in England
and France been just the reverse of its reception here? Why has
it been possible for my themes and ideas and explorations to be
so well understood overseas and so misunderstood here at
home? What kind of responsible journalism or criticism is represented when a writer like Bob Chesley must use a fatal disease
to attack me and my novel? What kind of repressive community
are we creating for ourselves when a critic can, as George
Whitmore did in *Body Politic,* implore his readers not to buy
or read my book? Or where a bookstore refuses, as the Oscar
Wilde Memorial Bookshop does, to sell my book? I ask in all
reasonableness: What have I written that is so awful that these
almost totalitarian acts can happen? That my novel can still
cause such controversy among our political spokesmen over
three years after its publication is amazing to me and only
supports the theories I've had from the very beginning of these
outcries: I have touched some essential painful truth that some

do not want to look at, and methinks those who protest protest
too much.

■ ■ ■

If these political spokesmen are our leaders, where are they
leading us? I see no one leading us in an organized plan to gain
our civil rights in New York. I see no one making our annual
march up Fifth Avenue to Central Park anything other than the
messy, straggly, uncoordinated, unconvincing mess it is. Many
people claim to speak for us in Central Park; but they are very
angry with each other and apparently out of touch with the
community that rambles through that park not listening to
them.

Unfortunately, all of our political critics haven't learned
that it's very easy to criticize and much harder to get anything
done.

What does it take for all of us to work together?

■ ■ ■

If KS were a new form of cancer attacking straight people, it
would be receiving constant media attention, and pressures
from every side would be so great upon the cancer-funding
institutions that research would be proceeding with great inten-
sity. The very government agency—the Centers for Disease
Control, in Atlanta—that is monitoring KS so slowly is the
same CDC that vigorously investigated Legionnaire's disease
when it was a national front-page story and Philadelphia was
clamoring for results.

Why is Bob Chesley attacking *me?* Why is he not attacking
the CDC for taking so long to prepare their epidemiological
studies? Why is he not attacking the National Cancer Institute
and the American Cancer Society for showing so little interest
in KS and forcing Dr. Friedman-Kien to wait months and possibly years for them to fund his research, which has already
produced interesting results?

Two new cases of KS are being diagnosed in New York each
week. One new case is being diagnosed in the United States
each day. Nothing is being done by the gay community to insist
that the straight community, which controls all the purse
strings and attention-getting devices, help us. Why is Bob Ches-

ley not chastising *The New York Times* for ignoring us? Why is he not going after CBS and NBC and ABC for not running any items whatsoever on their programs? A recent new strain of penicillin-resistant gonorrhea among straights made prime-time news headlines for a week.

Why is he not attacking the men on street corners and in sex and head shops who are selling bottles of popper so filled with impurities that a chemical researcher who has analyzed them said they represent "brother killing brother"? Why is he not dunning the pharmaceutical companies to discover less toxic cures more speedily for our most persistent health problem, amebiasis, which has made it almost impossible for us to make love with each other?

Why is he not criticizing our mayor, who is so shabbily two-faced in all his dealings with one of his largest minorities? Are there any gay men or women on the newly formed Mayor's Committee on Minorities? The city's Orientals now have their own local television channel. And why is the mayor not helping us with amebiasis and KS, both of which are public health problems?

And why is Bob Chesley not looking at the "eroticism" that has made gay health such a concern in New York that every gay doctor in this city is, as Dr. Mass puts it, "exhausted"?

Why is Bob Chesley attacking me? Why is he not asking every homosexual in this city: Why are we here? What are we here for?

■ ■ ■

If every homosexual in New York had voted against Edward Koch, he would not be Mayor of New York. How long must it take for this fact to sink in? I beg everyone to think of the power this should entitle us to. Isn't this a far more important issue to deal with than all these petty jealousies and political irrelevancies I read about week after week in our gay press?

And isn't it far more important to try to deal with the fact that more than 180 of us are suffering from potentially lethal cancers and our entire community is doing so little to help them and ourselves?

■ ■ ■

What is this dream world we inhabit? Why is our community so impotent and lethargic? Is everything *too* good for us? Do we need Dunkirks before we can organize and fight back? Until then, can we only hurt each other?

■ ■ ■

I am not glorying in death. I am overwhelmed by it. The death of my friends. The death of whatever community there is here in New York. The death of any visible love.

"Whom do we hate most?" George Steiner has asked. And answered: "We hate most those who ask of us more than we want to give, who suggest to us that we are far from stretching to the full height of our own ethical possibility."

I t can be imagined, the barrage of letters that filled the *Native* for weeks after this appeared. Happily, the vitriol was evenly divided, pro and con. I say "happily" only because it was good to get *some* public support. I was also beginning to realize the usefulness of controversy. It was controversy that helped sell so many copies of *Faggots;* it was, and is, controversy that helps an issue stay before the public, so that more people join in debate, in this process becoming, one hopes, politicized. At the least, it helps people think about the issues and perhaps even make up their minds.

In the year between this article and the next, Gay Men's Health Crisis was officially founded by Nathan Fain, Dr. Lawrence Mass, Paul Popham, Paul Rapoport, Edmund White, and me. In a retrospect that, sadly, only Larry, Edmund, and I are still alive to share, this year of 1982 and, for me, the year or so following, was an inspirational time.

Paul Popham—who was a close friend before we had our painful disagreements on the direction GMHC should take, disagreements that destroyed a friendship

that was not to be restored until he was on his deathbed—and I supervised the daily running of the organization. For both of us it became a consuming passion—helping, urging, nurturing, watching this small
group develop, at first falteringly, but then beginning to
grow as increasing numbers of dedicated men and
women came to join us. It was one of those rare moments in life when one felt completely utilized, useful,
with a true reason to be alive. But this very community
zeal, shared by growing numbers who often sought different goals, and who were to be unable to work together politically, was to become, also at first falteringly
but then increasingly, an enormous and painful and destructive problem that I don't think has been solved to
this day.

Where Are We Now?

Our second *Newsletter* comes to you at a time when the AIDS problem would seem to have reached a very dark day. Medical scientists cannot really tell us much more now than they could six months ago, when our first *Newsletter* came out. The signals we get from responsible medical authorities are confusing, in part because these authorities are confounded by AIDS and very few doctors like to say, "I don't know." Case numbers are doubling every six months. There is an almost 40-percent mortality rate. There are currently three new cases a day nationally and one and a half new cases a day in New York, which still is the city where 50 percent of all cases occur. Gay men still represent 74 percent of all victims. There is the woeful prediction that there will be ten thousand cases in two years' time.

It's very hard for us not to cry out in anger, frustration, fear, desperation, and utter bewilderment, "How many people must die before something happens!"

By "something" we mean a concerted, all-out effort by our community and by our country to make everyone recognize that we are in the midst of the worst epidemic to hit us since

---

* *GMHC Newsletter*, No. 2. Written October 1982, published February 1983.

polio and to mobilize ourselves into the great and effective agency for action and change that this country is capable of becoming in time of emergency.

For it is hard to imagine a worse emergency, or an enemy to match the stealth and horror of this insidious epidemic, an unknown disease that hides itself.

This being so, it seems to us at Gay Men's Health Crisis that there are still too many people who don't know what's going on, or, worse, who act as if they don't know what's going on.

1. The funding for an all-out research assault has been very slow in coming. Our epidemic is already a year and a half old. Although an earlier award provided $2 million to the CDC for AIDS, there is at this moment no money for specific AIDS research pending in either house of Congress.

The National Institutes of Health, which has an annual budget of four billion dollars, has said it will release— "sometime this year"—at least $3 million through their National Cancer Institute and at least $2 million through their National Institute for Allergy and Infectious Diseases. But they have already received $55 million worth of grant requests from hospitals, doctors, scientists, and institutions who have been clamoring to do research into AIDS.

Five million dollars doesn't buy much research these days, or represent much of a commitment on the part of our country, when you consider the number of victims we have sustained, which, as of January 13th [1983], totaled 333 AIDS deaths.

And when we read articles like the following from *The New York Times* of October 10th, 1982, we are angry about the priorities of our country: "The United States Ambassador . . . donated $25 million Friday on behalf of the Reagan Administration to aid relatives of fifty-seven [natives of a small foreign country] killed in a flood and landslide at a mining camp . . . along with a message from President Reagan saying, 'The American people join me in sending sympathy to those injured, their families and the families of those who lost their lives.' "

2. The straight media have been extremely negligent. Remember the almost daily sympathetic attention they lavished on Legionnaire's disease, toxic-shock syndrome, the Tylenol scare, swine flu—victims from all of which total far fewer than we have sustained from AIDS? Now that AIDS is appearing in more heterosexuals, and in babies, the media have recently paid more attention, but, strangely, only a little more.

Constant national media attention helps exert pressure in Washington to release the flow of funds. And without this media attention we have been deprived, for most of the past year and a half, of our nation's main network of communication: how word is spread, information disseminated, alerts sounded. (Six men recognized they had KS lesions from viewing slides that were shown at GMHC's Second Open Forum two months ago.)

Although the *New York Native* has been excellent in keeping its readership constantly apprised of what is happening, the total circulation of all gay publications is unfortunately tiny compared to our total numbers.

So how can we tell each other, *all* of us, that what's happening now is literally a matter of life or death?

3. There has been a great lack of communication between the gay community and the medical/scientific community. Studies are constantly announced and undertaken by people who have only the vaguest notions of how we live. A mere request in the *Native* for volunteers, with a promise of a complete physical examination or some free "test for AIDS," will net more than enough volunteers in a matter of hours. From these men, statistics are garnered, by heterosexuals unsophisticated in our ways, which are then publicized as fact in medical journals and the media. But the men who respond to these requests are most often those at higher risk, and do not necessarily represent a cross-section of the gay community.

4. We want to mention the complex issue of doctors who have felt unable to help guide us through this terrible period. Medical research and health policy must be shaped on local and national levels. It is this policy that will help determine how this epidemic—and our lives—will be han-

dled, as local and federal governments will have no choice but to become involved. The areas of gay health and sexual medicine are still very loosely defined. If we don't field our own experts, representing *us*, fighting for *us*, there is no telling what will happen to us as more and more pressure is brought to bear on officials to "find an answer" and who then might take the path of least resistance and scapegoat gay men.

Thus far, not enough doctors have stepped forward, identified themselves as gay, and pitched in to help on a public level.

5. Here in New York, the meetings GMHC instituted with City Hall have been very slow in achieving results. In no way have we gained the significant acknowledgment of crisis that San Francisco has, with that city's emergency bequest of $300,000 to its AIDS-related endeavors. Indeed, our top-priority request—that our city help us find space that AIDS patients can use for their own lounge and support-group sessions, to be with their own—remains unfulfilled. For lack of permanent space, AIDS and KS support groups have been forced to move around from week to week, often to top-floor walk-ups that KS patients lack the strength to climb.

Working with our city government is a very slow process. We are not discouraged yet, but we are a long way from receiving the recognition gay communities have achieved in such cities as San Francisco, Los Angeles, Houston, and Washington.

6. The gay community itself is not yet united on AIDS. There is one thing we must not allow AIDS to become, and that is a *political* issue among ourselves. It's not. It's a health issue for us. And it's a national public health emergency issue. This may be the hardest task of all for many of us. We've been too accustomed to fear, particularly the fear that our sexual freedom, so hard fought for, will be taken away from us. But we must realize that sex is not the fabric holding our community together; that's a very questionable assumption indeed about our commonality. We must realize that we are much, much more, that we have a sense of self and identity and relating such as exists

in any religion or philosophy or ethnic background, and in which sex plays no more a role than it does in heterosexual identity. And if it takes an emergency epidemic to teach us this lesson, then let this be one of life's ironies.

We all want this epidemic stopped immediately. GMHC is hardly pleased to report that no miracle drug or cure has shown itself. And all of us want to know how to live our lives now. All doctors everywhere dealing with AIDS are under immense stress, and the most stressed of all are the physicians of New York who treat large gay populations—a position of truly heartbreaking frustration. These doctors are telling us to lessen the number of sexual partners we come in contact with, so that, if a transmissable agent is the culprit, we will decrease our chances of getting or giving it. No doctor we know of is trying to make moral judgments with this advice. Quite the contrary. They cannot bear to see one more AIDS diagnosis, and so they are understandably in favor of seeing us live at the expense, perhaps, of our temporarily suspended sexual liberty. But GMHC believes that each individual must make his own decision.

Since, as of January 13th, there were 891 cases of AIDS in thirty-three states, 67 cases in thirteen foreign countries, and 426 cases in New York City, it is hard for us, for the moment, to refute this advice, though everyone is entitled to decide for himself.

All of us, however, must do everything in our power to make our community and our government and our country recognize the frightening implications of these rising numbers. We must orchestrate this concern, locally, nationally, in Washington, and pray that this country understands that what is happening to us, and is now happening to heterosexuals, demands immediate attention. How many of us are carrying within us the seeds of this mysterious disease? It is hard to live in New York now without the torment of this question. And how many of us must die before an effective national plan of attack is begun?

Listen to these words from Dr. James Curran of the CDC: "How are we going to spend the next ten years? That's how long it could take before a causal agent can be found, along with its cure. We don't have enough people worried about this yet."

■ ■ ■

Gay Men's Health Crisis is now one year old. We're certainly no longer the bunch of kids who got together and brought you a disco dance. From six men we have grown to more than three hundred men, each of whom is giving a portion of his weekly time to combating AIDS, and we are now a major social service organization without—as yet—any funding from any state, city, or federal sources, only from you, our community.

We have raised over $150,000; given away almost $50,000 to research; printed and distributed some 25,000 copies of our first *Newsletter* (which was so well received that it is used as a training manual in many hospitals and was even requested by the Library of Congress) and at least 100,000 of this one; prepared and distributed 300,000 Health Recommendation Brochures (in English, Spanish, Creole, and French) with a list of symptoms; fielded almost five thousand Hotline emergency calls, which included hundreds of referrals to doctors; created a Patient Service program that includes Crisis Intervention Counselors (who stay with a patient from immediately after diagnosis as having AIDS), individual and group support therapy, a network of buddies to visit and do chores for those who are ill, legal advisers, and financial aid guidance through the complexities of the welfare system; arranged Open Forums for the community to hear and question doctors prominent in AIDS care; arranged contact with representatives of our mayor and congressmen; helped institute measures to protect the community from unsuitably prepared research studies; investigated and registered complaints against improper medical treatment and hospital care; set up training seminars for doctors, psychiatrists, psychologists, social workers, health-care professionals, and concerned laymen in all areas of AIDS concerns, including how to deal with a friend or lover who may be terminally ill; served as a central source for the media so that most of that which has appeared has been accurate and sensitive. And all of the above services have been provided by volunteers and provided free.

That GMHC has accomplished all of this (and mostly in the last six months), and that so many responsible gay men have stepped forward to accomplish all of this, is one of the most inspirational developments ever to occur in the New York gay community. We have never encountered so much love between men as we have felt in GMHC, and watching this organization grow in response to our community's terrible new needs has been one of the most moving experiences we have ever been privileged to share.

We would not be here in such strength without you. You have been responsible as well. That you have continued to send in your checks and volunteer your services or stop a GMHC member in the street and say Thank You—this has been inspirational, too. There are few communities that, when asked, and within the space of one short month, would loan an organization $130,000, interest-free, as 130 men have done, so that we could effectively plan the greatest gay fund-raising event of all time. And, with $60,000 worth of tickets already sold to our Circus before we've even really started our sales campaign, it looks as though you're going to support that as well.

It goes without saying that we desperately need your support to continue. We need your contributions and we need your names for our mailing list and we need you to come to our Circus in Madison Square Garden on April 30. Like every other living, human being, we need you to keep telling us you approve of us and what we're trying to do.

We must not let this awful sense of unknowing that AIDS yet represents divide us. We might all—every one of us—be potential AIDS victims. More than ever before we must fight together now—to help those who are already ill with AIDS, and to help insure our own future on this earth.

—The Board of Gay Men's Health Crisis, Inc.

It's hard to believe now that there was so much opposition to printing the above lead article on the part of GMHC's Board. The Board, which now numbered eight men (Larry Mass and Nathan Fain, sensing that the fights that were becoming more and more divisive would become even worse, had left the Board to contribute their energy to GMHC as non-Board members), was so terrified to print it that it was circulated, behind my back, and a vote was taken not to run it "as is" unless a number of disclaimers and caveats were included. Since I was the editor of this issue and dealt with the printer myself, I managed to run most of it as I had written it, and got in much hot water for doing so.

Basically, Paul Popham and I differed philosophically on points that were soon to alienate us completely. He was, for a start, a closeted gay man, who was also now president of the board of a gay organization. He felt GMHC should not in any way *tell* people anything, not in any way make up their minds for them. All we could do was pass out the latest word of what was known and said officially about AIDS, which was very little, usually insensitive and homophobic, and quite often spurious.

At great cost to his own health and stamina, Larry Mass, as both a doctor and a writer, was heroic in his never-ceasing efforts to provide accurate medical information regularly in the *Native.* But as the *Native* became known as "the AIDS newspaper," fewer people wanted to read it. Larry, too, would have his fights with the Board to release his impeccable "Medical Answers About AIDS" publications more swiftly and more often.

Paul and the Board were determined not to issue sex recommendations. Or anything that in any way could be construed as moralizing. It must be remembered that this was long before any causative virus had been posited. What if it was discovered that nothing infectious was going around, he asked. We'd look like fools. And we could also have done a lot of damage: the gay community had fought for so long for the sexual freedoms it now enjoyed that any aspersions cast upon the validity of these were bound to be destructive. It had taken so long for gay men to feel good about themselves. Paul's position seemed to be shared by just about everyone else—in and out of GMHC.

I was out to attack every perceived enemy in sight.
If the mayor wouldn't meet with us, attack him publicly.
If *The New York Times* wouldn't write about AIDS, go
after them with pickets. Reagan, doctors, the NIH, the
AMA—you name it, I was after it. I'd go on TV and call
Koch a pig (I've never been subtle), and be identified
with GMHC, and Paul would get very angry at me. (I
remember being interviewed by Jane Pauley on
"Today" and considering whether I should say Koch
was a closeted gay and that was why he was ignoring
us, but chickening out and calling him a pig instead.)
Because Paul (and several other Board members) were
in the closet, and because no one wanted to do it anyway,
I did all the media appearances by default. (Not that I
didn't want to do so, or wouldn't have fought to do so.)
And pretty much everything I'd say, and how I said it,
would drive Paul and the Board crazy. Particularly
Paul.

He knew he was right and I knew I was right. He
was a much better team player than I'll ever be. I'd been
a film producer. I thought I was producing GMHC. He'd
been an army officer. Both of us were accustomed to
getting results and, in very different fashions, having
our own way.

Paul, and the Board, which was composed of many
of our mutual friends, felt that softer tactics were required. "You get more with honey than with vinegar"
was a modus operandi that was urged upon me regularly.

For the first year or so, there was plenty else for
Paul and me to do without having to face up to resolving
our differences. Many more of our friends were becoming sick and dying. We were also creating an organization that must look after *them*.

1,112 and Counting

If this article doesn't scare the shit out of you, we're in real trouble. If this article doesn't rouse you to anger, fury, rage, and action, gay men may have no future on this earth. Our continued existence depends on just how angry you can get.

I am writing this as Larry Kramer, and I am speaking for myself, and my views are not to be attributed to Gay Men's Health Crisis.

I repeat: Our continued existence as gay men upon the face of this earth is at stake. Unless we fight for our lives, we shall die. In all the history of homosexuality we have never before been so close to death and extinction. Many of us are dying or already dead.

Before I tell you what we must do, let me tell you what is happening to us.

There are now 1,112 cases of serious Acquired Immune Deficiency Syndrome. When we first became worried, there were only 41. In only twenty-eight days, from January 13th to February 9th [1983], there were 164 new cases—and 73 more dead. The total death tally is now 418. Twenty percent of all

* New York Native, Issue 59, March 14–27, 1983.

cases were registered this January alone. There have been 195 dead in New York City from among 526 victims. Of all serious AIDS cases, 47.3 percent are in the New York metropolitan area.

These are the serious cases of AIDS, which means Kaposi's sarcoma, *Pneumocystis carinii* pneumonia, and other deadly infections. These numbers do not include the thousands of us walking around with what is also being called AIDS: various forms of swollen lymph glands and fatigues that doctors don't know what to label or what they might portend.

The rise in these numbers is terrifying. Whatever is spreading is now spreading faster as more and more people come down with AIDS.

And, for the first time in this epidemic, leading doctors and researchers are finally admitting they don't know what's going on. I find this terrifying too—as terrifying as the alarming rise in numbers. For the first time, doctors are saying out loud and up front, "I don't know."

For two years they weren't talking like this. For two years we've heard a different theory every few weeks. We grasped at the straws of possible cause: promiscuity, poppers, back rooms, the baths, rimming, fisting, anal intercourse, urine, semen, shit, saliva, sweat, blood, blacks, a single virus, a new virus, repeated exposure to a virus, amoebas carrying a virus, drugs, Haiti, voodoo, Flagyl, constant bouts of amebiasis, hepatitis A and B, syphilis, gonorrhea.

I have talked with the leading doctors treating us. One said to me, "If I knew in 1981 what I know now, I would never have become involved with this disease." Another said, "The thing that upsets me the most in all of this is that at any given moment one of my patients is in the hospital and something is going on with him that I don't understand. And it's destroying me because there's some craziness going on in him that's destroying him." A third said to me, "I'm very depressed. A doctor's job is to make patients well. And I can't. Too many of my patients die."

After almost two years of an epidemic, there still are no answers. After almost two years of an epidemic, the cause of AIDS remains unknown. After almost two years of an epidemic, there is no cure.

Hospitals are now so filled with AIDS patients that there is often a waiting period of up to a month before admission, no matter how sick you are. And, once in, patients are now more and more being treated like lepers as hospital staffs become increasingly worried that AIDS is infectious.

Suicides are now being reported of men who would rather die than face such medical uncertainty, such uncertain therapies, such hospital treatment, and the appalling statistic that 86 percent of all serious AIDS cases die after three years' time.

If all of this had been happening to any other community for two long years, there would have been, long ago, such an outcry from that community and all its members that the government of this city and this country would not know what had hit them.

Why isn't every gay man in this city so scared shitless that he is screaming for action? Does every gay man in New York *want* to die?

Let's talk about a few things specifically.

■ Let's talk about which gay men get AIDS.

No matter what you've heard, there is no single profile for all AIDS victims. There are drug users and non-drug users. There are the truly promiscuous and the almost monogamous. There are reported cases of single-contact infection.

All it seems to take is the one wrong fuck. That's not promiscuity—that's bad luck.

■ Let's talk about AIDS happening in straight people.

We have been hearing from the beginning of this epidemic that it was only a question of time before the straight community came down with AIDS, and that when that happened AIDS would suddenly be high on all agendas for funding and research and then we would finally be looked after and all would then be well.

I myself thought, when AIDS occurred in the first baby, that would be the breakthrough point. It was. For one day the media paid an enormous amount of attention. And that was it, kids.

There have been no confirmed cases of AIDS in straight, white, non-intravenous-drug-using, middle-class Americans.

The only confirmed straights struck down by AIDS are members of groups just as disenfranchised as gay men: intravenous drug users, Haitians, eleven hemophiliacs (up from eight), black and Hispanic babies, and wives or partners of IV drug users and bisexual men.

If there have been—and there may have been—any cases in straight, white, non-intravenous-drug-using, middle-class Americans, the Centers for Disease Control isn't telling anyone about them. When pressed, the CDC says there are "a number of cases that don't fall into any of the other categories." The CDC says it's impossible to fully investigate most of these "other category" cases; most of them are dead. The CDC also tends not to believe living, white, middle-class male victims when they say they're straight, or female victims when they say their husbands are straight and don't take drugs.

Why isn't AIDS happening to more straights? Maybe it's because gay men don't have sex with them.

Of all serious AIDS cases, 72.4 percent are in gay and bisexual men.

■   Let's talk about "surveillance."

The Centers for Disease Control is charged by our government to fully monitor all epidemics and unusual diseases.

To learn something from an epidemic, you have to keep records and statistics. Statistics come from interviewing victims and getting as much information from them as you can. Before they die. To get the best information, you have to ask the right questions.

There have been so many AIDS victims that the CDC is no longer able to get to them fast enough. It has given up. (The CDC also had been using a questionnaire that was fairly insensitive to the lives of gay men, and thus the data collected from its early study of us have been disputed by gay epidemiologists. The National Institutes of Health is also fielding a very naïve questionnaire.)

Important, vital case histories are now being lost because of this cessation of CDC interviewing. This is a woeful waste with as terrifying implications for us as the alarming rise in case numbers and doctors finally admitting they don't know what's going on. As each man dies, as one or both sets of men who had interacted with each other come down with AIDS, yet more information that might reveal patterns of transmissibility is not being monitored and collected and studied. We are being denied perhaps the easiest and fastest research tool available at this moment.

It will require at least $200,000 to prepare a new questionnaire to study the next important question that must be answered: *How* is AIDS being transmitted? (In which bodily fluids, by which sexual behaviors, in what social environments?)

For months the CDC has been asked to begin such preparations for continued surveillance. The CDC is stretched to its limits and is dreadfully underfunded for what it's being asked, in all areas, to do.

■   Let's talk about various forms of treatment.

It is very difficult for a patient to find out which hospital to go to or which doctor to go to or which mode of treatment to attempt.

Hospitals and doctors are reluctant to reveal how well they're doing with each type of treatment. They may, if you press them, give you a general idea. Most will not show you their precise numbers of how many patients are doing well on what and how many failed to respond adequately.

Because of the ludicrous requirements of the medical journals, doctors are prohibited from revealing publicly the specific data they are gathering from their treatments of our bodies. Doctors and hospitals need money for research, and this money (from the National Institutes of Health, from cancer research funding organizations, from rich patrons) comes based on the performance of their work (i.e., their tabulations of their results of their treatment of our bodies); this performance is written up as "papers" that must be submitted to and accepted by such "distinguished" medical publications as the *New England Journal of Medicine.* Most of these "distinguished" publications, however, will not publish anything that has been spoken of, leaked, announced, or intimated publicly in advance. Even after acceptance, the doctors must hold their tongues until the article is actually published. Dr. Bijan Safai of Sloan-Kettering has been waiting over six months for the *New England Journal,* which has accepted his interferon study, to publish it. Until that happens, he is only permitted to speak in the most general terms of how interferon is or is not working.

Priorities in this area appear to be peculiarly out of kilter at this moment of life or death.

■   Let's talk about hospitals.

Everybody's full up, fellows. No room in the inn.

Part of this is simply overcrowding. Part of this is cruel.

Sloan-Kettering still enforces a regulation from pre-AIDS days that only one dermatology patient per week can be admitted to that hospital. (Kaposi's sarcoma falls under dermatology at Sloan-Kettering.) But Sloan-Kettering is also the second-largest treatment center for AIDS patients in New York. You can be near death and still not get into Sloan-Kettering.

Additionally, Sloan-Kettering (and the Food and Drug Administration) requires patients to receive their initial shots of interferon while they are hospitalized. A lot of men want to try interferon at Sloan-Kettering before they try chemotherapy elsewhere.

It's not hard to see why there's such a waiting list to get into Sloan-Kettering.

Most hospital staffs are still so badly educated about AIDS that they don't know much about it, except that they've heard it's infectious. (There still have been no cases in hospital staff or among the very doctors who have been treating AIDS victims for two years.) Hence, as I said earlier, AIDS patients are often treated like lepers.

For various reasons, I would not like to be a patient at the Veterans Administration Hospital on East 24th Street or at New York Hospital. (Incidents involving AIDS patients at these two hospitals have been reported in news stories in the *Native*.)

I believe it falls to this city's Department of Health, under Commissioner David Sencer, and the Health and Hospitals Corporation, under Commissioner Stanley Brezenoff, to educate this city, its citizens, and its hospital workers about all areas of a public health emergency. Well, they have done an appalling job of educating our citizens, our hospital workers, and even, in some instances, our doctors. Almost everything this city knows about AIDS has come to it, in one way or another, through Gay Men's Health Crisis. And that includes television programs, magazine articles, radio commercials, newsletters, health-recommendation brochures, open forums, and sending speakers everywhere, including—when asked—into hospitals. If three out of four AIDS cases were occurring in straights instead of in gay men, you can bet all hospitals and their staffs would know what was happening. And it would be this city's Health Department and Health and Hospitals Corporation that would be telling them.

■   Let's talk about what gay tax dollars are buying for gay men.

Now we're arriving at the truly scandalous.

For over a year and a half the National Institutes of Health has been "reviewing" which from among some $55 million worth of grant applications for AIDS research money it will eventually fund.

It's not even a question of NIH having to ask Congress for money. It's already there. Waiting. NIH has almost $8 million already appropriated that it has yet to release into usefulness.

There is no question that if this epidemic was happening to the straight, white, non-intravenous-drug-using middle class, that money would have been put into use almost two years ago, when the first alarming signs of this epidemic were noticed by Dr. Alvin Friedman-Kien and Dr. Linda Laubenstein at New York University Hospital.

During the first *two weeks* of the Tylenol scare, the United States Government spent $10 million to find out what was happening.

Every hospital in New York that's involved in AIDS research has used up every bit of the money it could find for researching AIDS while waiting for NIH grants to come through. These hospitals have been working on AIDS for up to two years and are now desperate for replenishing funds. Important studies that began last year, such as Dr. Michael Lange's at St. Luke's-Roosevelt, are now going under for lack of money. Important leads that were and are developing cannot be pursued. (For instance, few hospitals can afford plasmapheresis machines, and few patients can afford this experimental treatment either, since few insurance policies will cover the $16,600 bill.) New York University Hospital, the largest treatment

center for AIDS patients in the world, has had its grant application pending at NIH for a year and a half. Even if the application is successful, the earliest time that NYU could receive any
money would be late summer.

The NIH would probably reply that it's foolish just to throw
money away, that that hasn't worked before. And, NIH would
say, if nobody knows what's happening, what's to study?

Any good administrator with half a brain could survey the
entire AIDS mess and come up with twenty leads that merit
further investigation. I could do so myself. In any research, in
any investigation, you have to start somewhere. You can't just
not start anywhere at all.

But then, AIDS is happening mostly to gay men, isn't it?

All of this is indeed ironic. For within AIDS, as most researchers have been trying to convey to the NIH, perhaps may
reside the answer to the question of what it is that causes
cancer itself. If straights had more brains, or were less bigoted
against gays, they would see that, as with hepatitis B, gay men
are again doing their suffering for them, revealing this disease
to them. They can use us as guinea pigs to discover the cure for
AIDS before it hits them, which most medical authorities are
still convinced will be happening shortly in increasing numbers.

(As if it had not been malevolent enough, the NIH is now,
for unspecified reasons, also turning away AIDS patients from
its hospital in Bethesda, Maryland. The hospital, which had
been treating anyone and everyone with AIDS free of charge,
now will only take AIDS patients if they fit into their current
investigating protocol. Whatever that is. The NIH publishes
''papers,'' too.)

Gay men pay taxes just like everyone else. NIH money
should be paying for our research just like everyone else's. We
desperately need something from our government to save our
lives, and we're not getting it.

■   Let's talk about health insurance and welfare problems.

Many of the ways of treating AIDS are experimental, and
many health insurance policies do not cover most of them. Blue
Cross is particularly bad about accepting anything unusual.

Many serious victims of AIDS have been unable to qualify

for welfare or disability or social security benefits. There are increasing numbers of men unable to work and unable to claim welfare because AIDS is not on the list of qualifying disability illnesses. (Immune deficiency is an acceptable determining factor for welfare among children, but not adults. Figure that one out.) There are also increasing numbers of men unable to pay their rent, men thrown out on the street with nowhere to live and no money to live with, and men who have been asked by roommates to leave because of their illnesses. And men with serious AIDS are being fired from certain jobs.

The horror stories in this area, of those suddenly found destitute, of those facing this illness with insufficient insurance, continue to mount. (One man who'd had no success on other therapies was forced to beg from his friends the $16,600 he needed to try, as a last resort, plasmapheresis.)

■   Finally, let's talk about our mayor, Ed Koch.

Our mayor, Ed Koch, appears to have chosen, for whatever reason, not to allow himself to be perceived by the non-gay world as visibly helping us in this emergency.

Repeated requests to meet with him have been denied us. Repeated attempts to have him make a very necessary public announcement about this crisis and public health emergency have been refused by his staff.

I sometimes think he doesn't know what's going on. I sometimes think that, like some king who has been so long on his throne he's lost touch with his people, Koch is so protected and isolated by his staff that he is unaware of what fear and pain we're in. No *human* being could otherwise continue to be so useless to his suffering constituents. When I was allowed a few moments with him at a party for outgoing Cultural Affairs Commissioner (and Gay Men's Health Crisis Advisory Board Member) Henry Geldzahler, I could tell from his responses that Mayor Koch had not been well briefed on AIDS or what is happening in his city. When I started to fill him in, I was pulled away by an aide, who said, "Your time is up."

I could see our mayor relatively blameless in his shameful secreting of himself from our need of him in this time of epidemic—except for one fact. Our mayor thinks so little of us that he has assigned as his "liaison" to the gay community a man of such appalling insensitivity to our community and its needs that I am ashamed to say he is a homosexual. His name is Herb Rickman, and for a while our mayor saw fit to have Rickman serve as liaison to the Hasidic Jewish community, too. Hasidic Jews hate gays. Figure out a mayor who would do that to you.

To continue to allow Herb Rickman to represent us in City Hall will, in my view, only bring us closer to death.

When I denounced Rickman at a recent gay Community Council meeting, I received a resounding ovation. He is almost universally hated by virtually every gay organization in New York. Why, then, have we all allowed this man to shit on us so, to refuse our phone calls, to scream at us hysterically, to slam down telephones, to threaten us, to tease us with favors that are not delivered, to keep us waiting hours for an audience, to lie to us—in short, to humiliate us so? He would not do this to black or Jewish leaders. And they would not take it from him for one minute. Why, why, why do we allow him to do it to us? And he, a homosexual!

One can only surmise that our mayor wants us treated this way.

My last attempt at communication with Herb Rickman was on January 23rd [1983], when, after several days of his not returning my phone calls, I wrote to him that the mayor continued to ignore our crisis at his peril. And I state here and now that if Mayor Ed Koch continues to remain invisible to us and to ignore us in this era of mounting death, I swear I shall do everything in my power to see that he never wins elective office again.

Rickman would tell you that the mayor is concerned, that he has established an "Inter-Departmental Task Force"—and, as a member of it, I will tell you that this Task Force is just lip service and a waste of everyone's time. It hasn't even met for two months. (Health Commissioner David Sencer had his gallstones out.)

On October 28th, 1982, Mayor Koch was implored to make a public announcement about our emergency. If he had done so then, and if he was only to do so now, the following would be put into action:

1. The community at large would be alerted (you would be amazed at how many people, including gay men, still don't know enough about the AIDS danger).

2. Hospital staffs and public assistance offices would also be alerted and their education commenced.

3. The country, President Reagan, and the National Institutes of Health, as well as Congress, would be alerted, and these constitute the most important ears of all.

If the mayor doesn't think it's important enough to talk up AIDS, none of these people is going to, either.

The Mayor of New York has an enormous amount of power—when he wants to use it. When he wants to help his people. With the failure yet again of our civil rights bill, I'd guess our mayor doesn't want to use his power to help us.

With his silence on AIDS, the Mayor of New York is helping to kill us.

■ ■ ■

I am sick of our electing officials who in no way represent us. I am sick of our stupidity in believing candidates who promise us everything for our support and promptly forget us and insult us after we have given them our votes. Koch is the prime example, but not the only one. Daniel Patrick Moynihan isn't looking very good at this moment, either. Moynihan was requested by gay leaders to publicly ask Margaret Heckler at her confirmation hearing for Secretary of Health and Human Services if she could be fair to gays in view of her voting record of definite anti-gay bias. (Among other horrors, she voted to retain the sodomy law in Washington, D.C., at Jerry Falwell's request.) Moynihan refused to ask this question, as he has refused to meet with us about AIDS, despite our repeated requests. Margaret Heckler will have important jurisdiction over the CDC, over the NIH, over the Public Health Service, over the Food and Drug Administration—indeed, over all areas of AIDS concerns. Thank you, Daniel Patrick Moynihan. I am sick of our not realizing we have enough votes to defeat these people, and I am sick of our not electing our own openly gay officials in the first place. Moynihan doesn't even have an openly gay person on his staff, and he represents the city with the largest gay population in America.

I am sick of closeted gay doctors who won't come out to help us fight to rectify any of what I'm writing about. Doctors—the very letters "M.D."—have enormous clout, particularly when they fight in groups. Can you imagine what gay doctors could accomplish, banded together in a network, petitioning local and federal governments, straight colleagues, and the American Medical Association? I am sick of the passivity or nonparticipation or halfhearted protestation of all the gay medical associations (American Physicians for Human Rights, Bay Area Physicians for Human Rights, Gay Psychiatrists of New York, etc., etc.), and particularly our own New York Physicians for Human Rights, a group of 175 of our gay doctors who have, as a group, done *nothing.* You can count on one hand the number of our doctors who have really worked for *us.*

I am sick of the *Advocate,* one of this country's largest gay publications, which has yet to quite acknowledge that there's anything going on. That newspaper's recent AIDS issue was so innocuous you'd have thought all we were going through was little worse than a rage of the latest designer flu. And their own associate editor, Brent Harris, died from AIDS. Figure that one out.

With the exception of the *New York Native* and a few, very few, other gay publications, the gay press has been useless. If we can't get our own papers and magazines to tell us what's really happening to us, and this negligence is added to the negligent non-interest of the straight press (*The New York Times* took a leisurely year and a half between its major pieces, and the *Village Voice* took a year and a half to write anything at all), how are we going to get the word around that we're dying? Gay men in smaller towns and cities everywhere must be educated, too. Has the *Times* or the *Advocate* told you that twenty-nine cases have been reported from Paris?

I am sick of gay men who won't support gay charities. Go give your bucks to straight charities, fellows, while we die. Gay Men's Health Crisis is going crazy trying to accomplish everything it does—printing and distributing hundreds of thousands of educational items, taking care of several hundred AIDS victims (some of them straight) in and out of hospitals, arranging community forums and speakers all over this country, getting media attention, fighting bad hospital care, on and on and on, fighting for you and us in two thousand ways, *and* trying to sell 17,600 Circus tickets, too. Is the Red Cross doing this for you? Is the American Cancer Society? Your college alumni fund? The United Jewish Appeal? Catholic Charities? The United Way? The Lenox Hill Neighborhood Association, or any of the other fancy straight charities for which faggots put on black ties and dance at the Plaza? The National Gay Task Force—our only hope for national leadership, with its new and splendid leader, Virginia Apuzzo—which is spending more and more time fighting for the AIDS issue, is broke. Senior Action in a Gay Environment and Gay Men's Health Crisis are, within a few months, going to be without office space they can afford, and thus will be out on the street. The St. Mark's Clinic, held together by some of the few devoted gay doctors in this city who aren't interested in becoming rich, lives in constant terror of even higher rent and eviction. This community is desperate for the services these organizations are providing for it. And these organizations are all desperate for money, which is certainly not coming from straight people or President Reagan or Mayor Koch. (If every gay man within a 250-mile radius of Manhattan isn't in Madison Square Garden on the night of April 30th to help Gay Men's Health Crisis make enough money to get through the next horrible year of fighting against AIDS, I shall lose all hope that we have any future whatsoever.)

I am sick of closeted gays. It's 1983 already, guys, when are you going to come out? By 1984 you could be dead. Every gay man who is unable to come forward now and fight to save his own life is truly helping to kill the rest of us. There is only one thing that's going to save some of us, and this is *numbers* and pressure and our being perceived as united and a threat. As more and more of my friends die, I have less and less sympathy for men who are afraid their mommies will find out or afraid their bosses will find out or afraid their fellow doctors or professional associates will find out. Unless we can generate, visibly, numbers, masses, we are going to die.

I am sick of everyone in this community who tells me to stop creating a panic. How many of us have to die before *you* get scared off your ass and into action? Aren't 195 dead New Yorkers enough? Every straight person who is knowledgeable about the AIDS epidemic can't understand why gay men aren't marching on the White House. Over and over again I hear from them, "Why aren't you guys doing anything?" Every politician I have spoken to has said to me confidentially, "You guys aren't making enough noise. Bureaucracy only responds to pressure."

I am sick of people who say "it's no worse than statistics for smokers and lung cancer" or "considering how many homosexuals there are in the United States, AIDS is really statistically affecting only a very few." That would wash if there weren't 164 cases in twenty-eight days. That would wash if case numbers hadn't jumped from 41 to 1,112 in eighteen months. That would wash if cases in one city—New York—hadn't jumped to cases in fifteen countries and thirty-five states (up from thirty-four last week). That would wash if cases weren't coming in at more than four a day nationally and over two a day locally. That would wash if the mortality rate didn't start at 38 percent the first year of diagnosis and climb to a grotesque 86 percent after three years. Get your stupid heads out of the sand, you turkeys!

I am sick of guys who moan that giving up careless sex until this blows over is worse than death. How can they value life so little and cocks and asses so much? Come with me, guys, while I visit a few of our friends in Intensive Care at NYU. Notice the looks in their eyes, guys. They'd give up sex forever if you could promise them life.

I am sick of guys who think that all being gay means is sex in the first place. I am sick of guys who can only think with their cocks.

I am sick of "men" who say, "We've got to keep quiet or *they* will do such and such." *They* usually means the straight majority, the "Moral" Majority, or similarly perceived representatives of *them*. Okay, you "men"—be my guests: You can march off now to the gas chambers; just get right in line.

We shall always have enemies. Nothing we can ever do will remove them. Southern newspapers and Jerry Falwell's publications are already printing editorials proclaiming AIDS as God's deserved punishment on homosexuals. So what? Nasty words make poor little sissy pansy wilt and die?

And I am very sick and saddened by every gay man who

does not get behind this issue totally and with commitment—to fight for his life.

■ ■ ■

I don't want to die. I can only assume you don't want to die. Can we fight together?

For the past few weeks, about fifty community leaders and organization representatives have been meeting at Beth Simchat Torah, the gay synagogue, to prepare action. We call ourselves the AIDS Network. We come from all areas of health concern: doctors, social workers, psychologists, psychiatrists, nurses; we come from Gay Men's Health Crisis, from the National Gay Health Education Foundation, from New York Physicians for Human Rights, the St. Mark's Clinic, the Gay Men's Health Project; we come from the gay synagogue, the Gay Men's Chorus, from the Greater Gotham Business Council, SAGE, Lambda Legal Defense, Gay Fathers, the Christopher Street Festival Committee, Dignity, Integrity; we are lawyers, actors, dancers, architects, writers, citizens; we come from many component organizations of the Gay and Lesbian Community Council.

We have a leader. Indeed, for the first time our community appears to have a true leader. Her name is Virginia Apuzzo, she is head of the National Gay Task Force, and, as I have said, so far she has proved to be magnificent.

The AIDS Network has sent a letter to Mayor Koch. It contains twelve points that are urged for his consideration and action.

This letter to Mayor Koch also contains the following paragraph:

It must be stated at the outset that the gay community is growing increasingly aroused and concerned and angry. Should our avenues to the mayor of our city and the members of the Board of Estimate not be available, it is our feeling that the level of frustration is such that it will manifest itself in a manner heretofore not associated with this community and the gay population at large. It should be stated, too, at the outset, that as of February 25th, there were 526 cases of serious AIDS in New York's

metropolitan area and 195 deaths (and 1,112 cases nationally and 418 deaths) and it is the sad and sorry fact that
most gay men in our city now have close friends and lovers
who have either been stricken with or died from this disease. It is against this background that this letter is addressed. It is this issue that has, ironically, united our
community in a way not heretofore thought possible.

Further, a number of AIDS Network members have been
studying civil disobedience with one of the experts from Dr.
Martin Luther King's old team. We are learning how. Gay men
are the strongest, toughest people I know. We are perhaps
shortly to get an opportunity to show it.

I'm sick of hearing that Mayor Koch doesn't respond to
pressures and threats from the disenfranchised, that he walks
away from confrontations. Maybe he does. But we have *tried*
to make contact with him, we are *dying*, so what other choice
but confrontation has he left us?

I hope we don't have to conduct sit-ins or tie up traffic or get
arrested. I hope our city and our country will start to do something to help start saving us. But it is time for us to be perceived
for what we truly are: an angry community and a strong community, and therefore *a threat.* Such are the realities of politics. Nationally we are 24 million strong, which is more than
there are Jews or blacks or Hispanics in this country.

I want to make a point about what happens if we *don't* get
angry about AIDS. There are the obvious losses, of course:
Little of what I've written about here is likely to be rectified
with the speed necessary to help the growing number of victims. But something worse will happen, and is already happening. Increasingly, we are being *blamed* for AIDS, for this
epidemic; we are being called its perpetrators, through our
blood, through our "promiscuity," through just being the gay
men so much of the rest of the world has learned to hate. We
can point out until we are blue in the face that we are not the
cause of AIDS but its victims, that AIDS has landed among us
first, as it could have landed among them first. But other frightened populations are going to drown out these truths by playing on the worst bigoted fears of the straight world, and send
the status of gays right back to the Dark Ages. Not all Jews

are blamed for Meyer Lansky, Rabbis Bergman and Kahane, or for money-lending. All Chinese aren't blamed for the recent Seattle slaughters. But all gays are blamed for John Gacy, the North American Man/Boy Love Association, and AIDS.

Enough. I am told this is one of the longest articles the *Native* has ever run. I hope I have not been guilty of saying ineffectively in five thousand words what I could have said in five: we must fight to live.

I am angry and frustrated almost beyond the bound my skin and bones and body and brain can encompass. My sleep is tormented by nightmares and visions of lost friends, and my days are flooded by the tears of funerals and memorial services and seeing my sick friends. How many of us must die before *all* of us living fight back?

I know that unless I fight with every ounce of my energy I will hate myself. I hope, I pray, I implore you to feel the same.

I am going to close by doing what Dr. Ron Grossman did at GMHC's second Open Forum last November at Julia Richman High School. He listed the names of the patients he had lost to AIDS. Here is a list of twenty dead men I knew:

Nick Rock

Rick Wellikoff

Jack Nau

Shelly

Donald Krintzman

Jerry Green

Michael Maletta

Paul Graham

Toby

Harry Blumenthal

Stephen Sperry

Brian O'Hara

Barry

David

Jeffrey Croland

Z.

David Jackson

Tony Rappa

Robert Christian

Ron Doud

And one more, who will be dead by the time these words appear in print.

If we don't act immediately, then we face our approaching doom.

■ ■ ■

Volunteers Needed for Civil Disobedience

It is necessary that we have a pool of at least three thousand people who are prepared to participate in demonstrations of civil disobedience. Such demonstrations might include sit-ins or traffic tie-ups. All participants must be prepared to be arrested. I am asking every gay person and every gay organization to canvass all friends and members and make a count of the total number of people you can provide toward this pool of three thousand.

Let me know how many people you can be counted on providing. Just include the number of people; you don't have to send actual names—you keep that list yourself. And include your own phone numbers. *Start these lists now.*

L.K.

T his essay managed to create quite a stir, but more so in cities other than New York. It was reprinted in almost every major gay newspaper across the country. I told the Board of GMHC that I was writing it, and they told me to put in the disclaimer that I was speaking for myself and not our organization. When it appeared, they hated it.

The appeal for volunteers for civil disobedience was not successful. A group of about fifty managed to coalesce and meet for instruction with a straight black man who had worked with Martin Luther King, Jr. We called ourselves the AIDS Network Public Events Committee. Such a small number didn't augur well. But, as will be seen, it proved to be sufficient.

Although this article is dated after the letter to the mayor that follows, it's placed first for background. The repercussions from the letter to the mayor were to lead to the final break in my affiliation with Gay Men's Health Crisis, which this present article, along with all my media appearances, greatly exacerbated.

The AIDS Network Letter to Mayor Koch

3 March 83

Hon. Edward I. Koch
Mayor, City of New York
City Hall
New York, New York 10007

Dear Mayor Koch,

The AIDS Network, a gay community group of concerned health-care professionals, doctors, psychiatrists, psychologists, social workers, representatives of (including but not limited to) Gay Men's Health Crisis, National Gay Health Education Foundation, the Gay Synagogue, National Gay Task Force, Greater Gotham Business Council, New York Physicians for Human Rights, St. Mark's Clinic, and the Gay and Lesbian Community Council and all of its component organizations—having met together because of their growing concern over the alarming rise of serious cases of AIDS and the high mortality rate therefrom, and the general feeling that the City of New York, where 56.5 percent of all serious cases of AIDS cases are occurring, is not perceived as working swiftly enough to fight this fast-growing epidemic on all fronts—addresses the following requests to the Mayor of our City and to the Board of Estimate, along with the fervent plea that an immediate meeting be scheduled for a personal presentation.

It must be stated at the outset that the gay community is growing increasingly aroused and concerned and angry. Should our avenues to the Mayor of our City and the members of the Board of Estimate not be available, it is our feeling that the level of frustration is such that it will manifest itself in a manner heretofore not associated with this community and the gay population at large. It should be stated, too, at the outset, that as of February 25th, there were 526 cases of serious AIDS in New York's metropolitan area and 195 deaths, and it is the sad and sorry fact that most gay men in our city now have close friends and lovers who have either been stricken with or died from this disease. It is against this background that this letter is addressed. It is this issue that has, ironically, united our community in a way not heretofore thought possible.

The following points are urged upon the Mayor for his consideration and action:

1. PUBLIC ANNOUNCEMENT: The first and primary point is that the Mayor *publicly* pronounce to this City that it is in a state of extreme public health emergency. This announcement should be made to the press and all media so that its import can be immediately responded to. It is imperative that such an announcement be made and is indeed placed first among our demands since, in making this announcement, the Mayor is in fact placing into motion action on all the following points requiring immediate action.

2. EDUCATION: It is imperative that all sectors of the community be educated about the present emergency, including the populations at risk, which, at present, include gay men, Haitians, those populations liable to intravenous drug use, and hemophiliacs. It is imperative that such education inform people that the stricken communities not be stigmatized as the cause of AIDS, for they truly are the victims of this epidemic.

Health-care and hospital workers and mental-health providers of social and all public assistance services must also be educated immediately. It must be borne in mind that at present many hospital workers are simply not familiar with the problems of AIDS, how to care for AIDS patients, and the question of contagion. This applies to both city and voluntary hospitals. The number of complaints arising from all hospitals of improper patient care is rising.

3. CITY AIDS COORDINATOR AND OFFICE: That the Mayor establish the paid position of City AIDS Coordinator, together with a City AIDS Coordination Office. The appointment of this Coordinator is to be made in consultation with the stricken communities. The job of this Coordinator and this Office would be to oversee all AIDS activities and to be knowledgeable of everything that is transpiring in each department and organization in the AIDS Network.

4. INTER-DEPARTMENTAL TASK FORCE: MAYOR'S OFFICE REPRESENTATIVE: That there be a member of the Mayor's immediate staff appointed to join the monthly Inter-Departmental Task Force that the Mayor has already established and presently under the Chairmanship of Health Commissioner David Sencer.

5. INTER-DEPARTMENTAL TASK FORCE: BOARD OF ESTIMATE REPRESENTATIVES: That each member of the Board of Estimate have a representative on this Inter-Departmental Task Force.

6. INTER-DEPARTMENTAL TASK FORCE: MEETINGS: That this Inter-Departmental Task Force meet on a more regular basis and be empowered to achieve results.

7. ACCELERATION OF RESEARCH MONIES: That the Mayor contact the President of the United States personally, as well as the Governor of this State, and Congress, and urge that all use every power to accelerate the release of research monies already appropriated by the National Institutes of Health but still not granted to the many local and national doctors, hospitals, and laboratories clamoring to study AIDS. It is imperative that each of these parties be asked to locate and identify all discretion-

ary funds that might be immediately put to use to fight AIDS. All major New York hospitals and research facilities have been waiting in excess of one year for much needed monies to replenish their long-ago-depleted research funds.

8. RESEARCH: That the Mayor see to it that AIDS be represented in the new supplemental budget that the President will submit to Congress, and that the Mayor see to it that, in view of all new recent developments, the National Institutes of Health be funded to immediately process a second call of grant requests.

And that these funds be adequate to provide and support scientific investigation for: epidemiological research to determine risk factors and transmissibility, and to establish comprehensive national disease surveillance programs; socio-medical research to develop measures to assess social behavior, patterns of intimate contact, and characteristics of social support; immunological research to improve the medical and psycho-social treatment of patients. The combined goals of this research are to define and control this disorder. All of this is to be done in consultation and contact with the AIDS Scientific Review Board already established in this City.

9. IMMEDIATE REESTABLISHMENT OF SURVEILLANCE OF THE STRICKEN COMMUNITIES: That efforts be made to urge the Centers for Disease Control to join with Gay Men's Health Crisis and the AIDS Scientific Advisory Board in reestablishing epidemiological surveillance of, particularly, the gay community AIDS victims, which has presently been discontinued. This is imperative work that is not being done. An invaluable research tool is not being utilized.

10. PUBLIC ASSISTANCE AND PRIVATE INSURANCE CLAIMS: That the immense problems being encountered by patients and victims of AIDS in the areas of public assistance and social security and disability and Medicaid be addressed. There are increasing numbers of people unable to work and unable to claim various forms of welfare because AIDS is not on the list of qualifying disability illnesses. That the State Insurance Commission

also investigate private insurance companies' practices in rejecting claims for AIDS patients and victims.

11. SIGNIFICANT OTHERS: That a policy be adopted wherein and whereby patients are allowed to identify who their significant others are. Hospitals and health-care facilities should be advised that gay people consider lovers, partners, and friends as members of their primary family, and these should be judged as such and not refused admission to patients as not being family members, spouses, or blood relatives.

12. HEALTH-CARE EMERGENCY SPACE: A public health emergency requires space to administer to its problems, and Gay Men's Health Crisis, Inc., at present the organization most actively involved in tending to the many problems in the communities at highest risks, is without adequate space for its office and for the many patient services programs it performs, including Crisis Intervention Counseling, Individual Therapy and Group Support Therapy for victims of AIDS, Kaposi's sarcoma cancer, and *Pneumocystis carinii* pneumonia, and maintenance of its extensive community education programs that have resulted in hundreds of thousands of items of instruction and recommendation.

While it is the space problem of Gay Men's Health Crisis that is of most pressing immediate concern, it is the hope of the gay and lesbian community that all of its vital social services, both pertaining to AIDS, in organizations such as GMHC and St. Mark's Clinic, and in other areas, such as, but not limited to, SAGE (Senior Action in a Gay Environment), the Fund for Human Dignity, Lambda Legal Defense, and gay religious organizations, for the first time find a home under one roof to form a Gay Community Center, such as exists in the cities of Los Angeles, Philadelphia, and Houston. The old high school on West 13th Street would be ideal for this purpose.

Finally and in summation, while we are eager to speak for all at-risk communities, these points represent the concerns of the gay community mainly, though an effort to form a coalition of all at-risk groups has been made. A face-to-face meeting with the Mayor is requested with all dispatch so that the above can be attended to in as swift a fashion as possible, and so that the period of suffering for those stricken can be alleviated with all similar speed.

The favor of an acknowledgment is requested within thirty days from this date.

The AIDS Network was an ad hoc group that met, for several years, once a week at 8:00 A.M. It was formed by many who felt left out of GMHC, which unfortunately was gaining an "elitist" reputation. The remarkable fact about GMHC, that it was attracting many who had never participated in gay organizations or in anything having remotely to do with gay politics, worked against it in that many who had participated in the gay movement for years now felt disenfranchised and unwelcome at the most vital new center of gay activity. And these newcomers to "activism"—as it was becoming increasingly and tragically clear—were not "activists" at all; they were concerned citizens who wished to help quietly, in the pastoral sense. And so continued the concretizing of GMHC into its present state: that of a social service organization, rather than an advocacy one. While I supported the necessity for the former, I was passionately committed to the latter as well. GMHC, as far as I was concerned, was formed primarily to spread information and fight in every way to help the living keep living. And it was this fight to include my priorities in GMHC's agenda that I was losing, and was about to lose completely.

It was to the AIDS Network that these veterans of years of involvement in the gay movement came, as well as newcomers who shared their desires for more aggressive tactics of confrontation. I wrote the above letter with much input from those who attended an

emergency meeting I called. The letter was then signed
by representatives of some sixty gay organizations and
hand-delivered to the offices of the mayor and each member of the Board of Estimate. The mayor did not respond. On Sunday, April 10th, a very small group of
us—no more than twenty—picketed in torrential rain,
outside Lenox Hill Hospital, where the mayor was making an appearance at the historic AIDS Conference organized by Dr. Kevin Cahill (where he somehow
managed to induce appearances not only by the mayor
but by Cardinal Cooke as well, in addition to having a
statement from Senator Edward Kennedy read at the
opening).

This picketing was extensively televised locally, as
were the placards themselves, which included ones calling the mayor "blind" and "a coward" and one that said,
HEY, ED, COME OUT OF THE CLOSET AND HELP YOUR GAY
BROTHERS.

The very next morning, word was sent out from City
Hall that the mayor would finally meet with ten people
from the gay community.

When I arrived at the next meeting of the AIDS
Network, the ten people had already been chosen. Paul
Popham had, with the approval of GMHC's Board,
elected to take with him Mel Rosen, a graduate student
who was GMHC's part-time, volunteer, executive director.

I am not particularly proud of my subsequent behav-
ior, though I have come to understand it. I felt betrayed.
I had spent two years working full time to build GMHC.
I had called for the mayor's meeting and had arranged
the above petition. I told Paul that if I was not allowed
to attend, I would resign. He told me he had polled the
Board and they wished Mel to go. He said they were all
afraid I'd yell at the mayor and be an embarrassment.
I realized they wanted me to resign. That really hurt.
Petulantly, defensively, I resigned. Though I was implored by such gay leaders as Judge Richard Failla,
Virginia Apuzzo, and the late Peter Vogel, I stubbornly
refused to reconsider. Even when the AIDS Network

agreed to let me go as one of their representatives, I declined. I was furious and hurt and probably burned out. My friend Rodger McFarlane maintains that I was subconsciously preparing this break—that I wanted to write what was eventually to become my play *The Normal Heart,* and this was the only way I could allow myself to do so without feeling guilty.

Nevertheless, I did feel guilty, for quite some time, that I had so behaved. For many years I berated myself that, had I only stayed with GMHC, it would have included among its many activities the political-advocacy tasks that no one else was performing.

I was also to learn yet another lesson: When you are affiliated with an established organization, it's much easier to be taken seriously when talking to the media. Now I was disenfranchised, and I had lost my official soapbox.

Not one item of any substance was achieved at the mayor's meeting on April 20th. He listened, and did nothing. Matters remained as they were before. And as many of them still are now.

The Mark of Courage

I t is now more than two years since AIDS entered our lives. Every one of us has learned more in these two years than ever before about what it means to be gay—in all ways, good and bad.

I am prouder now of gay people than ever. We have never been closer together as a community than we are now. We are learning how courageous we are. To oppression, homophobia, discrimination, self-hate, religions that don't want us, and families that think we're freaks, has now been added an epidemic that kills. We have to be courageous to live through all of this. Gay men and lesbians are the most courageous people I know.

Courage is a wonderful quality, one of the best. But how do we take it and make it work for us?

We've all learned a few hard lessons during these past two long years. One is that AIDS represents how badly we're served by our medical system.

---

* Gay Pride Day speech, June 26, 1983, delivered at parade rally. Published in the *New York Native*, Issue 67, July 4–17, 1983.

Another is that, as a community, so far we still have very little political power.

It has taken two long years to get Congress to consider AIDS funding. It has taken two long years for the National Institutes of Health to consider to whom to give funding. It has taken two long years to get the media to pay attention to AIDS. It has taken two long years to get *The New York Times* to write with any regularity about an epidemic that's occuring in its very own city. And it has taken two long years to get our very own mayor to timidly acknowledge that we have an emergency here.

Who knows how many more people will die needlessly because of this unconscionable tardiness?

The official rate of AIDS cases is now up to seven a day. This is the *official* figure; it is low. Because names of patients go onto lists that enter government computers, many patients and their doctors are now refusing to report their cases to the Centers for Disease Control, which is unable to guarantee confidentiality.

We must find ways of making sure these atrocities never, never happen again.

The White House is threatening to veto the supplemental budget that contains $12 million for AIDS. Reagan's men have specifically identified the AIDS funding allotment as being unnecessary. While I've been told this money will probably be found somewhere, the threatened veto only serves as another delay: Now the NIH will not release any more money for research until next October or November. These research grants are for three-year periods, so we're now looking at 1987 before these research reports on AIDS will be due.

Yes, we have to be courageous to live through all of this.

We have to be courageous as we wake up each day, as we wait for whatever we pray will be discovered to be discovered, and we continue to face the fact that *time is not on our side.*

I'd like to ask some questions.

Can we afford to have a New York gay community that is disorganized, lacking recognized and designated leaders who can speak for all of us? We must be able to send our best, brightest, smartest, cagiest, wisest to represent our side at various bargaining tables. We must not get bogged down with petty internal squabbles.

Can we afford to be disorganized nationally, with little political networking from city to city, from state to state?

Can we afford to be represented in Washington by only one lobbyist? Today, special-interest groups of every size and description support large staffs in Washington. We 24 million gay men and lesbians are going to have to dig into our pockets and pay for better and more extensive representation in our nation's capital, where so much of what affects us is decided. I am proud to cite the recent decision by the Board of Directors of Gay Men's Health Crisis to help establish a Washington lobby for AIDS with $40,000 of the dollars you have already contributed.

Can we afford to support just one gay charity or one gay issue? I call upon all gay organizations that seek money from the community to distribute their complete financial statements and a tally of their total paid-up membership—in other words, to be fiscally responsible. I call upon all members of the boards of directors of these organizations to retain their positions because of their skills and abilities, not for reasons of tokenism or friendship. It is essential that each organization be run by people who are the best that we can find, without regard to superfluous distinctions.

Can we afford to have such a bad relationship with the mayor of our very own city, whom we helped install in that very office? It took us nineteen months even to be heard. His office promised us space for AIDS patients and activities nine long months ago. We still have nothing. San Francisco's gay community has received $4 million from its mayor, and Houston has a gay vice-mayor. We don't even have a liaison from the mayor to the gay community on non-health issues who is available to us on any regular basis—much less one who does an acceptable job of representing our community.

Can we afford to be ignored by *The New York Times?* Yes, that paper is finally reporting about AIDS, but that's all that's being written about us. Any newspaper that refuses to report on the activities of one million of its constituent population is irresponsible. I'd like to suggest a twenty-four-hour-a-day,

seven-days-a-week picket line outside the *New York Times* of-
fices. We should carry neat placards: ONE MILLION GAY MEN
AND LESBIANS WANT EQUAL TIME; ONE MILLION GAY MEN AND
LESBIANS WANT TO BE CALLED GAY.

Can we afford any longer not to start our own Anti-Defama-
tion League? This is an organization that the Jewish people
started with only a handful of volunteers in 1913, "to stop the
defamation of the Jewish people." In those days you could still
see ads that demanded: "No dogs! No Jews!" You don't see that
anymore because the Jews started an organization that protests officially every single time anything anti-Semitic appears
in public. It's time we started our own.

Can we afford duplication of energies and services? Do we
need a Gay Men's Health Crisis and an AIDS Network and an
ARC and a Gay Men With AIDS? Isn't there more strength in
unity? Do we need both a National Gay Task Force and a Gay
Rights National Lobby? If we do, could they not work together
more effectively? And if we don't, could the boards of directors
of these two organizations please join the rest of us in helping
Virginia Apuzzo become the one truly national leader we so
desperately need at this moment in history?

Can we afford not to have more support from our lesbian
sisters at this time of crisis and as this crisis unites the gay male
community?

Can we afford not to heal wounds and unite?

Can we afford not to have an openly gay member of the City
Council? I support Bill Hirsch's excellent idea that all the
money we collect at our local Human Rights Campaign Fund
Dinner at the Waldorf stay right here in New York to find,
nominate, campaign with, and elect our own openly gay candidate.

Can we afford to continue living under the tyranny of beauty
and muscles and big tits and big dicks and clonedom and youth?
Can we afford not to begin working hard toward eroticizing
intelligence, kindness, responsibility, devotion, achievement,
respect—skills and qualities that are far more sexy, far more
lasting, and far more important for our survival than big pecs
and biceps and a washboard stomach?

Compared to what we have lived through these past two

years, to work on any or all of the above should not be as frightening.

I know that each and every one of us is scared and frightened in ways we've never been before. But let our fear not lead to denial, to going back into closets, to pretending. Let our fear give us extra courage. We are each our own masters.

To see the miraculous growth and ascending maturity of Gay Men's Health Crisis is to know what we are capable of doing when we put our minds and hearts into it. I would like to pay tribute here to the man who is president of that organization, Paul Popham. This community will never know the incredible extent of this man's devotion or how much it will be forever in his debt. He has learned, as we all are learning, as we all must learn, how to grow from day to day, each day at a time, each moment and bit by bit, so that we soon find ourselves able to perform feats we never imagined or dreamed we were capable of the day before.

On a personal note, I would like to apologize to any of the people dear to me whose feelings I may have bruised these past two years. I have been very much the angry man. It seems that in my frustration at seeing AIDS ignored for so long I just couldn't shut up. I have perhaps tried in too clumsy a fashion to hurry things along. I am by nature an impatient man.

But I am also a hopeful man. We have never felt the love of our fellow gay men and lesbians so much as in these past two years. This most dire emergency in our history is giving us the chance to fashion a new community.

With and from such love we can perform miracles. With and from such love our courage can take us to our future. With and from such love visions are formed and made reality. Each of us must put aside our fear and recognize the great courage within us, and take this courage and turn it into action. We must do nothing less now than remake the soul of our time. It is incumbent on us, the living, to do so, to ensure the future for our gay children, the millions and millions of proud gay men and lesbians who will follow us.

Solzhenitsyn warns us: "If we perish and lose this world, the fault will be ours alone." But we shall not lose it. We shall not perish. Our people are marching. Our people are courageous. Our people will survive.

I missed GMHC terribly. After such a long period of furious activity, constantly ringing phones, a mountain of problems waiting for solutions, and the sustaining comradeship of so many devoted fellow workers as we all aspired to make something happen, I now found myself alone at home, and feeling very much a pariah. One day there weren't enough hours in the day and the next day I had nothing to do. My phone hardly rang at all. I attended a few GMHC social functions, where I stood on one side of the room and the Board, only weeks before my closest friends, stood on the other. On one occasion, I commandeered the microphone in the DJ's booth of a bar where volunteers were being thanked with a party, and attempted to rouse them into action against the Board. "Tell them they made a mistake in letting me go. . . . Tell them they must fight harder and not be so timid and afraid. . . ." That sort of thing. When I emerged from the booth (I've been told that the whole episode was like something out of *Dr. Strangelove*), I was accosted by one of the volunteers, who started screaming at the top of his lungs that I was out to destroy GMHC. It dawned on me that now I couldn't even criticize this organization—which I had come to look upon as my child—and certainly not publicly, without inadvertently hurting it, perhaps stunting its growth in these early years of its development.

I wanted very much to come back to it (and I would later expend a great deal of useless energy in three separate attempts to get myself back on the Board), but I had made the decision that it was time to attempt to write something about my experiences since the epidemic began. It's not often that writers are so placed on the front line of history in the making, and I felt an obligation as well as the desire. I had earlier attempted to do so in a novel, but I'd found this form not immediate enough to convey the urgency of my feelings. Also, it had taken me three years to write *Faggots*, and I

wanted whatever I wrote to be out in the world as
quickly as possible. I also knew that no film company
would ever finance a movie about either AIDS or any
other subject remotely dealing with homosexuality.
That left only a play, and the only time I'd tried a play
before, I'd failed.

Well, I'd decided to go to Europe for the summer.
Perhaps in wandering about, the matter would sort itself out. And indeed it did. It was while I was in Germany, while visiting Dachau, that the thoughts began to
coalesce into what would shortly become my play *The
Normal Heart.*

Paul Popham and I had made peace with each other
shortly after the *Dr. Strangelove* episode. Somehow we
were still able to do that then. Our friendship and respect for each other was still able to survive our huge
differences in personality and style. He was a gentle,
quiet man, accustomed to the rigors and structures of
the corporate world and of the army, where he'd been
a Green Beret. He'd never had to work with a loose
cannon like me before, and I think most of the time I
was, for him, an exotic creature from another planet.
(He once told me he'd never met a Jew till college.) My
problem with him was of a different nature: I was half
in love with him, which he sensed and which made him
uncomfortable. (Straight men, I believe, don't usually
have these added problems in running their organizations.) This made it even more difficult for us to handle
our philosophical disagreements equably.

The performance of the Ringling Brothers Circus
that GMHC had bought out on April 30th was a huge
success. It was, up to that time, the biggest, most successful gay fund-raising event ever held, clearing over
a quarter of a million dollars. Leonard Bernstein walking across the length of Madison Square Garden in his
white dinner jacket to conduct the circus orchestra in
the national anthem, while eighteen thousand gay men
and their friends and families cheered, was one of the
most moving moments I have ever experienced. (*The
New York Times* did not report the occasion, a cruel

oversight that Abe Rosenthal was later shamed into apologizing for.) Paul generously announced to this crowd that I was leaving to take a rest, and that the Board wished to thank me for all my efforts. And the crowd cheered again, which I also will long remember.

I stayed on until June 26th, because I'd agreed to speak on Gay Pride Day. The version of my speech printed here is a bit more polite than some of my additions on the spot; I was gratified, when I called Mayor Koch "a heartless, selfish son of a bitch," that resounding cheers were heard again. I rushed to the airport and took a plane to Europe. I thought the bastard might be sending someone after me.

2,339 and Counting

I've been away from New York City for three months. I left after two miracles: the sold-out Circus benefit that Gay Men's Health Crisis sponsored in Madison Square Garden and the biggest Gay Pride Day parade New York gay people and their friends ever marched in together. Eighteen thousand at the first and many hundreds of thousands at the second. I was proud to be gay when I left New York. I had never seen the New York gay community so visibly together. The epidemic of AIDS had, miraculously and ironically, brought us together like the English at Dunkirk.

How could so much progress have evaporated so quickly?

I return to New York to find much of the New York gay community back at its petty bickerings, at the mercy of loud-mouth do-nothings murderously tying up what passes for political process among our disparate groups. I return to find Gay Men's Health Crisis—for two long and woeful years the only AIDS game in town for accurate information, for a list of social services that matches the Red Cross, for providing loving and supportive care to over four hundred patients—suddenly the

* *Village Voice*, October 4, 1983.

butt of outrageous and bitchy criticism. What should be cherished and supported by this community as a prideful treasure—and believe me, all of you gay men who are open to the possibility of contracting AIDS, there is no one else in this city who gives or cares much for us—has suddenly become the community's newest, most fashionable victim of badmouth. I returned to find GMHC's next vital fund-raiser, the October 1st Rodeo at Madison Square Garden, less than one-third sold out.

I return to find something else going on, just as bad and just as dangerous. Somehow there are waves of rumor that the epidemic is waning, that figures have slowed down, that, as in some fairy tale, we're all on our way to a happy ending and we can now return to apathy and closetry.

How can we be so dumb and blind and ignorant? In March, I wrote an article for the *New York Native* called "1,112 and Counting." Six months later there are more than twice as many cases in our country—2,339. Of these, 945 are dead. New York City is the home of over 40 percent of all victims—975, with 392 dead. (In March, New York figures were 526 cases and 195 dead.)

In June, 67 new cases were reported in this city; in July, 88 new cases were reported in this city; in August, 102 new cases were reported in this city. (Back in March, there were 56.) How can anyone believe things are getting better?

Almost three out of four cases still occur in sexually active gay men. "Sexually active" is defined as having sex once (i.e., the opposite of sexually inactive). The early profile of extreme promiscuity among victims is no longer accurate. A nun in Haiti has died from AIDS after having had sex only once in her life.

(Women now account for 151 cases, 59 of them not IV drug users, Haitians, or hemophiliacs. Six percent of all AIDS cases are now occurring in what—in insulting James Watt-ese—is called "the general population," i.e., people who are not gay, Haitian, hemophiliacs, or IV drug users.)

I return to find five letters on my desk. One announces a memorial service for my thirty-first friend who has died. The four others are from leading doctors involved with the AIDS epidemic. Each conveys the same message: Each doctor is frightened that the community is returning to the sexual freedoms of pre-AIDS days and that there is no visible gay political leadership in New York City to fight with the mayor and the Department of Health to force them to treat this epidemic with the same responsibility they would if it was happening in any other community. One letter, from the leading oncologist treating AIDS patients in New York, begs me to implore GMHC to plead with the gay community to observe complete sexual celibacy until the epidemic is stemmed.

I return to find that, after a few weeks of miraculously responsible journalism, *The New York Times* has regressed to its former silence on the subject of AIDS, while a raging epidemic is decimating its city. Until the day I die, I will never forgive this newspaper and this mayor for treating this epidemic, which is killing so many of my friends, in such an irresponsible fashion. This newspaper, which purports to record what is going on here to a population that includes one million gay people, has yet to do one human interest story on AIDS, to profile one patient, to do an in-depth article on GMHC, which represents one of the most amazing grass-roots responses by a community to taking care of its own. Day after day I see articles on every other charity and community and sufferer you can imagine. Never is there anything that deals with the human side of AIDS. (Or, for that matter, the human side of anything gay: Have you read much in the *Times* on SAGE, on Lambda, on any gay person beside Harvey Fierstein?) To *The New York Times*, we are still freaks, the homosexuals. Compare this to the *Washington Post*, which runs three to four sympathetic and moving articles every week. (Washington has thirty-two cases of AIDS.) Or the *Philadelphia Inquirer*, which, with the *Los Angeles Times*, leads the nation for the quality of its AIDS coverage. (Philadelphia has thirty-six cases.) No, I will never forgive *The New York Times*, late to arrive and early to leave. And by not maintaining their reporting on this crisis, they have helped to nurture our community into this false sense of security. (To see, day after day, their page after page of ads featuring gay-designed fashions is as morally repugnant as if Hebrew National had advertised in Hitler's favorite newspaper.)

It is no secret that I consider Mayor Koch to be, along with the *Times*, the biggest enemy gay men and women have to contend with in New York. Why does our gay leadership always act as if they are frightened of him? The sum total of this city's

contributions to the AIDS epidemic to date is $24,500. That's it.
Along with two meetings a month thrown in by a Department
of Health that gives new meaning to the word "lethargy." Is
it any wonder that in my Gay Pride Day speech I called Mayor
Koch "a heartless, selfish son of a bitch?"

San Francisco's mayor, in a city that has 284 AIDS victims,
has given $4 million to the organizations that provide to her city
what GMHC provides for this one, including free buildings for
patient services and money to remodel them. GMHC has been
without a home for the two years of its existence, waiting,
waiting, for the space the mayor's office promised over a year
ago. When GMHC asked to use an abandoned and derelict high
school on West 13th Street, the mayor demanded $2 million for
it, cash up front, no terms, immediately. It would require an
additional $800,000 to make it habitable. GMHC does not have
this money, and in any event it considers it immoral to use
donations received for patient care to pay the city for real
estate the city should be providing free and would be providing
free to any other community that was enduring an epidemic of
death.

Because GMHC refuses to take advantage of the mayor's
generous offer, it is being accused by other gay organizations
of not being "community minded." Thus the mayor has suc-
ceeded in turning us against each other.

But GMHC must find larger quarters now. It has waited and
waited until its activities can no longer be contained in the five
tiny cubbyholes of a rooming house generously donated to it by
two loyal members.

From here, over four hundred patients are supervised by
over three hundred trained clinical volunteers each and every
day. From here, over 1,500 Hotline phone calls are logged every
week. From here, over 2 million pieces of printed literature
giving the most up-to-date information have been dispatched all
over the world. From here, twenty training sessions for doctors
and nurses and Open Forums for the entire state are arranged
each month.

And into these offices every week arrive ten new AIDS victims, seeking help. For them, GMHC provides crisis counseling,
group therapy, welfare guidance, recreational activities, and
hospital and home care. The demand for crisis counseling itself

is now so great that fifty new counselors must be trained each month to join the 160 men and women who each look after one or more patients—many of them, now, not gay—on a daily basis. This counseling is the only loving contact most of these victims ever receive.

To these tiny rooms come, each day, one hundred requests for some sort of GMHC service. I have never seen a more inspirational organization in operation anywhere in my life. I have never witnessed a more fiscally responsible organization in my life (certainly not in the gay community), and I have never seen an organization catering to an epidemic that is the worst in modern history treated so shabbily by a mayor, by a city, by a federal government—or taken so much for granted by the community it is trying to help.

GMHC comprises five hundred extremely active volunteers. There is a full-time staff of nine, two-thirds of whose salaries are paid for by state grants. Less than one-third of GMHC's budget is spent on administration. GMHC has raised over $500,000 from benefits and small-donor contributions. It has given away some $80,000 to local research that would otherwise have been stopped, $12,000 to the National Gay Task Force to help fund its own AIDS Hotline, $40,000 to help pay a Washington lobbyist to fight for AIDS attention, and $25,000 to the gay Community Health Project to continue its vital AIDS screening program and diagnostic testing. That this latter project is not being funded by the city or by the Department of Health is shocking and offensive.

How dare Mayor Koch deny these committed and passionate GMHC workers, desperately trying to care for an entire epidemic virtually by themselves, the necessary space and funding he would be providing to any other community—Jewish or Black or Poor or "General Population"—were AIDS happening to them?

And how dare the gay community not support the GMHC Rodeo in Madison Square Garden on October 1st? Where else is GMHC meant to find its money for all of these exhausting services if not from us?

I appeal to the moral sense of obligation, to the sense of what is right and must be done, of every gay person in this city to come to GMHC's Rodeo at Madison Square Garden on October 1st. AIDS is not going to go away. Its cause is still invisible and its cure is still unfound. Treatment trials on every front are not very hopeful or promising. By the failure of gay men and lesbians to pack Madison Square Garden on October 1st, a message goes out to our mayor that our vote is not important, that he can continue to ignore us and our health crisis, and to our President and Congress and the world that their support is not necessary, and to AIDS victims that their care and cure is no longer on our minds.

We are asking the world to help us, to give us huge amounts of money to investigate this scourge. If we cannot help ourselves, we do not deserve anyone else's help.

Let's make another miracle. We have four days to sell ten thousand tickets.

This was published as an ad in the *Voice,* paid for (it cost $4,000) anonymously at the time by Joe Paschek, GMHC's treasurer, and his lover and business partner Lee Hulko. Joe was the financial genius who, from the very beginning, gave GMHC the impeccable and responsible fiscal security it still has; even though he was unhappy with me, he recognized the need for this ad.

I wrote it at the request of Rodger McFarlane, who was now GMHC's first full-time, paid executive director. Rodger inherited the Rodeo, which was probably a bad idea—to attempt to so quickly repeat the Circus success—and he saw an empty, yawning Madison Square Garden threatening only days before the event. It was not well attended, but somehow it managed to make a $75,000 profit. Most of the tickets were sold at the last minute.

I had returned not only from Europe but from Cape Cod, where I had written the first draft of *The Normal*

Heart, and I was on my way south, to an isolated log cabin
in Little Washington, Virginia, loaned me by old friends,
to write the second draft.

Because of my closeness to Rodger (we were then
living together as lovers as well), I felt I still had at least
some closeness to GMHC. Anyway, I continued to fight
for it publicly as loudly as I could. Rodger's relationship
with me, however, presented him with unnecessary problems: Because of it, he was unable ever to truly win the
confidence of the Board, particularly of Paul Popham. Although he worked his ass off, and was responsible for
running GMHC, magnificently, during the period of its
biggest growth (1983–85), the Board, now increased to
include several more who also viewed me unkindly,
looked skeptically upon his total loyalty and trustwor-
thiness.

Paul became so distrustful of Rodger that at one point
he asked for a Board evaluation of his work. The Board
came back with the studied information that Rodger was
doing the work of ten people, and Paul had egg all over
his face. (When, in early 1985, *The Normal Heart* opened,
Rodger contributed a fact sheet on the current status of
the epidemic to be included with the program; Paul was
so furious at what he considered this gesture of support
of me that he recommended Rodger be fired.)

During the next year and a half I was fully occupied
in rewriting my play and somehow finding a way to get
it produced. It was turned down by some fourteen play
agents. It was turned down by any number of directors
and producers and New York City and regional theater
companies. It was turned down by American Playhouse
and PBS. But, with the help of Emmett Foster, who was
a personal assistant to Joseph Papp, and who was also a
GMHC volunteer, I was able to bring it to the attention
of this man who was to become so important in my professional life.

Equal to Murderers

11 June 84

To:

Mr. Abe Rosenthal, *The New York Times*
Dr. Lawrence Altman, *The New York Times*
Mr. Tom Morgan, *The New York Times*
Judge Richard Failla, Gay Men's Health Crisis
Mr. Rodger McFarlane, Gay Men's Health Crisis
Mr. Paul Popham, Gay Men's Health Crisis
Ms. Virginia Apuzzo, National Gay Task Force
Dr. David Sencer, Commissioner of Health
Dr. Roger Enlow, Office of Gay and Lesbian Health
Mayor Edward Koch

I am attaching an article from last Friday's *Washington Post* entitled "AIDS Epidemic Is Expanding, Not Shrinking, Experts Say." As you can see, this was a main, featured article, appearing on page A-3. It was sent to me by Tim Westmoreland, counsel to Representative Henry Waxman, who is Chair-

---

* *New York Native*, Issue 95, July 30–August 12, 1984.

man of the House Subcommittee on Health. Tim, like me, cannot understand why there is so little information passed on to
the New York community about the appalling continuation, the
march of this epidemic. After all, New York is still the worst
hit. There are now *over four* new cases every day in this area,
but you would not know it from reading *The New York Times*,
or any of the literature put out by the above offices. The worst
epidemic known to modern man is happening right here in this
very city, and it is one of the best-kept secrets around.

All that is asked for, from all of you, is to transmit information, to keep an endangered population informed. Why is that
so difficult?

That all of you listed above continue to refuse to transmit
to the public the facts and figures of what is happening *daily*
makes you, in my mind, equal to murderers, with blood on your
hands just as if you had used knives or bullets or poison. Because you continue to refuse to inform New York's population,
the perception by the average gay man on the street is that this
epidemic has disappeared or leveled off or improved. Because
of false hope (owing to the announcement that a virus has been
isolated) that a cure will come tomorrow, the average gay man
is back to living with his head in the sand. Because *The New
York Times* is not reporting this vital news, because the city's
Department of Health is not disseminating these appalling statistics, because the gay community's own organizations are too
cowardly to speak out and speak up—all of this perpetuates the
widespread ignorance that can only make for continued contagion, infection, and—at the present rate of increase—a minimum of 64,000 cases in two years' time.

In the name of God, Christ, Moses, whatever impels you to,
at last, perform acts of humanity, when will you address this
issue with the courage it demands?

D uring this week in June, gay health organizations
sponsored a conference of several days, held at New

York University, to discuss many issues pertaining to the health, both mental and physical, of gay men and lesbians, and, only tangentially, AIDS.

By now Rodger and I had split up. I had failed in all three of my attempts to get back on GMHC's Board. I'd fought with Paul again, and again we no longer spoke. I was taking out my anger on Rodger for not supporting me—even if it meant he had to threaten to quit unless I was reinstated (a tactic that had certainly failed when I tried it).

I was appalled that so little of the health conference was devoted not only to AIDS but to any discussion of political action. After all we were continuing to endure, still no one was going after our enemies. GMHC by now was completely entrenched as a purely service agency, which angered me to the point of irrationality. Why couldn't they take stands? Why couldn't they advise men to cool it sexually?

I stood outside the conference entrance and handed out this letter to those attending. Then I went inside and interrupted the conference, yelling at them that they were not talking about what was *really* important. My reputation by now was completely that of a crazy man.

My use of the words "equal to murderers" in attacking my own people, my former lover, some of my former best friends, was not new. I had called them the same when I had been thrice rejected for re-admission to the Board. Yes, my reputation by now was completely that of a crazy man.

We Can Be Together

How to Organize the Gay Community

H ere we are—another Gay Pride Day. We have a lot to be thankful for. We're still alive.

I have often been asked, "Okay, bigmouth, you're always yelling at us so much. Tell us what you think we should do. Be constructive."

So, at the risk of being yelled at even more, here is a list of Larry Kramer's suggestions: what we could be doing to get ourselves together for however many future years of gratitude we're going to be granted.

I

Organize. Okay, how do we organize? Well, you start with a few friends, and they get a few friends, and then you get all of them to get a few friends. You go from neighborhood to neighborhood, then from borough to borough, then from city to city, then from state to state, and then you've got the whole country. It is slow, thankless, necessary work, and until we do it—until we have one massive organization that represents *at least* one

* *Long Island Connection*, Vol. 4, Number 12, July 17, 1985.

million gay men and women—we'll still be victims of the system.

The biggest gay organizations in this country can only boast
membership lists of 20,000 (GMHC) or 8,500 (NGTF). That's
shocking. The National Rifle Association, Jerry Falwell's Moral
Majority—they get what they want because they can prove
they have mailing lists of millions of people. When they send
out requests to these millions to write letters to Congress,
those letters get written and responded to. That's how you get
things in this country. That's how democracy works. Visible
pressure from visible numbers. And there's not that much
wrong with the idea. What's wrong is our inability to put this
method into action ourselves.

Now we have a choice to make. Do we want to add our
names to the lists of already existing organizations—GMHC,
NGTF, Gay Rights National Lobby, all of which have very poor
records of fighting for us, and all of which are controlled by
boards of directors who are timid sissies, old ladies, old men, old
farts, useless—or do we, somehow, try to start a brand-new
organization from scratch?

I would dearly like to see the latter—something new is often
better than something tired. But something new, to be effective,
takes money, lots of money. I am talking about hundreds of
thousands of dollars, maybe a million. It also takes a leader, and
we have precious few of them. I would like to see such a new
beginning, but until a gay Rockefeller comes along and plunks
down the start-up funds, I don't see it happening. And we can't
afford to do it on the cheap again—that's the trouble with
NGTF and GRNL: They haven't got the funds to stay in shape;
they're in debt; and it's hard to do good work when you're in
debt.

Therefore, for the present, we don't have much choice but
to try to make our existing organizations better. Pump some
blood and energy into those sagging, wheezing carcasses. How
can we do this? Well, believe it or not, we accomplish this by
joining them. We get in touch with GMHC, with NGTF, with
GRNL, and we say to them: I will join your organization; here
is my contribution. *But*—and this is the biggest of big *buts*—I
am giving you this money and at the same time I am telling you
I don't think you are doing a good enough job. I am giving you

this money to *fight*. To establish as powerful a lobbying presence in Washington as you can. We simply must have our own people fighting for us in Washington, and you are not doing that. In taking my twenty-five dollars (or whatever it is) you must pledge to me that this money will be used for political fighting and only that. At a recent East End Gay Organization meeting, I was thrilled to hear my remarks met with a pledge by their president that they would try to raise, among themselves, part or all of the amount it costs to maintain one lobbyist in Washington—$60,000.

This gives rise to another possibility. That you and your friends could start fund-raising on your own to pay for a lobbyist's salary. If groups and organizations all over this country would each commit themselves to raising $60,000 a year, we would have a platoon of lobbyists in Washington that would be impressive. Don't worry about finding the right person. We have contacts in Washington that can locate him or her.

To give you an example of why lobbyists in Washington are our first priority, let me cite what not having them has meant. "The" AIDS virus was isolated in France fifteen months before Washington announced that our scientists had "discovered" it. The Centers for Disease Control in Atlanta wanted to put this French virus to work immediately, in those vital tests that will help us make progress toward a cure, a vaccine, and blood tests. But they were told, "Don't you dare use the French virus. We, the government, have poured millions of dollars into our own research; you wait until we discover our own virus." I put this simplistically, of course, but that's the essence. For fifteen months a virus had been isolated that could have helped research move ahead. If we had had lobbying power in Washington, we could have charged in and said: "No, sir, you use that French virus immediately, or I tell my membership of one million (2 million, 3 million) about the hanky-panky that's going on and some of you might not get reelected." (Why didn't GMHC fight for the use of the French virus?)

Did you know that the majority of the funds allocated to AIDS research goes not to finding a cure, but to finding a vaccine, producing blood tests—to almost anything but to improve the chances of the sick and dying? If we had people in Washington fighting for us, we could fight to right that imbalance. We could fight for our lives, which we must do now. Getting as many people as possible representing us in Washington—our people, paid for by us—is top priority. And our present organizations are not doing this, either fast enough or at all.

GMHC will give you the feeble excuse that it is a not-for-profit organization and is thus prohibited by law from participating in political action. You don't think the Catholic Church, the Salvation Army, the American Cancer Society haven't found ways to become political without losing their not-for-profit status? An organization is prohibited from spending *over a certain percentage* of its income on political activity. It doesn't take any money to have a troop of volunteers sit down and write letters—the cheapest, most effective way of making your voice heard. It doesn't cost any money to have a troop of volunteers picket City Hall for their inattention to the AIDS crisis. It doesn't cost any money to have a troop of volunteers flood switchboards with complaints when *The New York Times* runs something ignorant and hateful.

Ironically, appallingly, when you come to GMHC to offer your services as a volunteer, they will tell you, "We don't need any volunteers right now—we're all filled up." Can you imagine an organization with as much to do as it has, refusing the services of volunteers? That path only leads to stagnation and death. You must say to them: "I think this is the stupidest thing I have ever heard—but write down my name and phone number anyway, and when you are ready to form a political-action division, please call me." And when you haven't heard from them after a week or two, call them back and say: "I am still waiting to volunteer my services for a political-action division." After a while, they will get the message.

It is possible for you to let those foul boards of directors of GMHC, or NGTF, or GRNL know that they are all sitting on their hands. Simply call each organization directly and say you would like to have a list of their board members and their addresses. They are obligated to send such a list to you. Then write to each director and say: "If you don't care enough to fight harder, do you think you could relinquish your seat to someone who will and can?"

II

Organize. Okay, so now you have sent your membership donations to GMHC, to GRNL, to NGTF, and you have got a group of twenty-five of your friends to join with a group of twenty-five of somebody else's friends and the fifty of you are thinking about joining with another fifty that has similarly organized in Brooklyn. How do you keep the damn thing from falling apart? What's your agenda? How do you keep everyone active and busy and interested and committed—before they get bored out of their minds and return to the baths and drugs? How do you sustain energy?

My answer to that is that every one of us—women, too—must repeat to ourselves, like a catechism, over and over: *Each and every minute of my life, I must act as if I already have AIDS and am fighting for my life.*

It also means that each of the one hundred members that you now have can and should work at least one night a week at one of these organizations. (There is no local office of GRNL, but that does not mean there couldn't be.) When you work as a volunteer for an organization, get to know the other volunteers, the staff, and the board members. (Board members rarely show up at their organizations; some of them don't even know what their organizations do. But you're going to change all that.) Get to know the lay of the land. And as you do, let them get to know you and why you're there and what you stand for. *You stand for fighting.* Fighting to get lobbying power in Washington. Fighting to get Mayor Koch to do something, anything, for AIDS. Fighting to get *The New York Times* and every magazine and publication you read or come across to pay more attention to the tragedies that we as gay people face all the time but see so little written about: AIDS, immigration, discrimination in jobs and housing, the nerve of Archbishop—pardon me, Cardinal—O'Connor. There are many, many issues.

In fact, now that you have your own little organization going, one order of business could be each of you, there on the spot, sitting down and writing a letter to the same person. One hundred letters sent at one time to *The New York Times*, to Mayor Koch, to Senator D'Amato, are going to be seen and read. If they don't respond, write them again.

Establish goals. This can mean tracking down the person or persons you think responsible for some fault, or the person or persons you think might be able to help you do something about it. If a friend of yours who has AIDS has been treated badly in a hospital, find out who at that hospital can help you to see that it won't happen again. If you want to know what Senator Moynihan's or Senator D'Amato's position is on AIDS and how much they have done about it (next to nothing), locate someone working for them, both here in New York and in Washington, and establish a relationship on the phone with that person. You will find out that one phone call will lead to another—and, good detective that you are, you will pursue your goal like the best of bloodhounds. You will be paid attention to if you say "I represent the Long Island Chapter of Gay———; we have one hundred members in our chapter and we are affiliated with other chapters that bring our total membership to over one thousand, and we feel that you are not doing enough to fight for us."

Constantly keep your goals in view. Constantly reassess your goals, and your progress in reaching them. Be realistic, but also challenge yourself to try to do more and more, reach further, fight harder. Constantly remind yourself of what it's all about.

So now you have an organization going that has one hundred members and each of you also spends one night a week or one hour a week volunteering for GMHC or NGTF or some other gay organization that you are interested in putting into fighting shape, and each of you is also writing one letter a week to protest one of the many indignities we endure every day. Where do you go from here? Are you so tired now that you are fed up and disgusted, and have returned to your former state of Doing Nothing About It? *Just remember the old battle cry: Each and every minute of my life, I must act as if I already have AIDS and am fighting for my life.*

If this continues to give you energy, and I pray to heaven that it does, now you must try to connect your organization with another organization that has been growing in membership, too. This is called networking, and historically gay organizations have been terrible at it. We've simply never been able to get along, particularly in New York, the most competitive and brutal of cities. But once again, we simply have to grit our teeth, repeat our catechism, and try. It's do-or-die time, fellas and girls.

The most convenient way of networking locally is right under our noses. At present, it's a mess. But it's there, in place, and ready for rehabilitation. Once a month there meets a very peculiar organization. It is called the Community Council, and ostensibly it is composed of one representative from every existing organization in New York that has asked to join and has paid its dues. In its heyday, there must have been sixty or seventy constituent members. Now I understand there are less than a dozen. This is a pity. The Community Council is potentially a very good starting point for getting us some power in New York City. It really should be put back into shape—with reconstituted goals. Just think of how many gay organizations there are: GMHC, NGTF, Men of All Colors Together, the various choruses and music groups, Salsa Soul Sisters, the political clubs, gay alumni groups from Yale and elsewhere. These are groups with combined memberships that must approach at least fifty thousand. If every gay organization in the area got themselves back onto the Community Council, I think we could start something rolling.

In the past, this organization had no power, because it had no elected officers and chose not to take any strong stands. It was a monthly forum for screaming. Meetings of the full Community Council were, quite frankly, revolting. Nobody would listen to anybody else. To get a consensus on anything—even the time—was next to impossible.

So why am I offering up this den of vipers as something filled with hope and potential? Because it is there, it is in place. What is not in place is machinery to make the Community Council effective. It must change its modus operandi. It must elect officers, it must take political stands on all issues, and it must make these stands heard. It must organize, just as you have done.

That the Mayor of New York has ignored us for so long is something the new Community Council can take a stand on. You let City Hall know that the mayor is expected to march in our parade. It is appalling that he has refused to do so for so long. That Mayor Koch refused to give us, for free, a falling-down building for our community center is shocking. The Community Council, if it had teeth, could have demanded that we be *given* that building, for which we paid $1.5 million. It's still not too late. That Mayor Koch has continually assigned us a useless liaison to the gay community is equally unacceptable. First we had the hated Herb Rickman. Well, we did manage to get rid of him. Now we have sweet Lee Hudson, who is, I'm afraid, only a figurehead. She can't *do* anything. Who can blame her if she has trouble defending Koch's position on almost any gay issue you can think of? At a recent meeting, she put forth Koch's Office of Gay and Lesbian Health Concerns as a positive step that Koch has taken for our community. I said, "Indeed it was—but then why did he keep it without a head for almost a year?"

A strong Community Council could have a lot to say about who gets that job. And about seeing that the Office of Gay and Lesbian Health Concerns *does* something.

Ed Koch knows he is in trouble with the gay community. He was booed at the AIDS benefit at the Shubert Theatre. I consider him to be the one person most responsible for letting the AIDS epidemic get out of hand. He is now going around trying to "make nice" to us. He appeared at the gay synagogue, made a little speech, and answered questions. (It has taken him five years to accept their invitation.) This is the man who, in five years, has given a total of $75,000 to community AIDS services, compared with San Francisco's $16 million. A strong Community Council, with you and your group a part of it, could roundly and loudly protest this inhumanity.

If you have AIDS in San Francisco, you are eligible to enter one of the best hospital wards in this country—the AIDS section of San Francisco General Hospital. Visit a few AIDS patients in almost any hospital in New York, and you are liable to hear stories that make your hair stand on end. If you get AIDS in San Francisco, you are eligible for a whole assortment of services that you cannot get in New York—housing, crisis counseling of a kind that GMHC is no longer able to offer, a faster and more responsive welfare system. You don't get any of these things without fighting for them. Why hasn't GMHC fought Mayor Koch harder for these things? Why haven't we made GMHC fight harder? You could come down with AIDS tomorrow. Do you want to be treated like a San Francisco gay or a New York gay? *Each and every minute of my life, I must act like I already have AIDS and am fighting for my life.*

III

Organize. Now that you are on the Community Council, and it has been turned into a responsive, responsible organization, it is time to turn toward national objectives. You must locate the equivalent of the Community Council in every town and city that you can. And representatives must meet regularly to cement ideas on how to network area by area, region by region, across the country.

It is through this kind of network that we could plan a march on Washington and make it work. I am here to tell you that if one million gay people marched on Washington, they would see us and hear us. I am not talking about 10,000 or 100,000. These numbers march in Washington every other weekend. Political power comes from *numbers,* and numbers mean *visibility,* and optimum visibility is a march on Washington of one million women and men. Oh, Mother of God, would that not be a day of Glory! Hallelujah! Why is it such a dream? Why couldn't we bring it off? With you and your friends and their friends, it just might happen. And once we have marched on Washington, we must do it again. And again. And again. Like anti-war protestors did against our country's involvement in Vietnam.

I have for some time been putting forth the notion of a Summit Meeting. What I have in mind is that leaders from all over America would come to a central place and sit in a room and say, "Okay, for this meeting we are all going to get along together and work out some way to organize our national gay community into a working mechanism that can become a presence in Washington." Such a Summit Meeting would be fraught with every problem imaginable—people in groups have a hard time agreeing on anything. But I cling to the hope that with the threat of AIDS we might just be able to put on our crisis wardrobe and get on with it at last.

It is through a national organization that we could achieve most. Our very own organization, powerful, strong, with a huge mailing list, in Washington, on the spot, just like the

National Rifle Association, the Moral Majority, the American Red Cross, General Motors. Everyone who is anything has an office in Washington. And we don't. Some 24 million gay men and lesbians have no office in Washington. How ludicrous a situation. What a death wish.

An office in Washington, a building in Washington, a troop of lobbyists in Washington—these mean something. Just as *not* having any of these means something. Without them we are prepared to die, and without a whimper of protest. A recent issue of a powerful Washington newsletter, read on Capitol Hill, had a lead article that said, in essence: "You, the senators and representatives and power brokers who are reading this, don't have to worry about the gay vote, about the gay community, because they are unorganized, because they have no representatives in Washington, because they are powerless. Therefore you don't have to vote for anything pro-gay, and if you vote anti-gay, don't worry about it—they won't even know it or fight back." Many senators and representatives and lobbyists read this. Please God, may that scare the shit out of you and get you off your ass and into action.

I cannot overestimate the necessity of this desperately needed political presence in Washington.

IV

Organize. Here are two other things to think about:

Help force Ed Koch and Carol Bellamy into helping us. We are about to have a mayoral race between a "confirmed bachelor" and an "unmarried woman." Because both of them are so terrified of being perceived as gay, they bend over backwards to ignore us. They are going to be making a lot of campaign promises now. We must make Koch promise us everything he has denied us. If either of them wants the gay vote, they must be honest about gay issues. *Whoever opens the closet first gets my vote.*

We are fortunate in this area to have two gay newspapers that get better with every issue, the *Long Island Connection* and the *New York Native.* [The *Connection* ceased publication shortly after this appeared.] Make sure you and your friends read these papers. This is the best way I know of keeping up to date on what is happening about AIDS. If every gay man and lesbian reads them, these papers make a little more money, which means they can afford to extend their coverage. You might even write to Bloomingdale's or some other favorite store and ask them: "Why aren't you advertising in the gay press? I buy from you—why don't you support my papers?"

But other gay newspapers are not so good, and they should be told they are not so good. The *Advocate,* this country's leading gay newspaper in terms of sales, has its priorities in the wrong place, has had its head in the sand for too long. The *Advocate* lives in the Age Before AIDS. The mentality of this newspaper is strictly laid-back California est, Hawaiian shirts, and guest houses in Key West. Every article sounds as if it was written by the same person who engages in no serious discussions of anything controversial. You might write a few letters to the *Advocate* as long as you're writing.

The *Washington Blade,* as our presence in Washington, is equally as shocking in its lack of zeal, its reluctance to crusade in a city where it could do the most good. The *New York Native* has a woman in Washington, Ann Fettner, writing some of the best AIDS pieces around. How is it that the *Connection* can in one issue present more political news than the *Blade* can present in several months? Why can't we have a dynamic, fighting newspaper in our capital, exerting pressure where it's needed most? Another great opportunity tragically wasted.

How are we to know what is going on if we do not have an effective network of newspapers? If *The New York Times* and the *Chicago Tribune* and the *L.A. Times* aren't going to write about us, and if the *Advocate* and the *Blade* lack the interest or resolve to crusade, if the gay papers in almost every city other than New York fall far short of what we need, how are we going to get the word out—about anything?

The *San Francisco Chronicle* is blessed with an openly gay reporter, Randy Shilts. In the first ten months of 1984, the *Chronicle* ran 163 articles about AIDS. God bless you, Randy. Compare this with the puny, paltry numbers of thirty-seven in the L.A. *Times,* and twenty-four in the *Washington Post.* Why doesn't the *Advocate* raise a stink about this in its California pages? Why doesn't the *Blade* raise a stink about this in its

Washington pages? *Each and every minute of my life, I must act as if I already have AIDS and am fighting for my life.*

Okay, here comes the hardest question of all. How are we all going to get along with each other in order to get any of this done? I certainly include myself here. I have a bad temper; I am impatient with anybody who doesn't agree with me—and all of you are probably a bit of the same. I have no real answers to this. I have already fucked up once, woefully, in my relationship with GMHC. If we could only sit down together in the same room (which GMHC will not do with me), saying and thinking our catechism, putting up a few pictures in our mind's eye of our friends who have died, maybe we might be able to do it.

We gays are still as children in this political game. We are inexperienced. But day by day and month by month we learn a little more. And in learning we acquire skills. Perhaps, touched by political reality, after we've bitched each other to death, we will learn how to negotiate, how to compromise, how to give a little. I know I have said, "I will never forgive the Board of GMHC," and "I will never forgive Mayor Koch." But GMHC and I are both different entities now from what we were when we commenced our quarrels three years ago. Doesn't it make more sense to have your critics on your side? It seems to me the secret of a successful organization is the ability to accommodate all views—not closing out those in opposition. This, after all, is the secret of America. (GMHC has shut out all opposing voices—and they have systematically made certain that access to the organization was and is denied to anyone who does not think as they do. Ask me, ask Dr. Joseph Sonnabend, ask Michael Callen, ask Jim Fouratt.) If GMHC is to regain strength, if NGTF, GRNL, the Community Council, *all of us,* are to find new strength, it can only be in one room, together. Just as political enemies face each other daily in Congress. Being gay people, what if we tried to hug each other, even a little? (Imagine Koch and Kramer hugging. Well, stranger things have happened.)

Togetherness is numbers. Togetherness is unity. Unity is strength. Strength is power. Power is acceptance. Acceptance is a certain kind of Equality.

Let me say a few final words about leadership. Over the

years, we have had precious few leaders who stayed around long enough to achieve anything. It seems that no sooner does a good one come along than he or she has some hidden agenda: to use his or her gay leadership position to get a better-paying political job, for instance.

In most cases, however, the quality of our leadership has been second-rate. Good people do not want to get involved in gay politics—and who can blame them? It is, as I started this article by noting, a thankless job. But now is a time for sacrifice. These are the years of death and dying, the plague years, and they are here to stay.

So we must obey certain moral imperatives, commandments if you will, just as if we were devout practitioners of any religion that calls for service, for giving. We must give to the cause of Gay Rights all that we have to give. We must urge, beg, implore every potential leader we know to become actively involved. We know who among our friends is better able than others: who has valuable skills—for reasoning, for public speaking, for common sense, for passion. Or who has money. God, how money is needed. We know whom among us we respect, to whom we listen, to whom we go when we need advice. These are our potential leaders: your lawyer, your accountant, your professors, your doctors. Tell them they must devote their brains and skills and passions to helping make us stronger *politically.*

It is from among these people that we will find our leaders, our fighters. Many of them are still in the closet at work, perhaps even at home. We must implore them to hide no longer. It is up to each one of us to pass along this message: No longer will any excuse be tolerated for shying away from responsibility. Not if these people wish to continue enjoying our respect. Yes. Shame them into participation, if necessary. We simply must field a better qualified set of leaders to represent us in the coming years. We need them locally (New York has the most poorly organized gay community of any major city); we need them in Washington; we need them everywhere.

So help locate these men and women. Ask them to join your own group of twenty-five or fifty. Tell them to bring their colleagues, those they respect and admire. Make your group as tough and smart and agile as you can. Let us field our best fighting power—and we will be respected adversaries in due course.

All of this, I know, sounds exhausting. But which of us does not have a few spare hours a week? Or an evening? Which of us does not have a few hundred dollars? Or a piece of paper and a pen? Or a telephone?

And who among us does not have friends? Friends to join our first small organization?

Who among us does not know a potential leader—a doctor, a lawyer, a scientist, someone from Harvard or NYU? I do not mean to sound elitist, but with education comes responsibility, and if ever we needed responsible, well-educated, presentable leaders, it is now.

Every single one of us can and must answer all the above questions with "That's me. I do."

For every single one of us faces the possibility that he might be dead, very shortly, in a few years, perhaps in a few months.

Did you know that scientists and doctors are now thinking that the AIDS virus may have been around for as long as *twenty* years? That someone you fucked with twenty years ago could have transmitted the virus to you? So that even if you have lived in a monogamous relationship for nineteen years, you still might not be completely in the clear. We're all walking time bombs, waiting for whatever it is to set us off.

Each and every minute of my life, I must act as if I already have AIDS and am fighting for my life.

I devoted 1985 and 1986 mostly to *The Normal Heart.* I finally had a hit show. During and after the almost-year-long run at Joe Papp's Public Theater in New York, where it starred first Brad Davis and then Joel Grey, there were productions in Los Angeles (with Richard Dreyfuss), at the Long Wharf in New Haven (with Tom Hulce), at the Royal Court in London (with Martin Sheen), transferring to the West End (Tom Hulce again,

and then John Shea), and, after these, at just about
every major regional theatre in America and by companies around the world, including such unlikely places as
Poland, where a production was so successful that it's
being repeated on Polish television. Poland is a country
where homosexuality is so frowned upon that gay suicides are common. I rarely allow myself to feel good
about having written something that might help change
people's minds. I never think that happens. But it was
nice to have a success.

Some two years of negotiations with Barbra Streisand for the film rights (she was to produce, direct, and
play the part of Dr. Emma Brookner) came to nothing
but $20,000 in legal fees for me. People predicted from
the start we were two impossibly difficult people who
could never come to terms. When she first called me, she
was filled with excitement and passion, both for my play
and the problems it dramatizes. Her own agent, Stan
Kamen of William Morris, with whom I'd been told she
was exceptionally close, had just died from AIDS. I was
interested in her filming it mainly because I figured she
would draw a larger world audience to the film than
anyone I could think of. But I was soon forced into
realizing that her excitement and passion were an up
and down thing. It was not until I met her, some many
months after negotiations began (it takes a very long
time to deal with someone with so many lawyers, man-
agers, agents, partners, assistants, secretaries, and personal attendants) that she had decided to make another
film first, which I'd not been told originally. And this
film, *Nuts*, was one that not only suffered delay after
delay, but was awful when it finally came out, by which
time I no longer wanted her to film *The Normal Heart*.

But, for these two years, she had me in a bind:
Negotiations dragged on and on, never fully completed,
so I was not free to go elsewhere without fear of her
legal reprisals. In essence, she not only sat on me and
my play, but effectively saw to it that no one else could
bring this subject to the screen—an action that I think

was selfish and exceedingly inhumane. While I enjoyed my creative meetings with her (she is a very smart woman), she would not agree to guarantee that I would be the only screenwriter. I gave in on this point, and hated myself (and by extension, her) for doing so.

For a while, I toyed with the idea of directing the film myself. Many of the stars who had played Ned Weeks were willing to allow me to direct them, and the magnificent Linda Hunt agreed to play my Emma. But money was not so available for this novice director as I'd hoped, even with such a fine cast as I was able to assemble, and even with my old friend Paul Maslansky (who'd done so well with his many *Police Academies*) as the producer.

Just when the matter of a film appeared to be dead, another old friend, and former boss, David Picker (who, as head of United Artists, had been responsible for allowing me to script *Women in Love*), appeared once again in his role of White Knight. He is now setting up the film, and if all goes well, we may just make it to the screen at last.

By now I'd learned that no matter what I wrote and said and did, I was going to get flak from somewhere. But for the first time in my writing career, there wasn't much criticism against *The Normal Heart*. What little there was came from gay critics who accused me of writing "a self-serving revenge play" against the Board of GMHC, making myself the hero. I'm sorry they saw the play so narrowly. I tried to make Ned Weeks as obnoxious as I could. He isn't my idea of a hero. He fucks up totally. He yells at his dying lover and screams and rants and raves at and against everyone and everything else and gets tossed out of "the organization" on his ass. I was trying, somehow and again, to atone for my own behavior. I tried to make Bruce Niles, the Paul Popham character, the sympathetic leader he in fact was. I hoped Paul would come and see the play, which he would not do, and be honored.

But I also wanted to show that these were our fights that kept us diminished and divided. I think they're fights not dissimilar to those in any growing organization, gay or straight, and that they probably can't be avoided, or afforded.

One peculiar fallout from the play, and from my other political writing, is my being pegged as an advocate of celibacy. I don't think I've ever advocated that, or urged anything but caution, and "cooling it." Characters in *The Normal Heart* may have said other things (as they did and do in real life), but it's a selfish and vicious critic who can so yank a line or two of dialogue out of context to nail the author with it as his sworn message. I was against promiscuity long before *The Normal Heart;* I believe being gay offers much more than that. But proponents (even in this age of AIDS) of promiscuity—which is far different from sexual freedom, which I, of course, support—have made me their enemy. I do confess to not knowing where one draws the line between caution and disregard. That is everyone's personal decision to make when he or she is completely informed of all that is known. But I am not so dumb as to believe that an entire population can stop having sex. Nor do I think it's healthy for many that they do so.

After the main productions, I found it increasingly difficult to sit through the play any more. It contains too many unhappy memories. (It also contains too much clumsy writing.) I wrote it to make people cry: AIDS is the saddest thing I'll ever have to know. I also wrote it to be a love story, in honor of a man I loved who died. I wanted people to see on a stage two men who loved each other. I wanted people to see them kiss. I wanted people to see that gay men in love and gay men suffering and gay men dying are just like everyone else.

Second-Rate Voice

How sad that the *Village Voice* would not publish Anna Mayo's excellent AIDS article ("The Principle of Uncertainty," *Native*, 151). How much sadder *Voice* editor Robert Friedman's excuse, as reported in the *Native*, for not doing so: "I felt the end product was too speculative. It didn't convince me." If we had to wait for convincing evidence on practically any aspect of AIDS, we would have nothing to read at all. No—the major important job every publication should be performing for its readers (and the one the *Native* has been accomplishing better than any other publication in the world) is to allow all theories to be aired, crackpot as they may seem—*now*. Last week I would have considered any radiation theory crackpot; last night I watched a "60 Minutes" segment on radiation contamination as the cause of leukemia in children in Wareham, Massachusetts.

I think I know as much about AIDS as any layperson. I do not fully believe anything I have read or seen or heard about. I am not a hundred percent convinced about any theory or set of "facts" about anything beyond the fact that our lives are

* *New York Native*, Issue 152, March 17, 1986.

filled with such an unfair and inhuman tragedy as to propagate madness—of all kinds. I think every single person, *without exception,* who is making *major* decisions about AIDS, for this country, for this state, for this city, for the mainstream media— is second-rate. They are second-rate scientists, second-rate doctors, second-rate epidemiologists, second-rate journalists, second-rate intelligences. There is not a first-rate brain among them.

Therefore I think it is imperative that all theories be aired, so we can each listen, sift, combine, question for ourselves, and make our own decisions. It is incumbent on the editor of each serious publication to provide space and outlet for serious speculation.

Over the past five and one-half years, I have become so disillusioned with the concept of our "free press" that I can now read Solzhenitsyn as a brother and not as a foreigner. If we have to "convince" Robert Friedman, Abe Rosenthal, Ben Bradlee, and Dan Rather that there is a story going on here as atrocious as any atrocity story the Second World War produced, then we are in trouble.

We are, of course, in trouble. We are in great trouble. Our troubles become greater and more perilous with each second. I do not need to call New Yorkers' attention to what appears to be yet another wave of new deaths and diagnoses among our friends. I do not have to call any perceptive gay person's attention to the fact that we are as politically unorganized, both locally and nationally, as we have ever been, that we are still in no way equipped to face the horrors that are coming down the pike. I do not have to tell anyone how tired we all are— physically, emotionally, spiritually—as individuals and as a community. Quite frankly, I despair.

It is imperative that we know that we have no friends to help us in many quarters where we think we have them. We have no friends at the Centers for Disease Control. We have no friends at the U.S. Department of Health and Human Services. We have no friends at the New York City Department of Health. We have fewer friends at an increasing number of New York City hospitals. (A very dear friend of mine was turned away by a doctor at New York Hospital when he had a suspected case of AIDS, with the statement, uttered quite openly and baldly, "I no longer take any gay patients." At New York Hospital!)

And, it saddens me to say, we have no friends at the *Village Voice.* We must not forget that this paper has, quite possibly, as bad a record on AIDS coverage as any paper in America. It was May 1983, a grotesque twenty-three months after the epidemic was officially declared, before they ran their first major article (by Stephen Harvey). During this agonizing period, gay writers constantly submitted ideas and requests, only to be treated badly. "They were obnoxious" is how one free-lance gay writer remembers his treatment. Many of us simply couldn't believe the *Voice* was doing this to us. We understood *The New York Times* not writing about us; that we were accustomed to. Dr. Lawrence Mass, the award-winning medical journalist to whom the gay community owes so much for his pioneering reporting on AIDS in the *Native,* was actually commissioned by the *Voice,* in November 1982, to write an AIDS piece. "The Most Important New Public Health Problem in the United States" was the title of the article he submitted. After three months of sitting on it, the *Voice* refused to run it. "It's not a *Voice* piece," was what senior editor Karen Durbin told Mass, in no way allowing him the opportunity to rework or resubmit the article. The *Native* ran it immediately.

Voice coverage to this day is spotty, second-rate, unimaginative, out-of-date, or stuff we have read earlier elsewhere. In Richard Goldstein, their openly gay senior editor, we have a first-rate example of the Uncle Toms among us—openly gay people who do nothing to help us, when they are in positions where they easily could. I would not like to live with Goldstein's conscience, all these years of being at the *Voice* and not writing or assigning AIDS articles when he should have been. How an openly gay senior editor could sit on his ass for the first twenty-three months of an epidemic that was, and still is, decimating his brothers, defies comprehension. Not that his record has been all that much better since. No, we must not forget the shameful silence of the *Voice,* as we must not forget the shameful silence of *The New York Times* for not writing about the Final Solution when it happened.

I was greatly encouraged when, last year, the *Voice* was purchased by Leonard Stern, the business partner of one of my closest friends. I was even more encouraged when someone I knew, Robert Friedman, was appointed the new editor. Both Leonard and Robert promised me that AIDS would immediately become top priority. At Robert's invitation, I submitted to him (and continue to do so) lists of possible AIDS stories and lists of good writers to write them. Alas, if anything, AIDS coverage at the *Voice* is even less than it was during the previous regime. The paper that takes such delight and relish in exposing every latest juicy tidbit about the Koch administration refuses to write about what history will prove to be the biggest scandal in the Koch administration—their heinous handling of the AIDS crisis from day one until this very day. (Dr. Mathilde Krim released the most damning report on what Koch has not done on AIDS; why did no New York newspaper other than the *Native* report on this? Isn't this the stuff the *Voice* I used to love and respect—many long years ago—would trumpet to the skies?)

For the life of me, I don't understand why this situation continues. Stern is not out to kill us. Friedman is not a monster. Even Goldstein, much as I detest what he stands for, can do good work. I think each would consider himself to be a caring person, devoted to at least some of the principles of humanism. And yet, week after week, all they turn out are more issues filled with pointless tripe, filled with pages and pages of critics with their jerk-off reviews, sounding off on what's on the tube, what's playing in the latest loft, where you can buy the trendiest spaghetti or eat it, who was seen at what stupid movie preview, what undiscovered rock song/star/ballet/mixed media simply must be discovered, what film director/playwright/novelist/poet/painter has a career that's too big and overinflated or too small and underappreciated. Have you ever seen a publication that devoted so much of its valuable space to so many saying so little you care about reading? While we are dying. While the "Village" part of the *Village Voice* is dying.

One of the saddest lessons I have learned from this epidemic is that the true heterosexual liberal, for some unaccountable reason, is not necessarily the gay person's friend. He or she will fight for blacks, women, Hispanics, abortion, nuclear disarmament, keeping the Jefferson Library open all week. But when it comes to homosexuality, they get queasy. Figure that one out. I can't.

Just as, for the life of me, I can't understand why the *Village Voice* is so stinking awful on gay issues in general and AIDS in particular. I can see no reason for any gay person to read this paper; in fact, I think we should avoid it at present.

An Open Letter to Richard Dunne and Gay Men's Health Crisis

D ear Richard,

The Doomsday Scenario that many have feared for so long comes closer. Next week, 274 people will die from AIDS. Next week, 374 more will become infected with the killer virus. In four years' time, 270,000 people will have AIDS. Of these, 179,000 will have died. Around the globe, many millions already are infected. As many as 50 percent of these millions will die.

Two out of three AIDS cases in America are still happening to gay men.

For all the worthy Patient Services and Education that have been provided, the rate of infection and death continues unabated.

As presently constituted, organized, and managed, Gay Men's Health Crisis, Inc., of which you are Executive Director, is simply not equipped or prepared or able to deal with an emergency of this magnitude.

This letter is an urgent plea to you and your Board of Directors to wake up, look coldly and harshly at the realities you have been ignoring for so long, and reconstitute yourselves so

---

* *New York Native*, Issue 197, January 26, 1987.

that at last you perform the actions you were established to perform in the first place: to fight for gay men—that we may go on living.

For the past five years I have painfully watched as GMHC has attempted to be all things to all people, in so doing losing complete sight of the larger picture, of what is happening, of what you should be doing and are not doing.

I call for nothing less than a total reassessment of your goals and a rethinking of what you are there for, what we need you there for, and what you must accomplish for us.

This letter has been in my mind for some time. I have not written it before because I kept hoping someone up there would come to his or her senses. This has not happened, and the action that finally prompted this letter is this:

In *The New York Times* of January 10th, you are quoted (concerning the release by ICN Pharmaceuticals of its most promising ribavirin data at a press conference) as follows: "We cannot understand why they chose to raise the hopes of so many people by releasing their clinical trial information through a press conference instead of a more responsible manner such as an appropriate medical journal."

I prayed that you did not say this. I prayed that the Executive Director of the organization that is meant to fight for the rights of gay men—men and rights that have been constantly, continuously denied, with a disregard for us bordering on the murderous—did not say this to a newspaper and to a world filled with heterosexual connivance, bordering on collusion at the least and conspiracy at the most—ignoring us, treating us like so much offal fit to die in agony while tests, trials, delays, ignorance, inhumane uncaring, lying, and ass-dragging characterize the daily activities of just about everyone and everything in sight, particularly the "appropriate medical journals."

I do not give a flying fuck what the *New England Journal of Medicine* reports about AIDS, or *Science* or *Lancet* or the *Journal of the American Medical Association*. From the very beginning of this epidemic they have shown scant humane concern for us, for our rights, for our continued healthy survival on this planet. Indeed, one of the main reasons this epidemic became an epidemic was that the *New England Journal of Medicine*—that "responsible . . . appropriate medical journal"—would not accept papers of warning from leading doctors observing a new phenomenon that they wished to warn the world about quickly, when they had little clinical data or test results, only observation. For an entire year, doctors at New York University and UCLA Medical Centers could not get the *New England Journal of Medicine*—that "responsible . . . appropriate medical journal"—to publish their frightening observations. And, of course, during that year, that crucial first year, an epidemic that could have been controlled and contained got woefully out of hand. These "responsible . . . appropriate medical journals" have scarcely been better since. How dare you be so trusting and naïve—you who are head of Gay Men's Health Crisis!

Why could you not applaud them? The ribavirin data *is* promising, as Dr. Mathilde Krim had the good sense to remark in the *Times*, "but not conclusive" (which no one is stating it is). From such encouragement can come swifter action at the FDA level, can come swifter and further tests, can come the release and availability of this drug to a wider market—can come all the things those who are dying so desperately pray for: PROGRESS.

But what does Auntie GMHC say and sound like? You sound like my old great-uncle Herschel—whom we loved very much, but who was nevertheless an unimaginative, whining, superior, dried-up old stuffed shirt, who was smelly and had been around too long. We used to call my great-uncle Herschel "the old fart."

I speak metaphorically, of course, of the attitude that you represent and the philosophy GMHC has come to represent. I cannot for the life of me understand how the organization I helped to form has become such a bastion of conservatism and such a bureaucratic mess. The bigger you get, the more cowardly you become; the more money you receive, the more self-satisfied you are. No longer do you fight for the living; you have become a funeral home. You and your huge assortment of caretakers perform miraculous tasks helping the dying to die. I do not cast aspersions on these activities, but I ask you to realize how exceedingly negative this concentration of your energies is. Your words to *The New York Times* only confirm this negativism yet again.

I think it must now come as a big surprise to you and your Board of Directors that Gay Men's Health Crisis was not founded to help those who are ill. It was founded to protect the living, to help the living go on living, to help those who are still healthy to stay healthy, to help gay men stay alive. Mercifully, there are still far more of us who are yet alive. Patient Services were added almost as an afterthought. I do not deny the importance of some of these services, though in most cases I think it inappropriate for you to be providing them. (More on this below.) GMHC was founded to utilize any strength it might be fortunate enough to acquire along the way: to bargain with, to fight with, to negotiate with—to use this strength to confront our enemies, to *make* them help us. This is what political strength is all about. It is *all.*

In this city, our enemies include our mayor and our Department of Health. In this country, our enemies include our President, our Department of Health and Human Services, the Hitlerian Centers for Disease Control, the U.S. Food and Drug Administration, the Public Health Service, and the self-satisfied, iron-fisted, controlling, scientific frankensteinian monsters who are in charge of research at the National Institutes of Health and who, with their stranglehold grip of death, prevent any research or thinking that does not coincide with the games their narrow minds are playing. If, after six years of this epidemic and the years you have been in charge at GMHC, you can view any of these entities or personages as anything other than our enemies, then you are perversely unsuited for your job and should be replaced immediately.

These are a lot of enemies. It would appear to represent the entire "Outside World." I did not believe in 1981 that by 1987 I would sound paranoid; I consider myself to be blessed with hard-nosed, cold sanity, which becomes more objective and realistic day by day.

Most of GMHC's efforts are devoted to providing services the *city* should be providing and would probably be forced to provide if GMHC were not in existence. This is not to say you are not providing them better than the city would; you are. But in taking our money, you are, in essence, asking us to pay twice for what you are doing—once in our contributions to you, and once in our taxes to this city. Thus you should be providing for us additional services our city will never provide—gay services, gay leadership. You don't. You have become simply another city social service agency, and at the rate one hears about your inner squabblings, the rapidly declining quality of the staff you are hiring, and the increasing unhappiness of those who work for you, it will not be long before you are indistinguishable from any of the city departments—Health, Police, Parking Violations—that serve our city so tepidly.

1. AIDS patients in New York still receive care far inferior to that in San Francisco, Los Angeles, Houston, Boston, and Paris (to name only a few cities that come to mind). I would not like to get sick with AIDS in New York and be forced to deal with the lack of decent treatment facilities, particularly if I had no adequate health insurance. How have you let this happen? First-rate health care should be your highest priority. Houston has an entire new and gleaming hospital dedicated solely to AIDS patients. San Francisco, from the very beginning, had entire divisions of hospitals put aside for us. How dare you, your executive staff, and your Board not be the leaders in fighting for these decent treatment centers?

The mayor has seen to it that GMHC has been given just enough money to shut you up. But in buying your silence, this city has lost: coordinated AIDS care, decent hospital care, home care, housing, systematic public education programs, extensive risk-reduction education programs. Through no fault of your own, you are actually perpetuating misery.

2. Your role in demanding better city education has been lackluster at best. You may congratulate yourselves on the many brochures and pamphlets you have distributed, but as you well know, this is like throwing crumbs to only the few hungry birds. Why have you not pressured government, city, state, and federal, to educate more widely? It is appalling that, consistently, year after year, this is overlooked. And it is fully in your province to expedite it. The governments of England, France, Germany, and Norway are mailing to EVERY SINGLE PERSON IN THOSE COUNTRIES full educational infor-

mation, pamphlets with specific do's and don'ts. It is simply puerile and futile to believe that you can educate an entire city and an entire world yourselves with pamphlets and brochures. You can't. It is a gigantic and enormous task. That you do not fight for the education of everyone is a shocking waste of both your energies and an ignoble denial of your charter. How dare you?

3. And just who is it you are attempting to educate? You seem to go at it in such scattershot fashion. You are given a great deal of money to educate everyone, but you overlook with amazing aplomb the vast majority of women, blacks, outer-borough and inner-city residents, children—almost everyone except gay men. It is hard to defend you against charges of racism and sexism. If you are going to cater mainly to gay, white, middle-class males, then you should say so and accept only a percentage of your city and state grants. (Your recent sad and sorry attempt to provide an educational forum for women was a total embarrassment from beginning to end. Much of the best AIDS work in this city and country has been developed by women. Why were so many of them actually forbidden input?)

4. Why have you not been in the forefront of demanding the immediate availability of drugs on a "compassionate usage" basis to those who are in the throes of dying anyway? Even putting aside the (I think untenable) notion that false hope is being provided, the availability of these drugs could provide invaluable efficacy tests. I know few PWAs who are not begging somehow to be on some kind of drug protocol somewhere, anywhere, but who are turned away at every door. How dare you not use your strength and muscle to further these ends?

Why, in fact, are you not fighting for those who would administer drug trials? There are now many treatment modalities that are promising. You continue to pooh-pooh them all—a negativism beyond comprehension to those of us who have seen so many die. You possess the biggest captive pool of people with AIDS in the world. Such studies would be far more valuable than most of the studies you *do*. Why was it left to Dr. Mathilde Krim to crusade courageously for the release of AZT? How dare you not have supported her in this cause? And where are you now, when the government and Burroughs Wellcome have gone back on their word to release the drug widely, embarrassing Dr. Krim, who had been promised more than she was given? Why is it that whenever there is a fight for something substantive and controversial (in an epidemic where *everything* is controversial), GMHC is rarely to be heard?

Why aren't you pioneering the availability and use of antivirals as prophylactic treatment for those now carrying the virus? There is enough medical evidence that this will prove helpful, and each day that a virus carrier goes unattended is a day his T-cells can be declining. Studies in this area are desperately important—truly life-saving evidence may lie in their results, but they are overlooked and ignored by the NIH, by the CDC, by the FDA, and hence by hospitals and pharmaceutical companies who don't wish to finance them themselves. How can you be so retrograde and inhumane in this most important field?

And why isn't GMHC providing drugs that are unavailable, actually selling them to the needy at cost? Why must sufferers fly to San Diego, rent a car, drive to Mexico, and sneak drugs back over the border like common criminals, at a cost in money and energy they can ill afford? Ribavirin once cost three dollars for a box of twelve in Mexico; now it costs thirty dollars a box. It will undoubtedly increase now that Mexico knows its true value. Compassionate doctors in Texas and elsewhere are now buying the drug directly from the manufacturer at cost, picking it up in Mexico, and selling it to their patients at cost. Why aren't you providing services like these? So what if this is circumventing the law? A lawsuit brought by the government against you would be the best thing that could happen to underline the horror of how the FDA is attending to AIDS. When *People* magazine ran a story on the one courageous New York gay doctor, Dr. Barry Gingell, who brought back ribavirin from Mexico illegally, the FDA was roundly criticized. Confrontation helps! Why are you such sissies!

It is now reported that AZT is going to cost each patient $10,000 a year when it becomes available. What are you

doing to confront this abhorrent future in which few patients will be able to afford the very drug that might save
them?

How dare you ignore issues like these? These are the
things you should be doing.

5. Why do you not ride herd on Research—leaving it to
others—like the *Native*—to cry out in alarm when obvious
false trials are championed and legitimate avenues are
ignored? Why have you not pushed for an Office of AIDS
Coordination in Washington? Where is the systematic
Master Plan promised by Dr. Edward Brandt years ago,
when he was head of the Department of Health and
Human Services, and promised as well by Reagan, Cuomo,
and Koch? How can you be so infernally silent on this top
priority?

6. Why are you spending so much of your time, energy,
and money on these interminable "Safe Sex" pageants? I
find it ironic to find myself asking this. My initial fights
with the GMHC Board, which resulted in my being bru-
tally exiled from your organization, had to do with my
insistence, and your refusal, to say anything about sex at
all. Now you appear to have gone to the other extreme—as
if GMHC were a sort of sex clinic to compete with Masters
and Johnson and the hateful Dr. Helen Singer Kaplan.

It simply isn't cost-effective to teach eight hundred men
how to play with their pee-pees when millions infected are
playing with theirs.

7. What has happened to your presence in Washington?
There once was a network of AIDS organizations—of
which GMHC was and is the richest and most powerful—
that hired a lonely lobbyist—though you could afford
many more. He's gone, and I hear nothing about his soli-
tary replacement. Of all the areas that demand your
strong attention and support, and our money, at the very
top of the list is the necessity of establishing a power base
in Washington. I have said time and again until I am blue
in the face that it is appalling that some 24 million men and
women have no lobbying presence in Washington to speak
of. How do we expect to achieve anything at all? The
smallest unions, the tiniest of organizations, have staffs of

lobbyists, and that is how small-interest groups, minorities, accomplish things. That is how the National Rifle
Association is so powerful and achieves results that are
anathema to so many. They organize and fight and lobby.
They let Washington know they are there. You have the
money for this. How dare you not use it?

Again I state what may come as a surprise to you, your
Board, and readers, that GMHC WAS FOUNDED TO
FIGHT. How dare you not have some sort of political wing,
some sort of spin-off that would see to it that lobbying is
done by experienced hands? (Three years ago GMHC
Board member Bob Diario was supposed to be preparing
such a plan. What happened to it? Why is it taking so
long?) Every successful charity works this way, finds legal
ways to fight, pressure, lobby. You cannot tell me that the
Catholic Church is not one of the most politically savvy
organizations around, as is the Salvation Army, the American Cancer Society, Sloan-Kettering, you name it. Hiding
behind a tax-exempt status (your constant excuse for
being so cowardly every time you have to stand up and be
counted on any controversial issue—in an epidemic where
just about *everything* is controversial!) is simply no longer
tolerable. Cardinal O'Connor's got one of the biggest
mouths around. And he uses it. Just like Ed Koch. Where's
your big mouth? If you haven't got one—get one! How can
you justify having sixty case workers on staff and not one
lobbyist?

8. Since I left GMHC, your image, your sense of public
relations savvy, your visibility, to put it impolitely, sucks.
There is not a better way to increase your power than
through press visibility. Article after article appears, and
there is no mention of GMHC. Story after story, and no
longer is it centered, as it should be, on GMHC. Human-
interest stories must be created by talented and imagina-
tive public-relations people and press coordinators and
planted in the media. It is not a job for one person; it is a
job for a number of people. The papers should have GMHC
in every single AIDS story, every single day. That is how
you become stronger; that is how you get more money
from donations and from grants and foundations; that is

how you gain respect and acquire the power necessary to negotiate. That is how you make the mayor provide adequate treatment for everyone in this city. That is how you get the release of drugs to dying patients. That is how you get educational materials provided to everyone, in the mail, on TV. That is how you get TV stations to broadcast condom ads. How dare you not use adult methods to run an adult organization? How dare you not use the rudimentary tools of modern communications to bolster the power you have inherently been handed by the gay community, your constituents. In the past months there has been another burst of AIDS media attention, with many cover stories, many TV documentaries. In former times, GMHC was front and center. I am saddened to see how rarely you are even mentioned now.

You have more than enough money to hire these people. I don't think it's an accident that your public profile has declined. I think this comes from specific Board instructions. It is an appalling choice.

9. Yes, GMHC was founded to fight, to spread information to gay men, and to fight for them. It was *not* founded, believe it or not, to provide Patient Services of any sort. This came later—and it has come to dominate you. It has provided you with the excuse to be cowards. It has provided you with a cover so that you can say, anytime something controversial requires attention: "We are too busy taking care of patients."

The time has come to rethink this devotion. As cases increase so horrendously day by day, there is no way on this earth that you can continue to provide Patient Services to the whole world. Already the quality of that service you are providing is suffering—how could it be otherwise? Soon you will drown and be totally useless.

If you were the fighting organization, negotiating from the strength that our numbers and our contributions have provided you with, you would use these numbers, this strength, this money, to force the system to provide these services. It is no mystery why San Francisco has services paid for by the city. GMHC was founded to fight for these services. Instead, like some hurt little boy, it has cowered in fear, avoided the fight to get them, and decided that "we'll take care of our own, ourselves." Well, now there are too many to take care of, and you must demand help. You must learn how to demand help.

It is no secret that the gay community in New York is not strong. The gay community in New York is invisible and weak. The gay community in New York is, I believe, in the worst shape it has ever been in politically for as long as I have been in New York, ironically just as the Gay Rights Bill has finally passed.

Since we appear to be a community that is incapable of organizing itself with strength, cohesion, unity, or networking, but only one that is capable of dealing with each other in combat, backbiting, and distrust (I am no exception to this), the services GMHC was founded to provide are more essential than ever. You have had millions of our dollars. You have a mailing list of over sixty thousand—by far the largest mailing list any gay organization has ever had.

You are the strongest organization we have, and our only hope.

Numbers and dollars equal power. How are you able, day by day, week by week, month by month, year by year, to deny this power, to ignore the fact that you have it, and to continually hide from it, as a sissy runs away from a fight? I have in the recent past referred in print to your Board of Directors as "a bunch of nerds." Any issue that is remotely controversial is certain to be turned away from your Board's table. I am ashamed of the whole lot of you. I did not spend two years of my life fighting for your birth to see you turn into a bunch of cowards. I did not spend two years of my life fighting to establish Gay Men's Health Crisis to see it turn into the organization it now is.

Get off your fucking self-satisfied asses and fight! That is what you were put there for! That is what people give you money for!

10. You continue to deny the political realities of this epidemic. THERE IS NOTHING IN THIS WHOLE AIDS MESS THAT IS NOT POLITICAL! How can you continue to deny this fact and assert that your role must remain unpolitical?

You have shut out every dissenting voice. You have effectively cut yourselves off from much of the gay community. If anyone doesn't agree with you, he or she is ignored. The list of your victims is endless—strong voices that, were they a part of your organization, would give you more strength and additional power. Because you would not harbor them, splinter groups were forced to take their issues and start their own homes—a splintering that only weakens, only makes everyone less strong. AIDS Resource Center, the PWA Coalition, AmFar, the once powerful and most useful AIDS Network (so sadly missed, now more necessary than ever as you continue to shilly-shally)—these and innumerable individuals are unwelcome at GMHC. Year after year, I wonder when someone up there will be man enough to offer peace—will try to heal the wounds—if only in the name of efficacy.

11. The world needs to know who dies from AIDS. This is essential if we are to underline the horror of what is happening. When Perry Ellis, Roy Cohn, Terry Dolan dies from AIDS, we must not allow this to be hidden or denied. (In the case of Perry Ellis, not only should we not allow the conglomerate that controls his company to put out lies to the press, but we should encourage a boycott of Perry Ellis products to rebel against the shame of their acts, just as we should not fly Delta Airlines now that it has ruled that a gay man's life is not as valuable as a straight man's.)

Why are you not fighting constantly with the Obituary Department of *The New York Times* to see that AIDS is listed as the cause of death, when it is? (The *Washington Post* reported Terry Dolan's death as from AIDS, as did *Newsweek;* the *Times* and *Time* magazine were the liars. Why did you not set the record straight?) And to insist that lovers be identified as lovers—not as one of the battery of stupid euphemisms they come up with. It has been proved that the *Times* will eventually respond to pressure. You are never there to pressure. Every time you keep your mouth shut, you tacitly claim the shame.

12. GMHC is what its Board of Directors wants it to be. Therefore, if any major changes are to be made, they will have to emanate from that holy table.

But GMHC has also placed itself in thrall to forces other than its Board. Somewhere along the line, the organization was completely taken over by Professional Custodians—social workers, psychologists, psychiatrists, therapists, teachers—all of whom have vested interests in the Sick, in the Dying, in establishing and perpetuating the Funereal. You help people to the grave, to face death. GMHC was founded to fight for life. But the fighters have been shut out, banished, as I have outlined above. Why is it not possible to do both!

Now—what can we do?

1. The fighters must be allowed to return. A branch of GMHC devoted to political fighting, to advocacy (if you must find a nice word to satisfy your tax-exemption excuses), must be established immediately and money poured into it. Your mailing list must be used for fighting. Congresspersons respond to the number of letters they receive, as do mayors. Your volunteers must be utilized for these outreach activities. They, too, must cease hiding behind their nurses' pinafores.

Professor Philip Kayal has done excellent research that has uncovered the fact that your volunteers identify their motives in working for you as more humanitarian than political. They must be made to realize that these two are intertwined, that we will have no future for them to be humanitarians in if they are not political. You have more volunteers than any gay organization has ever had. You have so many you cannot process them efficiently. Many are turned away because they do not have social service or welfare skills. You would have hundreds upon hundreds more if there was an arm of GMHC that allowed for advocates and their tactics. How dare you delay this any longer?

2. You must commence a complete rethinking of your goals and cease in your futile attempts to be *THE* AIDS SERVICE AND EDUCATION FOUNDATION. You are uncomfortable providing services to anyone other than gay men; perhaps you should concentrate your services just upon gay men. You have become weaker mainly as

you have tried to take care of everyone. The addict population is the fastest-growing AIDS category, and you are
simply out to lunch in this area. There is nothing wrong in
becoming a special-interest group. Indeed, that is what
you were first established to be.

3. Weed out the wimps on your Board of Directors and
among your staff. Replace them with fighters, with men
and women who are unafraid, who have connections in
high places they are not afraid to use. I am constantly
appalled that at least two members of your Board are on
close personal terms with the mayor, and that this has
produced absolutely zilch in tangible results for GMHC.

4. Begin the healing process. Draw back to yourselves
the splinter AIDS organizations dealing with gay men.
Draw back to yourselves the many in our community that
you have alienated and exiled. Educate your staff on the
history of GMHC, who founded it and what they fought
for and went through to make it the organization you
inherited.

5. I call upon your hundreds of volunteers to mobilize
and discuss what I am writing about. I hear so many stories of volunteer discontent. Now is your chance to make
your voices heard. You are, in essence, GMHC's slaves—
the oil for the Board's machinery—you do what they allow
you to do. But, as with all forms of slavery, the masters
could not exist without you.

6. As for everyone reading this:

We are all exceptionally tired. We are all AIDSed out.
In our exhaustion we allow the tendency to Let Someone
Else Do It. In our exhaustion we foster our continued
ignorance: We don't keep up with what is going on; we
don't want to know. We should read the *Native;* we should
read every article on AIDS. In this ignorance and exhaustion is our destruction. There is no one to do anything but
ourselves, each individual one of us. If the Board of GMHC
has been cowardly, we have allowed it to become so. If
GMHC is on the wrong course, we have allowed it to drift.
If Reagan has not uttered the word AIDS, we have abetted
this. We have given much money to GMHC with the hope
that they would leave us alone, with the notion They

Would Take Care of Everything for Us. But it does not work that way. Yes, they need our money, and will need it now more than ever. But they also need to be told you agree with what I am writing about.

To sum up:

GMHC cannot hope to provide Patient Services for the dying at the rate they are dying, or preventive education for the potentially infected at the rate they are becoming infected. The only way to force the system to provide these services across the board is by political pressure.

Our only salvation lies in aggressive scientific research. This will come only from political pressure. Every dime for research that we've had has come only from hard political fighting.

Thus all our solutions can only be achieved through political action. All the kindness in the world will not stem this epidemic. Only political action can change the course of events.

I challenge you and your Board to lead us. I challenge you and your Board to initiate the process that will bring about your metamorphosis into the organization that will fight for us in all the areas I have outlined above. It is a major challenge and I fear for our continued survival if you fail and we let you fail. GMHC is the only organization strong enough and rich enough and potentially powerful enough. There is no one else. You can no longer shirk your responsibilities, and we cannot let you. I pray that all those reading this will register their support either by writing to the *Native* or to Richard Dunne. I pray that many will agree, that you will not remain silent. I pray that GMHC will respond to this challenge. I am prepared to sit down so that jointly a list of community leaders can be formulated and an agenda drawn so that we can once again attempt to form a united stand against this horrific threat.

I beg the Board of GMHC to hear me. I beg the community of gay men and women in New York to hear me and join me in pressuring for action.

The worst years of the AIDS pandemic lie ahead of us. We are woefully unprepared. There are millions of us yet to die. Please etch this thought on your consciousness: THERE ARE MILLIONS OF US YET TO DIE. Three out of four AIDS cases are still occurring in gay men. Many millions of people carry the virus. Three out of four AIDS cases are gay men. THERE ARE MILLIONS OF US YET TO DIE.

With *The Normal Heart* safely launched, and while I was beginning to write several new plays, I found time to start agitating publicly again. And also the energy. In retrospect, I've realized my ups and downs of energy. Earlier I'd always denied any susceptibility to "burnout," but now I see that of course "burnout" came and went and came back again. When it came, I vowed, depressed, never to become politically active again. There had to be others out there to scream and yell; let them do it now.

But it seems that after a rest, my anger always reappears. There was (and still is) no single area of this awful epidemic that is being properly attended to. My list of dead acquaintances and friends grows and grows and grows. More men I once loved, or had sex with, have become ill and died. A continuing barrage of "definite" statements of facts from official authorities are contradicted days, weeks, or months later. I believed (and still believe) little of what I hear to be completely reliable. Anal intercourse was trumpeted (and still is) as *the* most likely cause of transmission. I know too many dead men who could not tolerate anal intercourse. A close friend of mine who has just been diagnosed last had anal intercourse *ten* years ago. That's equally terrifying to me when I read those obituaries of men I'd been with years before 1981.

The above bitter criticism of GMHC came about inadvertently. I received a confidential phone call from a GMHC Board member who was very upset. (The Board had of course grown and experienced a number of changes.) He gave me a list of his complaints, many of which I deal with above. He claimed there was great dissatisfaction among staff and volunteers, and he gave me specific grievances, which I then investigated and found to be true. At first I considered airing these more specifically—mentioning names and slipups. But that seemed to be unwise and petty; there is always backbiting and unhappiness and griping in any organization, and in any event, I realized that the complaints were symptomatic of much larger problems.

GMHC by now was a large and rich organization. I figured they could now withstand criticism and scrutiny I'd been reluctant to air publicly before, when it might do more harm than good. Although Paul Popham and I had not yet spoken or made our peace, I had been told that he, too, was unhappy about most of the matters I raised, particularly the leadership of Richard Dunne.

Paul was no longer actively involved with GMHC. He had been diagnosed with AIDS as early as December 1984, though it was not generally known until the following year, and by then he was quite weak. When this article appeared, I asked mutual friends what he thought of it. I was told he supported my stands almost entirely.

Since his diagnosis, he'd changed radically in his feelings about political actions; indeed, as he came closer to death, he became more impassioned publicly, even going to Washington to testify before congressional hearings. I was proud of him, though infinitely sad that his metamorphosis had come at such a price.

The letters column of the *Native* was filled with responses for weeks. There were the predictable attacks and the gratifying agreements.

There were also to be a few salutary results.

An Open Letter to Tim Sweeney

4 February 87

Mr. Tim Sweeney
Deputy Director for Policy
Gay Men's Health Crisis, Inc.

Dear Tim,

I am grateful for our recent meeting in response to my *Native* article. It has not been easy for me to reach anyone's ears at GMHC; indeed, when I am asked why I write at such a high pitch of invective, my response is that this seems to be the only way I can get anyone there to hear me. Calmer letters always go unanswered. It is too bad that so often in our community we are almost forced into insult before we hear each other. (Well, perhaps it is like that in other communities, too.) Thank you for being the first GMHC official willing to speak to me in some time. I am sad that your executive director, Richard Dunne, has refused my offer of a meeting and I am sad that your Board president, Nathan Kolodner, has

* *New York Native*, Issue 200, February 16, 1987.

117

not returned my phone call or responded to a similar offer for a meeting.

In any event, I think you and I did good work in preparing a list of six proposals for action. I was thrilled that you agreed with all of them. I was heartened to hear that some of these points are already under development or discussion at GMHC. I was pleased that your opinion of GMHC's Board was more positive than mine; and your assessment that they are indeed ready to forcefully move ahead toward strong, definite acts of politicizing GMHC sounded, to put it mildly, almost too good to be true.

In subsequent conversation with you, I began to feel that my initial enthusiastic reaction to our meeting should perhaps be touched with a little caution. You are only one man, with only the strength of one man—great though I know your strengths to be, and your passion, and your commitment. (I was particularly touched during our three-hour meeting when you spoke so movingly about how much your new job at GMHC meant to you, and the challenges and the opportunities it presented to you.) I know you to possess that rarest of skills—the ability to negotiate and maneuver in difficult and often treacherous waters. I guess I feel that if anyone can help turn GMHC around, it is you. But you cannot do this without the cooperation of your Executive Director and your Board.

I am always amazed at the strong reactions my *Native* articles arouse. I am told by the *Native* that these issues are among their highest-selling. I know that my phone does not stop ringing, that my mail brings many letters, that people stop me in the street. I am overwhelmed with positive support for my stands. It seems to me that I am saying things that must touch a sympathetic nerve in many people. Even if they respond negatively, they do so with the vigor that can only come from some important button having been pushed. I feel that I am saying what many feel but don't know how to say themselves.

As I told you in our discussions, I have been uncertain how best to respond to your letter. I want very much to provide all support to you in your efforts to bring about the vital necessary changes in GMHC's posture. I want very much for my letter, our meeting, the many supportive calls and letters, to somehow serve as some sort of pressure to move your Board and your

Executive Director forward quickly and forcefully and positively.

I have tried over the past weeks to get a consensus from the many people I have spoken with. I have called or been called by several dozen members of our community whom I know to be active and involved. I have called or been called by current and past GMHC staff, volunteers, and Board members. Quite frankly, I was amazed at how many volunteers and staff members wanted to talk; what troubled me was how frightened they were of speaking for attribution, as if some reign of terror existed in the homeland. Too much of what I found out was distressing. Some of it broke my heart. The inescapable fact confronting me everywhere I turned was this: GMHC is definitely experiencing abnormally glaring and traumatic growing pains.

Many urged me to continue vigorously to pursue my objectives by releasing full details of all this disenchantment. Much to my surprise, I found myself making the decision that—for the moment—it would not be productive to get into a screaming match, or to wash dirty linen quite so publicly as the recent GLAAD debacle that has wounded that organization, founded on principles as lofty as GMHC's. As you yourself said, we have so much hard work and energy invested in our organizations—we *must* make them work. And I love GMHC as much as, if not more than, most. After all, it was founded in my living room, I gave it its name (for better or worse), I arranged for my brother's law firm to be its legal counsel pro bono, which they still are, and I gave it two years of my life, full time. I am very proud that the organization is there partly because of me, and I am conscious of the many fine deeds it has accomplished over the years. If I have pain and anger and frustration as well, it is very much like that of a parent toward a wayward and unfocused child who is not growing up the way I want it to.

Therefore, for the moment, I think it best mainly to put on record what our six points of discussion were. In this way, the community has a guide to what you and I feel needs to be done immediately, and has a yardstick, as well, against which to measure your progress and that of your Executive Director, Mr. Dunne, and your Board's progress in bringing these points into living actuality.

1. Of top priority is our joint acceptance of the fact that GMHC must immediately establish a distinct division that is totally and wholeheartedly devoted to advocacy.

I am aware that there is some indecision as to whether this division should be within the structure of GMHC, as it is presently constituted as a 501-C (3) tax-exempt organization, or whether a separate division must be established with a 501-C (4) structure, which would allow for total political activity under your supervision, but not allowing for tax-deductible contributions. This is an issue that has been plaguing various Boards since GMHC was founded, and I beg that it not be allowed to drag on unresolved any longer. With the new tax laws, as I understand them, tax deductions for charitable contributions are not going to be as meaningful as formerly in helping to reduce the contributors' income taxes; therefore it would seem to me that a 501-C (4) non-tax-exempt division of GMHC should be established forthwith. This would have the further advantage not only of allowing Operation Outreach to function politically, but of allowing GMHC to utilize $175,000 of every $1 million of its (tax-deductible) contributions for advocacy.

I wish there were not so much constant worry about your holy tax-exempt status. You are an organization that should be pledged to obsolescence, not empire.

a. This advocacy division would be staffed with as close to 1-to-1 parity with the client services division, both in staff and volunteers, as possible. In other words, it would be a distinct partner with client services.

b. This advocacy division would have its very own lobbyists, as distinct from the lobbyists GMHC can hire on its own, and the lobbyist GMHC helps to finance via its participation in the AIDS Action Council. You would immediately hire one lobbyist for Washington, one for Albany, and one for New York City.

c. This advocacy division would hire immediately one full-time person whose sole job would be to increase the number of lobbyists in Washington. This person would go around the country working with other gay organizations and gay communities, the goal being the funding by said

organizations and communities of all or part of the cost of
one lobbyist. It costs anywhere from $60,000 to $100,000
a year to fund a good lobbyist in Washington. It would be
no big deal for the gay community in Houston or Dallas or
Philadelphia or San Francisco to have annual fund-raisers
just for this cause. Each city could, in effect, be responsible
for raising the salary of one lobbyist (several years ago,
EEGO—the East End Gay Organization—was considering
doing just this, but somehow it got sidetracked into participating with the AIDS Action Council). Within a year or so,
we could have a group of ten or fifteen lobbyists in Washington and, for the first time in our lives, begin to have
power in the place where it makes the most difference.

   d. This advocacy division would have volunteers devoted to increasing the size of the GMHC mailing list. The
more names on a mailing list, the more power the organization has to barter with. I am told the GMHC list is about
forty thousand names, not sixty thousand, as I wrote.
Well, it should be at least a million. There are many ways
to increase a list—from buying other lists to getting letter-
writing campaigns going, getting everyone you know to
add names for this cause.

   e. This advocacy division would involve itself in the
many aspects of advocacy—protests, civil disobedience,
organized mailings to members of Congress and government, the forthcoming March on Washington, visible displays of both coalition and disapproval. The blacks
mounted a very swift and effective march on Koch's Village apartment after Howard Beach. It has been a long
time since our Candlelight March of, was it 1984?

   2. Public Relations: Further staff members experienced
in this very special skill should be hired to work with Lori
Behrman (who was a most effective spokesperson on
"Channel 4 News" of February 3rd). Good PR is basically
about taking important people to lunch, making contacts
everywhere, and learning how to use them. It also requires
imagination—dreaming up new angles for stories and not
giving up until they are placed. Money must be found for
such schmoosing-up. Also, GMHC should issue public

statements on every issue concerning AIDS; in every possible article or media mention, there should be a GMHC quote or mention.

That most noble and courageous of protesters, Andrei Sakharov, has proved to us time and time again that, as *The New Yorker* wrote of him, "the main weapon in the struggle for human rights is publicity."

3. Drugs: We talked about the possibility of GMHC plugging into the pioneering and magnificently enterprising San Francisco organization, Project Inform, or providing essentially the same services here. Project Inform has an 800 number (800-822-7422; in California 800-334-7422) where anyone can get the most recently available information on all current drugs and treatments, how and where they can be obtained, and how they are doing in trials, to the best of their knowledge. I am in no way suggesting that GMHC recommend any particular drug or treatment. Results on all present drugs and treatments are still perplexingly unclear. Many patients do better not taking any treatment at all. But it should be a matter of individual choice whether or not someone wishes to undergo a particular treatment. In order for this decision to be intelligently made, the individual should have available to him, with a minimum of fuss and bother, the latest information concerning the efficacy, availability, and cost of whatever is going on around the world. Few patients have the energy, physical or psychic, to be Sherlock Holmes because doctors aren't telling them what they need to know. Your already existing Hotline would seem a perfect place to plug this service in.

4. The addition to the Board of Directors of four or five new members who are politically adept and active and vocal. I am glad to hear from you that you think the Board is now at last ready for political activism; but the truth is that, as a group, the Board is conservative, and unfortunately a conservative board tends to keep perpetuating conservative boards. They keep voting in people just like themselves.

I would like to interject here advice I had from a dear

friend and very wise woman. I called her for advice on all
of this. Her name is Dr. Gloria Donadello; she is a thera-
pist, a Ph.D., a lesbian, Professor of Social Service at Ford-
ham, a director on one of the earliest Lambda Legal
Defense boards, and a member of the advisory board of
SAGE:

"A board is supposed to be the liaison between the
organization and the community it serves. A board is supposed to be the representative of the community it serves.
It is lousy communication, listening only to your own
voice, if differing opinions are not heard. No organization
can be served well that way.

"People who work for an organization or are served by
an organization have to feel they have access to the power
that is running that organization. They are not going to
feel very good about themselves, or about their organization, when they don't. The leadership is making them not
feel good. And you can't expect people who have the least
amount of power to make the changes. For instance, poor
people can't pull themselves up by their own bootstraps.
Power is with those who have the power. If the board and
the executive director have the power, and they don't use
it, it's very difficult for the line workers, or the community,
to make the changes.

"What GMHC is going through—well, it is unfortunately predictable because this happens at about this time
in the growth of any service organization. I don't know
that it can be prevented, but when it is happening, you
must be very much on guard, and aware.

"It is always the danger that the grass-roots organization gets co-opted by the very system it was formed to
make accountable. Social work started out to reform—to
effect social change. Sadly, now, it's all maintenance of the
status quo.

"Part of the answer is to foster a conviction that rests
in a value that the system must be held accountable all the
time. But that takes courage. The organization has to be
willing to stick its neck out. Unfortunately we place too
much value in our society on the status quo. Challenging
the system is a no-no. For instance, an organization says,

'We're now a respectable organization providing respectable services'—but really nothing much has changed with respect to the rights of gay persons. So, in essence, the organization hasn't changed anything."

5. The establishment of a Standing Community Advisory Board. Some modest method must be found for outside dialogue to get the ears of the power structure of GMHC. This is just good simple community relations and, had it existed, there would perhaps not now be such ill feeling about your purchase of an expensive new building.

6. Fund-raisers like the 1983 Circus event at Madison Square Garden. This certainly is not such an important item as any of the first four points, and I offer it more for the morale of the community than for any notion of a cost-effectiveness I know to be less than that of other ways of raising money. But there was something so special about that night at the Circus (the idea was Paul Popham's—GMHC's first Board president) that everyone who attended will never forget it. We could see ourselves in all our magnificent strength—what we were capable of bringing off. How about Bruce Springsteen at Shea Stadium?

At our meeting, I asked you what you thought your timetable might be. You mentioned there were various committee approvals necessary before a full Board vote. Being an impatient sort, I bristled at the notion of committees and lengthy delays. Who among us does not know how often the very process of trying to get anything done gets nothing done? I understand the next full Board meeting is at the end of February.

I look forward to hearing from you about how quickly we can count on a schedule, an agenda, a plan. How long will it take before lobbyists can be hired, this advocacy division established? I hope you will do the community a courtesy by writing a short note to the *Native* to keep us abreast of progress.

AIDS MAY DWARF THE PLAGUE is the small headline that appeared on page A-24 (the real-estate page) of *The New York Times* on Friday, January 24th, 1987. N.Y. AIDS PLAGUE— 150,000 DOOMED screams out the headline of the February 4th *New York Post.* "A worldwide death toll in the tens of millions a decade from now" is what Secretary of Health and Human Services Dr. Otis R. Bowen is predicting. His numbers are a bit smaller than those of Dr. C. Everett Koop, the Surgeon General, who says "100 million people could be dead by the end of the century." That 100 million could be infected with the virus within five years is the prediction of Dr. Halfdan Mahler, the head of the World Health Organization. The current issue of *Atlantic* says that for every reported case there are sixty unreported.

I close again, as I did before, with the plea that you, your Board, and your executive director accept this challenge to become the true heroes our community so desperately needs. I close, as I did before, with the startling fact that two out of three official AIDS cases are still happening to gay men. Four million people may now carry the killer virus. The number of new cases is doubling every six to eight months. There are millions of us yet to die.

I do not think that any point or issue I raise in this letter is unreasonable or difficult to put into action. Please beg your Board and your Executive Director not to let us down.

I finally called Richard Dunne and we had a relatively uncommunicative lunch together. However, Nathan Kolodner, the president of the Board, called me and we established a working relationship that has now matured into a friendship. It turned out we shared many similar views of GMHC's problems.

It was to take too long a time, but several new members were added to the Board; they are not as politically forceful as this rabble-rouser would like, but they seem to be committed and intelligent. Lobbying in Washington still languishes, but a New York State lobbyist was finally added. The Public Relations department was modestly expanded, and attempts were made to improve the morale of the staff and volunteers.

Perhaps the most important addition has been the hiring, at my suggestion, of my friend Dr. Barry Gingell, to be head of the new Office of Medical Information. Barry, who is a person with AIDS, knows more about AIDS treatments than anyone else in the world, and he has been an invaluable resource that the AIDS community has come to rely on and revere. He immediately began *Treatment Issues: The GMHC Newsletter of Experimental AIDS Therapies,* which is, I think, as honest and fact-filled a publication as is available on this subject. Barry and a new Board member, Judy Peabody, have joined various NIH drug committees, so that our opinions can at least be heard, if not considered, at that ignoble Valhalla. Of all the voices in all the AIDS bureaucracies, I think Barry's alone has been the most willing to openly criticize and castigate the foul NIH AIDS program headed by Dr. Anthony Fauci, and the equally foul FDA AIDS program headed by Dr. Frank Young, constantly bringing this issue up to the press and at various conferences in Washington, where to criticize the NIH or FDA is to blaspheme God. He has been wonderful.

The Beginning of ACTing UP

On March 14th, 1983, almost four years ago to this date, I wrote an article in the *New York Native*. There were at that time 1,112 cases of AIDS nationwide. My article was entitled "1,112 and Counting," and through the courtesy of *Native* publisher Chuck Ortleb, it was reprinted in seventeen additional gay newspapers across the country. Here are a few of the opening sentences from this article:

"If this article doesn't scare the shit out of you, we're in real trouble. If this article doesn't rouse you to anger, fury, rage, and action, gay men may have no future on this earth. Our continued existence depends on just how angry you can get. . . . I repeat: Our continued existence as gay men upon the face of this earth is at stake. Unless we fight for our lives, we shall die. In all the history of homosexuality we have never before been so close to death and extinction."

When I wrote that, four years ago, there were 1,112 cases of AIDS nationwide. There are now officially—and we all know how officials count—32,000 with 10,000 of these in New York.

---

* Speech given at the Gay and Lesbian Community Center in New York, on March 10, 1987, to a group of approximately 250 men and women.

We have not yet even begun to live through the true horror. As it has been explained to me, the people who have become ill so far got ill early; the average incubation period is now thought to be five and one-half years, and the real tidal wave is yet to come: people who got infected starting in 1981. You had sex in 1981. I did, too. And after.

Last week, I had seven friends who were diagnosed. In one week. That's the most in the shortest period that's happened to me.

I would like everyone from this right-hand side aisle, all the way to the left-hand side of the room—would you stand up for a minute, please? [They do so.] At the rate we are going, you could be be dead in less than five years. Two-thirds of this room could be dead in less than five years. Please sit down.

Let me rephrase my *Native* article of 1983. If my speech tonight doesn't scare the shit out of you, we're in real trouble. If what you're hearing doesn't rouse you to anger, fury, rage, and action, gay men will have no future here on earth. How long does it take before you get angry and fight back?

I sometimes think we have a death wish. I think we must want to die. I have never been able to understand why for six long years we have sat back and let ourselves literally be knocked off man by man—without fighting back. I have heard of denial, but this is more than denial; it *is* a death wish.

I don't want to die. I cannot believe that you *want* to die.

But what are we doing, *really,* to save our own lives?

Two-thirds of you—I should say of *us,* because I am in this, too—could be dead within five years. Two-thirds of this room could be dead within five years.

What does it take for us to take responsibility for our own lives? Because we are *not*—we are not taking responsibility for our own lives.

I want to talk about a few specific things.

I've just come back from Houston. My play *The Normal Heart* was done at the Alley Theatre there. I did not want to go to see it, but a very insistent woman who works with AIDS patients there would not take no for an answer. Thus I had the opportunity and the great privilege to visit our country's first AIDS hospital, which is called the Institute for Immunological

Disorders. I've finally discovered the place I want to go to if I get sick.

You know how the topic of conversation in New York always turns to: Where would you go if you got sick? Which hospital? Which doctor? Quite frankly, I don't want to go to *any* hospital in New York. And I don't want to go to most of the doctors. They pooh-pooh everything new that comes along; they don't know anything about any new drug or treatment. They don't want to know. They throw you into the hospital, give you a grotesquely expensive workup, pump you full of some old drug that they've heard about from another doctor, and your insurance company pays for it, if you're lucky enough to have insurance. These doctors won't fight for anything, they won't go up against the FDA, they don't want to hear about any new theories or ideas. Why are they always so negative about everything? These doctors are making a fucking fortune out of us. They ridicule anything new that comes along, without even trying it. The horror stories emanating from almost every hospital in this city, with the possible exception of NYU, are just grotesque—all the way from an attempted murder of an AIDS patient at New York Hospital to a friend of mine who lay in the emergency room at St. Vincent's for seventeen hours, just last week, before anyone looked at him. No, I don't want to go to any hospital or any doctor in New York.

The Institute for Immunological Disorders is run by Dr. Peter Mansell, who is one of the top AIDS doctors in America. It has space for 150 patients. There are only sixteen patients there. This most wonderful AIDS hospital in the world—you probably don't even know about it; some of you are hearing about it for the first time. How can it happen that it only has sixteen patients? Only in America.

I'm going to tell you—it's not explicitly germane to us, but it is interesting—Texas is the only state in this country where if you don't have insurance, where if you're indigent, the state will not reimburse you or a hospital for the cost of your care. Most of those with AIDS in Houston don't have any insurance. They can't afford to go to Dr. Mansell's hospital. Mansell treats 150 patients every week, as outpatients, for free. Dr. Mansell's hospital, which is owned by a for-profit corporation, is losing a great deal of money. This hospital must not be allowed to die.

Dr. Mansell has found out some very interesting things. He has found out that 90 percent of all AIDS problems are better treated at home, and this includes home treatment for PCP. He has found that he can treat patients for two-thirds less than it costs anywhere else—an average of $11,000 vs. $33,000. He has found that the average length of hospital stay of his patients is ten days, versus thirty days anywhere else. The hitch, of course, is that no insurance policy covers outpatient care. The very insurance companies that are threatening to take away our insurance because we cost them too much won't pay for cheaper treatment. That doesn't make much sense, does it?

But the real horror stories that Dr. Mansell told me have to do with drugs and the FDA. Dr. Mansell has five drugs waiting to be tested. I never heard of four of them. He tells me that each has been shown to prove as promising as AZT was when it was approved. Each has passed what are called Phase One Safety Trials, which show them to lack noticeable side effects. The drugs are called Ampligen, Glucan, DTC, AS 101, and MTP-PE (for KS). He cannot get near the FDA. When one of the top AIDS doctors in the United States can't get protocols through the FDA, we're in big trouble. He showed me the protocols that he submits, and he showed me how they're sent back—the FDA asking for one sentence rewritten, three words revised—nothing substantial—each change causing a delay of six to eight months. Ampligen is a drug that has been around for a long time. Concerned citizens of Houston have formed a foundation and bought $250,000 worth of Ampligen, so neither the hospital nor the government had to pay for it—and the drug remains unused and untested because of FDA quibbling.

You know—each step of this horror story that we live through, we come up against an even bigger brick wall. First it was the city, then the state, then the CDC, then the NIH. Now it's the FDA. Ann Fettner wrote last week in the *Village Voice* about the FDA: "It is a bureaucratic mess, they aren't even computerized, things 'are likely to get stuck in the mailroom,' says Duke University economist Henry Grabowski—which means that much of our pharmaceutical talent diddles with refinements of approved drugs while many that are desperately needed are put on hold." A new drug can easily take ten years to satisfy FDA approval. Ten years! Two-thirds of us could be dead in less than five years.

In 1980 the then head of the FDA said, "Ribavirin is probably the most important product discovered during the intensive search for antiviral agents." It's 1987 and we still can't get it. Fettner says, "It's astonishing that ribavirin wasn't chosen before AZT." Leading researchers I have talked to explain this one way: The FDA doesn't like the difficult, obstreperous head of ICN Pharmaceuticals, which manufactures ribavirin, while Burroughs Wellcome, which makes AZT, is smooth, politically savvy, with strong PR people. The fast introduction of AZT was described to me in one word by a leading doctor: "Greed." He thinks little of AZT, refers to it as "yesterday's drug, that Burroughs Wellcome is trying to make their fortune out of before it's too late. I have too many patients on it who are becoming transfusion-dependent." I have a few friends who seem to be doing well on it. I have some who aren't. It's certainly not our savior.

AL 721 isn't even a drug—it's a food! How dare the FDA refuse to get it into fast circulation when it has proved promising in Israel at their famous Weizmann Institute? Indeed, Praxis Pharmaceuticals, which holds the American rights to it, could put it out as a food; but they apparently are gambling for big bucks by waiting for FDA approval to put it out as a drug, which is going to take forever, because Praxis doesn't appear to have much experience in putting out drugs at all. Rumor has it, also, that Praxis has forbidden the Weizmann Institute and Israeli doctors from giving AL 721 to any non-Israelis who go to Israel to get it.

What's going on here? To quote Dr. Mansell: "The FDA makes me froth at the mouth." We have reached a brick wall. There is a fortune being tossed at AIDS, but it's not buying anything. To quote Dr. Mansell: "A lot of money, a lot of energy—and very little to show for it." He runs one of the NIH-designated AIDS treatment centers and he has a hospital with *sixteen* patients! And we have ten thousand cases in New York City. He has an empty hospital, and he is one of the smartest men in this epidemic. How can this country be so wasteful!

Another researcher: "The NIH is too slow and too

determined to maintain central control. It is hugely bureaucratic, much like your own GMHC and other AIDS organizations have become." Not my words. Dr. Mansell again: "Many
of the drugs that the NIH is testing have already proved useless and ineffective somewhere else. Why do they insist on
testing them? Why do they refuse to test any of these new
drugs that are brought to their attention?"

Let's talk about double-blind studies that we're forced to
endure. Did you know that double-blind studies were not created originally for terminal illnesses? I never knew that. Did
you know that? How dare they, then, make us endure double-
blind studies? They are ludicrously inhumane when two-thirds
of this room could be dead in less than five years.

Double-blind studies are also exceptionally foolish, because
PWAs lie to get the drugs. I'd lie. Wouldn't you? If they told
me what to say to get a promising treatment, I'd say it, whether
it was true or not. I have friends who have forged their medical
records, who have gone to medical libraries to learn the correct
terminology to fill in the blanks. So all the results from all these
double-blind studies aren't going to tell anyone a thing. We're
willing to be guinea pigs, all of us. Give us the fucking drugs!
Especially if Dr. Mansell has five drugs that he says may have
fewer side effects than AZT.

Almost one billion dollars will be thrown at AIDS, and it's
not buying anything that will save two-thirds of the people in
this room. I just heard about a college on Long Island that's
been awarded a $600,000 grant from the Centers for Disease
Control—an organization I have come to loathe—to study
AIDS stress on college students. I can tell them right now and
save the government $600,000. I know what it's like to be
stressed. So do you.

I called up the offices of our elected officials and asked them
to send someone here tonight. Cuomo, D'Amato, Moynihan,
Koch. Every single one of them treated me as if I was ungrateful. "We have been on the front line of getting you your
money," each one of them said. "Leave us alone. You got your
money. What else do you want?" That was from Moynihan's
office: "What else do you want? We got you your money." When
I try to tell them that this money isn't working right, isn't

buying us anything, isn't properly supervised—once again, they don't want to know. I find the offices of Moynihan and D'Amato particularly insensitive to gay issues. Our only friend in Congress, and he's getting real tired, is Ted Weiss. And, of course, from Los Angeles, Henry Waxman.

So what are we going to do? Time and time again I have said—no one is going to do it for us but ourselves.

We have always been a particularly divisive community. We fight with each other too much, we're disorganized, we simply cannot get together. We've all insulted each other. I'm as much at fault in this as anyone.

I came back from Houston and I called people I haven't spoken to in many years. I called Paul Popham. Those of you who are familiar with the history of GMHC and with *The Normal Heart* will know of the fights that he and I had and the estrangement of what had once been an exceptionally close friendship. Paul is very ill now. He and I spoke for over an hour. It was as if it were the early days of GMHC again, and we were planning strategy of what had to be done. We talked not about the hurts that each had caused the other. He supported me in everything that I am saying to you tonight, and that I have been writing about in the *Native* in recent issues. He would be here tonight, except that he had chemotherapy today. He asked me to say some things to you. "Tell them we have to make gay people all over the country cooperate. Tell them we have to establish some way to cut through all the red tape. We have to find a way to make GMHC, the AIDS Action Council, and the other AIDS organizations stronger and more political."

We talked a lot about GMHC, the organization that represents so much of our joint lives. As you know, I have been very critical of GMHC recently, and wrote a rather stinging attack on them. Paul and I both feel that GMHC is the only AIDS game in town in this country, and, like it or not, they have to be made to act stronger in the areas of lobbying and advocacy. There are no other organizations with as much clout, with as much money, with as much staff. San Francisco's AIDS organizations still have not even put their pledged contributions into the AIDS Action Council, our joint lobbying effort in Washington, which is an appalling act on the part of San Francisco's gay community. "We have to shame them into their contributions," Paul said.

The people administering GMHC are running what amounts to a big corporation. We cannot fault them for running such a sound ship, such a fiscally sound ship.

But we desperately need leadership in this crisis. We desperately need a central voice and a central organization to which everything else can plug in and be coordinated through. There isn't anyone else. And in this area of centralized leadership, of vision, of seeing the larger picture and acting upon it, GMHC is tragically weak. It seems to have lost the sense of mission and urgency upon which it was founded—which Paul and I fought so hard to give it.

In my recent article attacking them, I asked GMHC for very specific things: lobbying; an advocacy division; more public-relations people to get the word out; a change of their tax-exempt status to allow for increased political activities; fighting for drugs; more strong members put on their Board. I was promised everything. I couldn't believe it; it was too good to be true.

Two months later, precious little has been done. The tax-exempt status has been changed. A lobbyist has been identified for Albany. A *part-time* PR person is about to be hired. When I asked why they were not hiring a full-time PR person, *six* full-time PR persons, the excuse I was given was "We don't have a desk." Two-thirds of us could be dead in five years, and this rich organization is not hiring people to get the word out because they haven't got room for a desk. [Cries from the audience of "Shame, shame!"]

No advocacy plan has emerged from GMHC, despite the fact that we have been promised one for six months. Paul Popham himself told me that the "Mission Statement" that was prepared by GMHC's executives is one that he never would have accepted when he was president of the Board.

This morning's front page of *The New York Times* has an article about two thousand Catholics marching through the halls of Albany today. On the front page of the *Times*. With their six bishops (including one whom we know to be gay). Two thousand Catholics and their bishops marching through the halls of government. That's advocacy! That's what GMHC has to plan and facilitate and encourage. That's what all of us have to do. Southern Methodist University gets on national television protesting something about their football team. Black people marched on Mayor Koch's apartment only days after Howard Beach. Why are we so invisible, constantly and forever! What does it take to get a few thousand people to stage a march!

Did you notice what got the most attention at the recent CDC conference in Atlanta? It was a bunch called the Lavender Hill Mob. They got more attention than anything else at that meeting. They protested. They yelled and screamed and demanded and were blissfully rude to all those arrogant epidemiologists who are ruining our lives.

We can no longer afford to operate in separate and individual cocoons. There cannot be a Lavender Hill Mob protesting without a GLAAD mobilizing the media, without a National Gay and Lesbian Task Force and AIDS Action Council lobbying in Washington, without a Human Rights Campaign Fund raising money, and without a GMHC and its leaders leading us. That's coordination. Without every organization working together, networking, we will get nowhere.

We must immediately rethink the structure of our community, and that is why I have invited you here tonight: to seek your input and advice, in the hope that we can come out of tonight with some definite and active ideas. Do we want to reactivate the old AIDS Network? Do we want to start a new organization devoted solely to political action?

I want to talk to you about power. We are all in awe of power, of those who have it, and we always bemoan the fact that we don't have it. Power is little pieces of paper on the floor. No one picks them up. Ten people walk by and no one picks up the piece of paper on the floor. The eleventh person walks by and is tired of looking at it, and so he bends down and picks it up. The next day he does the same thing. And soon he's in charge of picking up the paper. And he's got a lot of pieces of paper that he's picked up. Now—think of those pieces of paper as standing for responsibility. This man or woman who is picking up the pieces of paper is, by being responsible, acquiring more and more power. He doesn't necessarily want it, but he's tired of seeing the floor littered. All power is the willingness to accept responsibility. But we live in a city and a country where no one is willing to pick up pieces of paper. Where no one wants any responsibility.

It's easy to criticize GMHC. It's easier to criticize, period. It's harder to do things. Every one of us here is capable of doing something. Of doing something strong. We have to go after the FDA—fast. That means coordinated protests, pickets, arrests. Are you ashamed to be arrested? I would like to acknowledge one of the most courageous men in this country, who is with us here tonight. He is so concerned about the proliferation of nuclear weapons that he gets arrested at the expense of his own career. He uses his name and his fame to help make this world a better place. Martin Sheen. Stand up, Martin. The best man at Martin's wedding, his oldest friend, died today, from AIDS.

Look at this article from the *San Francisco Chronicle*, written by openly gay journalist Randy Shilts (just about the only reporter and the only newspaper in this entire country covering AIDS with proper thoroughness and compassion). Look who is our friend: the Surgeon General, C. Everett Koop. A fundamentalist is our friend. Koop said, "We have to embarrass the administration into bringing the resources that are necessary to deal with this epidemic forcefully." He said a meeting has been arranged with the President several times, and several times this meeting has been canceled. His own Surgeon General is telling us that we have to embarrass the President to get some attention to AIDS. Why didn't any other paper across this country pick up this story? You sure didn't see it in *The New York Times*.

It's our fault, boys and girls. It's our fault. Two thousand Catholics can walk through the corridors of Albany. The American Foundation for AIDS Research has on its board Elizabeth Taylor, Warren Beatty, Leonard Bernstein, Woody Allen, Barbra Streisand, Michael Sovern (the president of Columbia University), a veritable *Who's Who;* why can't they get a meeting with the President—their former acting buddy? Why don't we think like that?

Well, until we all bend over and pick up all those little pieces of paper, I don't have to tell you what's going to happen.

Nora Ephron had canceled at the last moment, and the Gay and Lesbian Community Center asked me to fill in for her at their monthly speakers' series. I had no idea what I wanted to talk about. I didn't particularly want to make a speech at all. I thought I'd said everything I had to say or could say—too many times. There didn't seem to be anything new to talk about.

For the previous month or so I'd been receiving persistent, pestering calls from a charming but determined woman in Houston. Her name was Mary Lou Galantino and she was Physical Therapy Coordinator at the Institute for Immunological Disorders. She simply would not take no for an answer. I must come to Houston to see my play, and I must come to see the Institute. Finally, when she managed to get the theatre to pay my plane and hotel expenses, I gave in. As I look back on it, it seems, like my appointment with Dr. Alvin Friedman-Kien at NYU in 1981, one of those fateful journeys. I wonder, if I hadn't gone to Houston and visited Dr. Mansell's Institute, what I would have spoken about. I wonder, if I hadn't gone to Houston, whether ACT UP would have been founded. Luck has been twice on my side: As with GMHC, I've been able to help coalesce already existing energy that is out there and help find a focus for its outlet.

There was much discussion following my speech, and the result was a decision to hold a further meeting, two days later. The gay grapevine functioned remarkably well, for some three hundred or more showed up that Thursday night, and the result was the establishment of ACT UP—the AIDS Coalition to Unleash Power—an ad hoc community protest group that, originally, was pledged to concentrate on fighting for the release of experimental drugs. (I say "originally" because its interests have now broadened to include other items and I feel they've lost a bit of focus on the drug issue, which for me is just about the main issue of paramount importance.)

A mass demonstration was planned for Tuesday morning, March 24th, on Wall Street, against the FDA. Joseph Papp contributed an effigy (built in his workshops) of Dr. Frank Young, the head of the FDA, who was "hung" in front of Trinity Church. Some 250 men and women tied up traffic for several hours and passed out tens of thousands of fact sheets about the FDA horror show, as well as copies of my *Times* op-ed piece (which follows). The demonstration and subsequent arrests made the national nightly newscasts, and when, several weeks later, Dr. Young made some promises (which he has yet to keep) about speedier drug testing and release, Dan Rather gave credit to ACT UP. It was a wonderful beginning.

Since then, ACT UP has grown to several thousand members and has inspired many chapters all across the country. It often seems that not a week goes by in which a protest is not going on somewhere. In New York, just about every possible target has been zapped, and many of these demos have made the papers and the TV news.

While these two organizations, GMHC and ACT UP, have given me a certain pride in that I helped to start them, I've discovered from both experiences that I'm better as an idea man than as someone easy to have around after that. The kind of energy that helps start organizations, and fuel them in the tentative early days, is also the same kind of energy that becomes embarrassing to organizations once they become healthy, large, and, in the case of GMHC, bureaucratized. I'm simply too opinionated, and impatient to move faster. GMHC became timid very quickly, and my speaking out so boldly and so violently against my list of perceived wrongs and enemies terrified the early members. With ACT UP, there has been a different set of problems: *Everyone* is very opinionated, and very angry. When I found, once again, that what I had learned to recognize, at last, was my style, was once again going to get me in hot water (what I have come to call the "fuck the founding father" syndrome), I quietly withdrew from active ACT UP participation, (although I try to join as many demonstrations as I can). I didn't want to repeat the GMHC experience.

I also now accept, albeit reluctantly, that, once started, there is little any one individual can do to control or affect an organization's development. It's like a person: It's more or less going to be what it's going to be. And, like a person, it wants to do it and get there on its own. And when I found that my suggestions were coming to be resented, not because of their content but because *I* was making them, I returned home to get back to my writing.

ACT UP became strong and healthy very quickly. The group is, for me, infinitely moving to witness, because it is composed mostly of such young people. These are men and women, some barely in their twenties, who have a comfort with their homosexuality that I never had at that age, and a desire to be politically active that, at such a young age, for such large numbers, is actually historically new and important in the ongoing struggle for gay rights.

The FDA's Callous Response to AIDS

Many of us who live in daily terror because of the AIDS epidemic cannot understand why the Food and Drug Administration has been so intransigent in the face of this monstrous tidal wave of death. Its response to what is plainly a national emergency has been inadequate, its testing facilities inefficient, and access to its staff and activities virtually impossible to gain. One private doctor, anticipating the FDA's release of the drug AZT, said that it would amount to a "sop to the gay community—so they'll shut up. They can't say they haven't been given *something.*"

Indeed, these are understatements. There is no question on the part of anyone fighting AIDS that the FDA constitutes the single most incomprehensible bottleneck in American bureaucratic history—one that is actually prolonging this roll call of death. This has been only further compounded by President Reagan, who has yet to utter publicly the word "AIDS" or put anyone in charge of the fight against it.

As cofounder of Gay Men's Health Crisis, America's first

---

* The Op-Ed page of *The New York Times*, March 23, 1987.

and largest community self-help AIDS organization, I have talked with doctors across the country. Most are reluctant to speak for the record—an act that often jeopardizes their grants from governmental agencies such as the National Institutes of Health, or even further impairs their relationship with the FDA.

But here are some of the things that privately infuriate them:

1. Dr. Frank E. Young, the FDA's commissioner, said that because of new rules and procedures, the FDA might now be able to shave two to three years from the seven to nine years of testing now required before drugs are released for general use. AIDS patients do not have that long to live. In New York City, the grotesque statistics now predict that upwards of two-thirds of all those infected (about a million people in America, according to the Centers for Disease Control) could be dead in less than five years. And it is not just men who are involved. In New York City, Acquired Immune Deficiency Syndrome is now the number-one killer of women between twenty-five and twenty-nine years old, the number-two killer of women between thirty and thirty-four years old, and the number-three killer of women between fifteen and nineteen. Heterosexual women who are not intravenous drug users have the highest rate of increase of any group.

2. Doctors everywhere are waiting to put into immediate use a battery of drugs that have passed Phase One safety trials—that is, drugs that are perceived to have no or few serious side-effects. All of these are considered much less toxic than AZT, which the FDA has now rushed into circulation and which is proving unsatisfactory in many trials, making numerous patients, in the words of one doctor, "transfusion-dependent."

No one can understand why AZT (the brand name is Retrovir) was released Friday, when ribavirin, a less toxic and many think a more promising drug, has not been made available. Food and drug authorities in Britain are preparing to release ribavirin widely.

3. In addition to ribavirin, why is the FDA withholding

Ampligen, Glucan, DTC, DDC, AS 101, MTP-PE, and AL 721? AL 721 is not even a drug but a food—a form of lecithin—that has proved promising at the Weizmann Institute in Israel. Ribavirin, at least, is available at black-market prices in Mexico for those who have the strength and money. None of the other drugs are available anywhere. Doctors wishing to test them have showed me the thick protocols they have submitted to the FDA, only to have them returned again and again with petty requests for the rewriting of one sentence, or the reversal of the order of several sentences, or the elimination of two words.

4. AIDS sufferers, who have nothing to lose, are more than willing to be guinea pigs. If all of the drugs listed here are thought to be less toxic than AZT, and AZT is available (albeit at the unconscionable rate of $10,000 per year per patient), we cannot understand for the life of us, or for what life in us many of us still cling to hungrily, why the FDA withholds them—especially when the victims are so eager to be part of the experimental process.

5. The FDA's continued insistence on double-blind studies (in which some patients receive the drug and others placebos—no one knowing which until the study is over) is incomprehensible.

Double-blind studies were not created with terminal illnesses in mind. It is, again, inhumane to withhold drugs from terminally ill patients willing to take them, Phase One trials having been completed safely. In the past, the FDA has authorized the "compassionate usage" of certain drugs. Why deny the same courtesies today to those with AIDS?

6. Indeed, there is no way the FDA, or anyone else, can set up genuinely "controlled" studies. Such studies require people to certify that they have or have not suffered from certain diseases in the past. But people with AIDS will say and do anything to obtain a drug or join a test. They forge their medical records, and because the FDA bureaucracy is so entrenched, every doctor I know also lies for them.

7. Why is antiviral therapy denied infected people whose immune systems have yet to be destroyed? Why do we withhold treatment and research until people are terminally ill? How many must die before this obvious mistake is corrected?

8. Finally, all of our federal AIDS-monitoring agencies, including the FDA, the National Institutes of Health, and the Centers for Disease Control, perversely refuse to cooperate with each other and with other countries as well, particularly France, whose scientists are making important strides with a fraction of our financial resources.

In its own inimitable and profligate fashion, the United States is hurling hundreds of millions of dollars at AIDS—but in a completely unorganized and unfocused way. A college on Long Island received a half-million-dollar grant to study "AIDS and Student Stress" but NIH-designated AIDS treatment centers are denied promising drugs and in some cases don't even have any patients. This is true at the Institute for Immunological Disorders, the magnificent new hospital in Houston devoted solely to AIDS, which can hold 150 patients but currently houses only eight.

The Institute's director, Dr. Peter W. A. Mansell, is more despondent than ever. His friends have personally raised $250,000 to purchase a supply of Ampligen for him. Dr. Mansell is one of our leading AIDS experts, and has been since the beginning. If he thinks Ampligen is safer than AZT, why can't he be allowed to test Ampligen? If he thinks all of the other treatments I have listed are safer than AZT, why can't he be allowed to use them all immediately? It makes no sense at all.

Our Surgeon General, Dr. C. Everett Koop, a Christian fundamentalist who has turned out to be a man of high honor and integrity, has been quoted as saying he is trying to "embarrass the administration into bringing the resources that are necessary to deal with this epidemic forcefully." He said he has tried to see the President several times—without success.

It's little wonder that the FDA flounders so grotesquely. From the first day of what now has become a national epidemic, the uppermost levels of the federal and New York City governments have chosen not to acknowledge AIDS. And when the histories of the Koch and Reagan administrations are truthfully written, this scandal will dwarf the political corruption in New York and the foreign-policy blunders in Washington. We need humanitarianism from our President and mayor—and heroism from the FDA.

Message Queen

A few years ago, I heard myself being referred to, behind my back: "He's that message queen."

I wrote *The Normal Heart* for one main reason: the world must know about the saddest thing I would ever know. I felt I had an obligation: Because fate had placed me on the front line of this epidemic from the very beginning, I was a witness to much history that other writers were not. That alone would not have forced me to write about it if I wasn't interested in it. But I was and I am, and I doubt I shall be interested in anything else for quite some time. A writer—this writer, anyway—can only write well about what he's interested in.

I don't consider myself an artist. I consider myself a very opinionated man who uses words as fighting tools. I perceive certain wrongs that make me very angry, and somehow I hope that if I string my words together with enough skill, people will hear them and respond. I am under no delusion that this will necessarily be the case, but I seem to have no choice but to try.

I am no longer particularly interested in plays and movies

* Speech given at "Epidemic, Center Stage: A Forum on the Role of Theater in AIDS," sponsored by Gay Men's Health Crisis, April 27, 1987, Washington Irving High School.

and books that are not *about* something meaningful and important. I no longer enjoy going to a movie for entertainment or escape. My mind wanders—why are they doing all those silly, inconsequential acts up there? I don't look down on purveyors of entertainment, indeed I envy them, particularly the ones who make millions of dollars from musicals about roller skaters or movies about outer space or the secret of my success or novels about I'll take Manhattan. But I don't know how much longer I have to live, and I would like to devote what time I have left to trying to contribute something more personally meaningful to this strange, perplexing world, filled with so much horror and so many selfish people.

However, I don't think it is the playwright's or the novelist's or the filmmaker's responsibility to deal in ideas or rhetoric or political meaningfulness. These people can express themselves any way they see fit. No, I hold no Marxist views about the creative responsibility, even though I might seem to live by them. I only know that at this stage of my own life, with death so palpable and continuously close, I only have time, with whatever professional authority my years of living and experience have given me, to be—a message queen.

As I said, I have no choice. I've tried, in the past few years, to write other things: plays and screenplays about non-AIDS matters. But I can't seem to. They seem unimportant. Nothing else seems as important as AIDS—and what gay men are living through.

With the exception of Hitler's Nazi Germany, I have never perceived so much utter wrongdoing in my life. Because of this, I can't understand—and have less tolerance for—why every so-called "artist" in the world is not dealing with the horrors of contemporary life—if not homosexual AIDS, then the AIDS of South Africa, the AIDS of racism and misogyny, the AIDS that is Ronald Reagan and Ed Koch and Phyllis Schlafly and Paul Cameron and Lyndon LaRouche and Jesse Helms and Governor Deukmejian and Representative Dannemeyer and Jerry Falwell and our Supreme Court. You do not have to have AIDS to have acquired a system deficient and immune. If writers everywhere were to write about these horrors, then perhaps there would be no AIDS and I would be free, we would all be free, to think about something else.

But most contemporary art has little relevance to the lives
we lead. Perhaps that is why I'm not interested in calling myself an artist. I just wish that those who do call themselves
artists, or those who traffic in art—the novelists and the paint-
ers and the critics and the professors and the rock groups and
the *New York Review of Books* crowd and the Yale English
Department crowd and all those many, many arts councils and
arts endowments and state councils for the arts and commis-
sioners of cultural affairs and the playwright's festivals and
that annual joke called the Eugene O'Neill Theatre Center and
all the bland dramaturges and committees who choose plays all
over the country for their blind audiences in their bleak
theatres and the crass men and women who run movie studios
and TV networks and national magazines and control the media
and all those self-styled expert judges who give Pulitzers and
Nobels and Guggenheims and Ford Foundations, and Tonys
and Oscars and Obies and Emmys and Grammys—what silly
names they all have!—that somehow all of these who call themselves artists or understanding of art would call themselves
artists less and become message queens more.

Finally, I would like to acknowledge the irony of both the
offering and the acceptance of this invitation from Gay Men's
Health Crisis, this now sturdy and entrenched organization
that I founded some six years ago with five other men. It is an
organization that I am both enormously proud of and enormously ashamed of—if it is possible to feel both so strongly,
and it is. How this organization—which was formed to be our
chief congress of message queens—can continue, day by day,
week by week, month after month, to be more and more sub-
sumed into the very bureaucracy it was founded to fight to
make accountable is a particular galling tragedy to its cofounder. I think it is truly appalling that GMHC has invited Ed
Koch to speak at its Walkathon on May 17th: that this organization and this community can continue day after day and year
after year to kiss the ass of the one person who has done so
little for this epidemic and even less for this organization—
indeed he is the one person in this entire world who is more
responsible than anyone for allowing this epidemic to get so out
of hand—is as criminal as his own acts (which still continue; he
does not change).

I can only pray—no, prayers are useless, as we all know by now, for there is no God anywhere who could allow such as is now transpiring—I can only hope—no, there is precious little of that left either, particularly for gay men, as day by day we in the gay community continue passively to participate in our own genocide—so what is there left? I don't know. I simply don't know. I can only go on writing what I write, if not as an artist, then perhaps as an historian. We simply must not allow whatever future world there might be to forget the acts of the Hitlers among us who try to destroy us. I no longer feel so certain that we will survive, even with this knowledge. If only each one of us could say to himself or herself: If I'm going to go, at least I'm going to go out fighting. Perhaps—perhaps— we just might survive if only each of you could become a message queen too.

The Plague Years

Tonight, the President of all the American people is finally going to make his *first* AIDS speech.

He will address a fund-raising dinner of the American Foundation for AIDS Research. He will speak on the eve of the Third International Conference on AIDS, which is expected to draw six thousand attendees to Washington, twice last year's attendance in Paris.

He will tell us that AIDS is awful and that it's his administration's No. 1 health priority, hollow assertions that have been voiced by somebody or other in his administration since 1983. He may talk about his new advisory commission on AIDS, about "education," and about testing.

But what will really count is how long and how seriously Ronald Reagan addresses the issues of research and treatment—the launching of an all-out federal war to find a cure for this plague. Even if he mentions these subjects, it is perfectly clear to me that no matter what Reagan says tonight, it's not going to alter the sorry journal of these plague years.

As a Reagan AIDS bureaucrat told me recently: "God help

---

* *Newsday* and *New York Newsday,* May 31, 1987.

us with the AIDS epidemic, because the U.S. government won't. Washington, D.C., is not interested in AIDS." The aide spoke in a very low voice—obviously ill at ease. "Why are you so nervous talking about AIDS?" I asked him.

"Are you kidding?" he replied. "If you don't say what they want you to say, you get reassigned to the Indian reservations."

Choose your favorite horror movie:

The World Health Organization estimates that a total of 100 million will test positive for Human Immunodeficiency Virus (the presumed cause of AIDS) in five to ten years. Estimates vary as to how many of the infected will succumb to AIDS, but there's increasing evidence that almost all infected people will fall ill, and the great majority will die.

The federal Department of Health and Human Services says that in three years our annual health-care bill for AIDS will be $16 billion. In a one-year span, full-blown AIDS cases attributed to heterosexuals who aren't intravenous drug users rose from 1 percent of all AIDS cases to 4 percent.

The numbers of AIDS patients hospitalized increased from 10,000 in 1984 to 23,000 in 1985. Fifteen percent of all acute-care hospital beds could be AIDS-occupied in four years (an 800-percent increase over current levels), according to Rodger McFarlane, the head of AIDS Professional Education at the Memorial Sloan-Kettering Cancer Center in Manhattan.

Says Dr. Mathilde Krim, co-chair of the American Foundation for AIDS Research (AmFar): "Everything about this epidemic has been utterly predictable, utterly, utterly and completely predictable, from the very beginning, from the very first day. But no one would listen. There are many people who knew exactly what was happening, what would happen and has happened, but no one of importance would listen. They still won't listen. This is an epidemic that could have been contained. We definitely could have contained it."

But now the AIDS epidemic is seven years old, has killed 20,798 people in the United States alone, is spreading uncontrollably throughout the population—heterosexual as well as homosexual—and will soon bankrupt the American health-care system.

And now Ronald Reagan is finally making a speech about AIDS.

Will he finally explode the myth that most Americans need not fear AIDS?

"A virus does not discriminate. A virus does not know the difference between black and white or straight and gay or male and female," Rodger McFarlane tells each and every class he addresses. "Why doesn't anyone believe that, even now?"

One answer is offered by a congressional aide who deals with health issues: "Never has such a bunch of second-rate people been put in charge of such a first-rate problem."

One of those in charge is Gary Bauer, forty-one, a former Under Secretary of Education, who is now Assistant to the President for Domestic Policy and head of the Office of Policy Development. He has been in his White House office a scant few months and is credited with helping Reagan put on the new makeup that's going to be worn tonight.

Recently, I asked Bauer if there had been a conscious decision to ignore AIDS. "I've never heard of anyone," he answered, "or even seen anybody wink, or even with body language, suggest that—look, if a lot of people die, hey, you know. . . . Now maybe when I'm not around, they let their true emotions hang out. . . ."

I begged Bauer to ask Reagan to consider his place in history, to institute some noble action before it was too late. Bauer's answer was: "I have not seen enough evidence that this is the Black Plague . . . I think only time will tell. . . ."

Why isn't there a forceful, clear-headed administrator in charge of AIDS—of coordinating research into its cause and developing a vaccine against it, and a cure for it, and of educating the public?

"Our belief is that the President is that already, the AIDS czar," is Bauer's answer.

The boss of the several contending government agencies that deal with AIDS is Dr. Otis R. Bowen, the Health and Human Services secretary. His flock includes HHS, the Food and Drug Administration, the Public Health Service, the National Institutes of Health, and the Centers for Disease Control.

It's the CDC that charts the numbers. The CDC's leaps to

conclusions about who was vulnerable to AIDS delayed an attack on AIDS for years. Since the syndrome (it was not yet named AIDS) was first seen in 1980 and first described in the CDC's *Morbidity and Mortality Weekly Report* on June 5th, 1981, the CDC has been the source of continually changing dicta about who is at risk. (First it was gays and Haitians. Now it's everybody.)

I asked Bauer why Reagan hadn't met with Surgeon General C. Everett Koop, the administration figure who is most outspoken about AIDS.

Bauer replied: "I saw a story where Koop was quoted as saying he had not been able to meet with the President. Let me tell you this: Dr. Koop would not normally meet with the President. . . . The fact that Dr. Koop has not met with the President is really not significant, although it's become some sort of symbol of something, I'm not sure what." Koop is a born-again Christian. His insistence that AIDS be dealt with as a medical, not a moral, problem has made him a pariah not only at the White House, but also to his former brethren in Christ who now boycott dinners in his honor.

Reagan has admitted that he hasn't read the forceful AIDS report that he asked Koop to prepare for him and that was published last October, just ahead of the equally discouraging report of the National Academy of Sciences.

It is Bowen who talks to the President about the state of the nation's health. Bowen declined to be interviewed for this essay.

Jim Gottlieb, staff director to Representative Ted Weiss (D.-N.Y.), said of Bowen: "I can't recall anything substantial he has said on AIDS."

The congressional aide I spoke with said Bowen's pet interest is catastrophic health insurance, which would be available only to those over sixty-five or those disabled for more than two years—qualifications AIDS patients don't live long enough to meet. "A messenger can go to the [presidential] well only so often," the aide said. "Bowen has chosen not to carry AIDS."

The next-highest-ranking federal health official is Dr. Robert Windom, the Assistant Secretary of Health. Windom, in office less than a year, had never before worked in Washington, or in government, or directed a large bureaucracy. A successful Sarasota, Florida, internist in private practice, Windom was chairman of the Reagan-Bush 1984 reelection committee in Florida, Georgia, and Alabama. Federal records show that Windom gave about $55,000 to Republican candidates between 1979 and 1984.

Bowen has handed Windom the AIDS crisis. Earlier this month, I asked Windom why more drugs weren't being tested. "We have a task force for that," was his answer. I asked why appropriated AIDS treatment money wasn't being spent. He answered, "We have a committee for that." I asked him about the most talked-about AIDS treatment, AL 721, "I'm not familiar with the details on that," he replied.

Such responses may be why a leading AIDS lobbyist called Windom "just plain dumb." A congressional aide says, "If his IQ were any lower, you'd have to water him." One of his co-workers did describe him as "a warm, affable, back-slapping fellow." Then his colleague sighed, "But he's out of his league."

Next "in command" of AIDS is Dr. Lowell Harmison, who is Windom's Deputy Assistant Secretary for Health and who also declined to be interviewed. One of Harmison's own colleagues explained Harmison's inaction on AIDS thus: "Lowell's philosophical framework is more 'How do we keep the bastards from getting us?' instead of 'How can we maximize our influence?' "

It took the CDC six long years to admit that it was dealing with an equal-opportunity virus. It has taken the FDA the same amount of time to accomplish something positive.

AIDS drugs are to be given "fast-track" attention when it comes to authorizing their use, FDA chief Frank Young announced this month. (It usually takes six to nine years for a drug to be approved.)

Huge drug companies such as Burroughs Wellcome (the owners of the antiviral drug AZT) seem to have an advantage at the FDA. Small, undercapitalized, or inexperienced companies that might be in the possession of potentially first-rate treatments may not get first-rate treatment from the FDA.

An example is Praxis Pharmaceuticals of Los Angeles. Praxis has the world license to produce AL 721, which was developed by the prestigious Weizmann Institute in Israel. It has taken two years for the FDA to take notice of AL 721, which is derived from egg yolks and could just as easily be distributed without FDA approval as a health food.

There's obviously more potential profit for Praxis in waiting to please the FDA; the price of AZT has gone from $8,000 to $14,000 per patient per year in less than four months since FDA approval. Before approval, Burroughs Wellcome had to give the stuff away.

Patients are now so tired of waiting for AL 721 (it's been two years since a favorable mention in the *New England Journal of Medicine*— and supplies in Israel have been mysteriously cut off) that they've had it analyzed, have passed around the recipe from coast to coast, and now whip it up in their own kitchens. A New York group has ordered $200,000 worth of a Japanese knock-off (one kilo, good for about a month, costs $200) and it's now being consumed. Dr. Craig Metroka of St. Luke's-Roosevelt Hospital Center has advised some of his patients to get it wherever they can: NIH trials of AL 721 are at least a year away.

Patients are also learning to duplicate or obtain other drugs that haven't received FDA approval. They include DTC (a French drug), Foscarnet (from Sweden), and ribavirin, on sale legally in more than twenty countries, including Mexico.

There are plenty of other reasons to go drug-shopping. The few drugs that the NIH and FDA have elected to test have either been busts, like Suramin, or, like AZT, have toxic side effects for many.

(Bauer, by the way, didn't seem well acquainted with AZT— which he mistakenly calls "ACT," although it has received more media attention than all other drugs combined.)

It's no wonder that patients have more faith in their own underground information network than in any establishment sources. There is still no official, central, computerized registry of AIDS information. A doctor in Santa Barbara, California, recently lost a patient to cytomegalovirus, one of the many opportunistic infections that afflict AIDS sufferers, according to Dr. Nathaniel Pier, an AIDS specialist. The California doctor could have learned to treat CMV by calling a doctor in New York.

The NIH is currently everybody's least favorite place. *Newsday, The New York Times,* and *The Wall Street Journal* have questioned why some $47 million appropriated a year ago for the testing of AIDS drugs has actually remained unspent, and why nineteen AIDS Treatment Evaluation Units, established with great hoopla almost two years ago, are either not functioning or are greatly under-utilized.

For example, most of the 150 beds at the Institute of Immunological Disorders in Houston, this country's first hospital devoted solely to AIDS, are empty because none of the $47 million has trickled down to Texas. (Additionally, Texas is the only state in the Union that does not reimburse hospitals for taking care of indigent patients. Administrators of the profit-making Houston institute say it's too costly to hospitalize uninsured AIDS patients.)

"The honeymoon with the NIH is over," is how Representative Weiss put it, as his office prepares to instigate through oversight hearings on NIH delays.

The NIH may be in charge of medical research in this country, but it was none too eager to embrace AIDS. One of the first evidences of the deadly syndrome were unusual cancers in otherwise healthy young men. For this reason, the AIDS question was first tossed to Dr. Vincent T. Devita, director of the National Cancer Institute at NIH. (Neither Devita nor his boss, Dr. James Wyngaarden, who is lord of the twelve institutes of the NIH, had time to speak to me.)

In 1981, Devita was in the possession of almost a billion dollars of research money; nevertheless, he decided that the as-yet-unnamed AIDS, which includes such cancers as Kaposi's sarcoma and various lymphomas, really belonged to the National Institute for Allergy and Infectious Diseases (NIAID), which had one-quarter the budget of the Cancer Institute. NIAID's director, then, Dr. Richard Krause, didn't want AIDS either, but Allergies didn't have as much power as Cancer.

Today, major and painful rivalries between the Cancer Institute and NIAID and inside both institutes are hampering the AIDS fight. Two figures at the NCI, Dr. Robert Gallo and Dr. Samuel Broder, have certainly found new meanings in competitiveness. According to one pharmacologist involved, Broder attempted to disparage Gallo's championing of AL 721 (in that

New England Journal report), mainly because Broder, who's in charge of developing new treatments, hadn't noticed it first. This gave rise to the NIH being condemned by the pharmaceutical community for rarely championing anything "Not Invented Here."

It's also said that Broder and Dr. Anthony Fauci aren't on such hot terms either. Fauci is director of NIAID and chief administrator of the nineteen AIDS Treatment Evaluation Units and of AIDS research and testing for the entire country, and no major decision can be made without him. He is being asked to do more than any human is capable of doing, with predictably human results.

He works eighteen-hour days; he must summon committees, preside over meetings, supervise the selection of drugs to test, monitor their results, deal with pharmaceutical companies, keep up on all the latest information (a new drug application can run to 100,000 pages of evidence), attend conferences all over the world, and put up with complaints from absolutely everyone.

Instead of screaming and yelling for help as loudly as he can, he tries to make do, to negotiate quietly.

Only after intense questioning does Fauci quietly admit that he desperately needs "somebody to cut through all the government red tape." But he doesn't want a larger research staff. "I've got no place to put them," he explained.

It is apparently *verboten* for a new lab to be built on the supremely manicured campus of NIH.

It should also be noted that the beds in Fauci's AIDS ward are, save two, empty. A whole floor in America's state-of-the-art hospital, $47 million given him to fund the testing of new treatments, and his beds are empty! Critics charge that Fauci is so in love with AZT, which he administers on an outpatient basis, that he is not interested in testing other drugs.

The battling over who's going to get the credit in the AIDS fight extends to the international arena. French scientists at the Pasteur Institute announced that they had isolated "the AIDS virus" and developed a test to detect it during 1983. A year later, NCI's Gallo claimed the same discovery as his own.

A recent British television documentary questioned the

honesty of Gallo's assertions and research. The Granada TV documentary also said: "The effects of the row are far-reaching. Senior scientists are refusing to talk to one another. Laboratories fear to exchange samples without watertight legal guarantees. The search for a cure has inevitably been set back."

The bitter U.S.-French dispute over "the AIDS virus" discovery was resolved in March with an agreement to share the patents for the AIDS blood test. But the bitter aftertaste lingers on the international scene, and few European scientists will attend this week's NIH-sponsored meetings.

Dr. Don Francis, a CDC scientist who was reassigned from the CDC headquarters in Atlanta, after criticizing Gallo, told Granada TV that the fight "has truly inhibited the progress necessary to combat this really, really dangerous virus that's now all over the world. Now there are two camps that are divided and therefore make the field a relatively unpleasant one to get into—and that keeps some of the best scientists out."

"You have smart men out there," said Dr. Krim, of the American Foundation for AIDS Research, "who know certain things are not working at the NIH; but it's difficult to expect an investigator to bite the hand that feeds him—the NIH."

Outspoken AIDS doctors have a difficult time at institutions beyond NIH, too. Take the case of Dr. Michael Gottlieb, AmFar's co-chair. Gottlieb, who has been working with AIDS since 1980, recently quit a full-time post at UCLA because, he said, he couldn't obtain tenure. The university claims he resigned before a tenure decision was reached.

The quality of NIH research and American research overall can be judged by the recognition that most AIDS breakthroughs have come from abroad: the discovery of "the virus" at the Pasteur Institute in Paris; the discovery of a second (West African) AIDS virus at the Pasteur Institute; the vaccine studies and experiments under way by Dr. Daniel Zagury at the University of Paris; the possible genetic predisposition toward AIDS susceptibility announced in London by Dr. Anthony Pinching; AL 721 from Israel; CSF, a new immune-stimulating drug, controlled by Sandoz, a Swiss company; and, indeed, AZT itself. Although American-discovered, it is now owned by Burroughs Wellcome, a British bunch.

Who is fighting all this American inertia?

Only two elected officials in Washington sounded the alarm early and have been courageous enough not to run away: Representatives Henry Waxman (D.-Calif.) and Ted Weiss. They've been joined by Senator Lowell Weicker (R.-Conn.)

Senators Daniel Patrick Moynihan and Alfonse M. D'Amato, as elected representatives of New York, the state most under siege by AIDS, have betrayed their constituents by the banality of their response. Nor has the occupant of Gracie Mansion been a Profile in Courage. "It is disgraceful that the mayor of New York does not provide sufficient leadership on this issue," says Nathan Kolodner, president of Gay Men's Health Crisis.

Edward I. Koch was so roundly booed at the recent GMHC Walkathon (which raised $1.6 million to help defray costs of services the city should be providing but isn't) that he ripped up his speech and sat glaring out at the audience, facing signs that proclaimed him THE WORST. WOULD YOU TRUST THIS MAN? one of the signs under his picture asked.

The city recently announced that it has drafted, but not implemented, a five-year plan to deal with AIDS by expanded care for those already afflicted, promotion of research, and expansion of education programs and voluntary testing.

This sounds like the plan Koch announced three years ago that never happened.

Reagan will talk tonight about mandatory testing and "education," and there will be much yelling and screaming from opponents and supporters of both.

It is imperative that the American people realize that while all the heat and fury from the religious right and its equally vocal supporters on the political right continue about the naughtiness of condoms and sex education and homosexuality and intravenous drug use, the presumptive virus continues to spread and kill.

Every stalling tactic costs lives.

They *know* this. Anyone who has watched the numbers of dead grow and grow knows this.

The record convinces me that no matter what Reagan says tonight, no substantial battle for a cure will be mounted while he is in office. There's only one word to describe his monumental disdain for the dead and dying: genocide.

In April 1987, the thought occurred to me that I could perhaps best put my writing skills and my knowledge of the AIDS epidemic to optimum use by writing a regular column, "Journal of the Plague Years." I submitted this proposal to Max Frankel at *The New York Times,* Robert Gottlieb at *The New Yorker,* and David Laventhol (an old childhood and college friend), the president of the enormous Times-Mirror newspaper empire. Frankel turned me down, which was to be expected, but Bob Gottlieb and David both were interested in proceeding. While vanity urged me to accept *The New Yorker,* I thought that being syndicated by the huge *Los Angeles Times–Washington Post* network of newspapers, which is what David was offering, presented the best opportunity of reaching a big audience in the fastest way. Hence I accepted their offer, went to Washington to research the article, came back to New York, wrote it, submitted it, had it edited to shreds of its former self—and then became bitterly disillusioned as it was turned down by every single one of the over three hundred papers the *Los Angeles Times–Washington Post* Syndicate telexed it to, *twice*—including David's own flagship, the *L.A. Times* itself.

The unedited version of the article I submitted, with the tone I was hoping to be allowed in print (magnified now a few decibles higher), forms the core of the speech I made in Boston, which is included as the next piece.

Reagan's first AIDS speech was received with boos. There were many of us in that audience who sat there listening, waiting for him to say something, anything, of import. It was not enough of a gesture for us that he was just *there,* for which we'd been told we must be grateful. He did not use the word "gay" or "homosexual" once. He praised heterosexual AIDS service organizations, but he could not say "Gay Men's Health Crisis." He announced that he was in favor of mandatory testing (the first round of booing), particularly for

marriage-license applicants, prisoners, and immigrants
(the second round of booing), and then he finally sat
down (the final cascade of booing). He'd not said one
word about *doing* anything positive. Elizabeth Taylor,
who had introduced him and who, word has it, was instrumental in getting this stupid man to address this
evening sponsored by the organization of which she is
co-chair, was obviously embarrassed and attempted to
make nice. But Reagan's face told it all. He is not accustomed to being booed in public and he was mad. Dr.
Mathilde Krim, AmFar's other co-chair, who had stated
beforehand that she would walk off the stage if Reagan
recommended mandatory testing, stayed put.

When he spoke at the opening ceremonies the next
day of the Third International AIDS Conference at the
Washington Hilton, George Bush was booed even
louder. "It's those gay activists," he was heard to say.
Well, a lot of it certainly was. But a lot of it certainly
wasn't. At last.

I'd no sooner arrived in Washington to begin researching the above article than I received word from
our mutual friend Craig Rowland that Paul Popham had
just died in Sloan-Kettering. And that *The New York
Times* was hedging on writing a special obituary, complete with photograph. I called Max Frankel's office and
found myself yelling and threatening that if this man
was not properly honored I would do everything in my
power to bring down the wrath of the entire gay community on *The New York Times* forever. Many others also
called, and Paul was given a short, obviously grudging,
few inches, with a photograph.

Then I sat down and, as so often happens these days,
tried to cry. There aren't any tears left. Only infinite
sadness. For all our losses. For the tragedy of all our
fights. For lost friends and lost friendships and lost
opportunities. At least I was grateful that Paul and I
had spoken, as friends, twice more in the past few
weeks, from his deathbed. We both apologized for all
the hurts we'd caused each other. His mind wandered in
and out, and the silences were long between his

thoughts. He repeated himself. "Keep fighting." "Keep fighting." "Keep fighting."

And so the man with whom I had spent so many of the early hours and days and months and years of this horrible plague fighting, too often with each other, to make GMHC a reality, was gone.

I Can't Believe You Want to Die

We have little to be proud of this Gay Pride Week.

One by one, we are being picked off by the enemy.

They are killing us.

I don't think you are going to like what I am going to say. It is the last time I am going to say it. I'm making a farewell appearance. I am not overly tired. I am certainly not suffering from burnout. I have a lot of piss and vinegar left in me—too much, in fact. No, I'm not tired.

Not physically tired, at any rate. I am, of course, as are you, very tired of many things. I am tired of what *they* are doing to us. I am tired of what *they* aren't doing for us. I am tired of seeing so many of my friends die—I'm exceptionally tired of that, as I know you are too.

I'm also tired of people coming up to me on the street and saying, "Thank you for what you're doing and saying." They mean it as a compliment, I know. But now I scream back, "Why

* Speech delivered on June 9, 1987, to the Boston Lesbian and Gay Town Meeting, held in Faneuil Hall, to kick off their Gay Pride Weekend. It was reprinted in many of the major gay newspapers across the country.

aren't you doing it and saying it, too?" Why are there so few people out there screaming and yelling? You're dying too!

I'm telling you they are killing us! We are being picked off one by one, and half the men reading this could be dead in five years, and you are all still sitting on your asses like weaklings, and therefore we, the gay community, are not strong enough and our organizations are not strong enough and we are going to die for it!

I have come to the terrible realization that I believe this gay community of ours has a death wish and that we are going to die because we refuse to take responsibility for our own lives.

Yes, most of all, I'm tired of you. I'm tired of the death wish of the gay community. I'm tired of our colluding in our own genocide. I'm tired of you, by your own passivity, actively participating in your own genocide.

How many of you have given a thousand dollars or more at any one time to any gay organization or gay charity? Ten thousand? (For the rich readers: one hundred thousand dollars? A million?)

How many of you have left anything in your wills to anything gay?

How many of you have spent at least one hour a week volunteering for a gay organization? Ten hours?

And if you don't like any of the gay organizations, how many of you have spent how much time to make any of them better? Instead of just bitching them into further weakness? Or helped them raise money to make themselves better?

How many of you have bothered to consider that by helping to raise $80,000 a year, you could fund a lobbyist in Washington to fight for us all year long—to join with a network of other gay lobbyists, paid for by groups in other cities, so that we could have as many lobbyists as General Motors or the National Rifle Association or the National Council of Churches or the American Medical Association, all of whom get what *they* want?

Is it such a big deal to get a group together to raise $80,000 to save your lives? (Did anyone notice that when Paul Popham died, he asked that contributions be made to AIDS Action Council, a lobbying group, and not Gay Men's Health Crisis, which he cofounded, and in whose ability to do anything but look after funerals he had lost confidence and faith?)

How many of you have written consistently or even irregularly to an elected official or testified at an official hearing on the subject of AIDS, or regarding treatment, or official lethargy in this city and state and country?

How many of you really trust the NIH to be capable of coordinating research around a crisis of this scope?

How many of you even know what the NIH is, or how important it is in your life? And that your very own life is in its hands? You didn't know that, did you? That your very own life is in the hands of an agency you don't know anything about.

How many of you believe there is sufficient education to contain what is happening?

How many of you have children? How many of you have spoken to a school board about sex education?

How many of you have had sex with more than one person in the last ten years?

How many of you have protested actively against mandatory testing?

How many of you are willing to face up to the fact that the FDA is fucked up, the NIH is fucked up, the CDC is *very* fucked up—and that, entering the seventh year of what is now a pandemic, the boys and girls running the show at these organizations have been unable to make whatever system they're operating work?

How long are you prepared to wait for these systems to work?

How long are you prepared to wait before our own AIDS organizations provide us with adequate information on available treatments?

How many hours and days are you prepared to spend on the phone attempting, in vain, to find out what is going on where and how it's doing and why your dying friends can't get it immediately?

How many of you believe you have no responsibility to take action on any of these matters?

How many of you need to die or become infected before you feel you can take action on why every single branch of government in charge of AIDS, both local and federal, is dragging its ass?

What's the number of dead friends at which you can decide to stop just sitting quietly like the good little boys and girls we were all brought up to be—and start taking rude, noisy, offensive political action? One? Ten? *One hundred?*

It always amazes me when I tell people they have power, and they answer me, "Power? Me? What power?" How can you be so conservative, dumb, blind? You know what is going on better than anybody, and yet you are silent, you constantly, consistently, and continuously sit on your collective asses and refuse to use your power.

Your voice is your power! Your collective voices! Your group power! Your political power! Your names all strung together on one long list is your power. Your bank accounts are your power, if you weren't all so devastatingly stingy when it comes to funding anything gayer than a Halloween costume. Your bodies are your power, your *living* bodies all strung together in one long line that reaches across this country and could reach to the moon if we only let it.

You know that this country is not responding on a national political level or a local political level, and yet you sit by along with everyone else and watch our men being picked off one by one by one by one by one.

No one is in charge of this pandemic, either in this city or this state or this country! It is as simple as that. And certainly no one who is compassionate and understanding and knowledgeable and efficient is even anywhere near the top of those who are in charge. Almost every person connected with running the AIDS show everywhere is second-rate. I have never come across a bigger assortment of the second-rate in my life. And you have silently and trustingly put your lives in their hands. You—who are first-rate—are silent. And we are going to *die* for that silence.

You know, it's not even a question of government funding anymore. For six long years we fought so hard to get the money. Finally Congress has appropriated masses of money. *Can you believe me when I tell you that it is not being spent?* Two years ago, nineteen official AIDS treatment centers, called

ATEUs (AIDS Treatment Evaluation Units), were set up by the NIH—and they still aren't being utilized beyond a fraction of their humane possibilities and intentions. One year ago the NIH was given $47 million just for testing new AIDS drugs—*and they aren't spending it!* Why didn't we know that? Where have we been for these long two years? Why didn't we know that this precious, precious time—during which how many dear friends of ours died—was being thrown out in the garbage because we didn't get on the phone and inquire politely: "Please, sirs, can you tell me what you're doing with all that nice money Congress gave you last May?" How could we have been so lazy and irresponsible—and *trusting?* We, of all people in this world, should know better, and know how not to trust. Where were our gay leaders? Where were all our AIDS organizations? Where were our people in Washington? Where was I? For I blame myself more than I blame anyone else. God fucking damn it, I trusted too!

When I found out about three months ago that $47 million was actually lying around not being used when I knew personally that at least a dozen drugs and treatments just as promising as AZT and in many cases much less toxic were not being tested and were not legally available to us, I got in my car and drove down to Washington. I wanted to find out what was going on. Like most people, I have no notion of how the system works down there, who reports to whom, which agency is supposed to do what. What I found out sent me into as profound a depression as I have been in since this epidemic started.

My first meeting was at the White House, with the President's Domestic Policy Adviser, Gary Bauer, who advises Ronald Reagan on AIDS. I asked him if ignoring AIDS was intentional. He answered me that he had not seen enough evidence that the Black Plague was going on yet. He was particularly interested to hear from me that the current evidence indicates that the gay male population of the major cities is on its way to becoming totally exposed to the virus. He asked me if I thought female-to-male transmission was as potent as male-to-male. I said the statistics were about the same. He said his advisers told him otherwise. I asked him if gay people who were AIDS experts could be on the President's Commission, and he told me No. I asked him why the President had refused to put anyone in charge—to appoint an AIDS czar? He told me the President *was* the AIDS czar. I asked him why the President had not only not read Surgeon General Koop's AIDS report, or the National Academy of Sciences AIDS report—both of which were then over six months old and both of which beg for immediate, all-out action—but he hadn't even met with Koop personally, his own Surgeon General, and he answered me that the chain of command dictates that, in matters of health, the President talks only to his Secretary of Health and Human Services, Dr. Otis R. Bowen. It turns out that Dr. Koop has absolutely no power; his position is simply that of figurehead. They do not like what he is saying, and I think that if you listen to what he is beginning to say now, you will see that Dr. Koop is being pulled back into line.

Dr. Otis R. Bowen would not see me. He is Reagan's *third* Secretary of Health and Human Services, and he is supposed to be in charge of AIDS. Until he appeared as the closing speaker at the Third International AIDS Conference, where I am happy to say he was roundly booed—were any of *you* there to boo him?—he had not been heard to say anything substantial at all about AIDS. The Secretary of the main department of your government in charge of AIDS—the one single man who can report to the President on the state of this nation's health—had yet to be heard saying anything about AIDS, at the beginning of the seventh year of this pandemic.

I discovered that Dr. Bowen had passed the AIDS buck over to his Assistant Secretary of Health and Human Services, Dr. Robert Windom. Dr. Windom has been in his job all of one year. He's never worked in government before. He was a private physician in Sarasota, Florida, and I figure he got his wonderful opportunity to work so close to his idol, Ronald Reagan, by contributing $55,000 to Republican candidates between 1979 and 1984. He is exceptionally ill-informed about AIDS. On a recent NBC Radio coast-to-coast call-in show, he answered two of his questions incorrectly. My favorite description of Dr. Windom comes from a top legislative congressional aide: "If his IQ were any lower, you'd have to water him."

You laugh—and Dr. Windom is in charge of your life! An uncaring, dumb stooge who knows next to nothing about any of the drugs or treatments or research is in charge of your life, and you are laughing! Over half the men here could be dead in less than five years, and you are laughing at this crack about Dr. Windom!

Dr. Windom reports to Dr. Bowen who reports to the President.

Dr. Windom has passed the AIDS buck to his assistant, Dr. Lowell Harmison. Dr. Harmison is sort of the power behind the power behind the throne. Dr. Harmison does not like gays. Dr. Harmison has been described to me by several congressional contacts as "evil." "You cannot say enough bad things about Lowell Harmison," I was told by more than one. He is so frightened of gay people that he was terrified we would intentionally give blood in order to pollute the nation's blood supply—*on purpose.*

Dr. Harmison reports to Dr. Windom who reports to Dr. Bowen who reports to the President.

Bauer, Bowen, Windom, Harmison. These are the four top men in charge of AIDS in the United States government, the government of all the American people. Your government. God (if there is one) help us—because these four idiots won't.

I am here to tell you that I know more about AIDS than any of these four inhumane men, and that any one of you here who has AIDS or who tends to someone with AIDS, or who reads all the newspapers and watches TV, knows more about AIDS than any of these four monsters. And they are the four fuckers who are in charge of AIDS for your government—the bureaucrats who have the ultimate control over your life.

Next I went to the National Institutes of Health. The National Institutes of Health receives $6.2 billion *each and every year* to look after the health of the American people. "To improve the health of the American people" is how the U.S. Government Manual describes the NIH's mission. How many of you can tell me the name of the head of NIH?

You don't know the name of the man who is given $6.2 billion each and every year to help make you better if you have AIDS? You should be ashamed of yourselves.

His name is Dr. James Wyngaarden, and he has never been heard to speak out publicly about AIDS either. He is given $6.2 *billion* every year, and not only doesn't he speak out about AIDS, but you don't even know his name!

Dr. Wyngaarden reports to Dr. Windom who reports to Dr. Bowen who reports to the President.

The NIH is like a college campus. It looks like Amherst, or like something from an old MGM musical. It's really made up of twelve institutes, which are sort of like dorms, or fraternities, all part of the whole. The grounds are manicured and you can't see any shit on the ground.

Seven years ago, when AIDS was first noticed, and you would have thought NIH would jump on it fast, this is what happened. You would have thought that because there was a cancer involved, called Kaposi's sarcoma, it should have gone to the institute in charge of cancer, the National Cancer Institute of the National Institutes of Health. The National Cancer Institute is the richest fraternity at NIH. In 1981, when AIDS first showed up and should have gone into this rich fraternity, the head of this fraternity didn't want it. So he blackballed it. He had $1 billion of research money "to improve the health of the American people," and the head of NCI didn't want it. Now, how many of you can tell me the name of the head of NCI, then and now?

The man who is in charge of the most important cancer research institute in the entire world—and you don't know his name? You should be ashamed of yourselves.

His name is Dr. Vincent T. Devita. In 1981 he didn't want AIDS, he didn't like the smell of it, and he didn't want to spend any of his institute's $1 billion a year on it, so he too passed the buck.

Dr. Devita reports to Dr. Wyngaarden who reports to Dr. Windom who reports to Dr. Bowen who reports to the President.

Dr. Devita passed the buck to a poor relation, a much smaller institute named the National Institute for Allergy and Infectious Diseases of the National Institutes of Health, which had a budget one-fourth of his and which was not nearly so popular a fraternity to rush and was then run by a man named Dr. Richard Krause, who didn't want AIDS either. He must have smelled the shit about to hit the fan because he quickly resigned as head of NIAID, and he was replaced by—now I am sure you can tell me the name of the man who is now the director of NIAID, the man who reports to Dr. Wyngaarden who reports to Dr. Windom who reports to Dr. Bowen who reports to the President—the single most important name in AIDS today, the name of the man who has probably more effect on your future than anybody else in the world.

How many of you know this man's name?

His name is Dr. Anthony Fauci. He's real cute. He's an Italian from Brooklyn, short, slim, compact; he wears aviator glasses and is a natty dresser, a very energetic and dynamic man. After a recent meeting a bunch of us from New York had with him, during which absolutely nothing was accomplished, he asked me what we thought of the meeting. I told him: "Everyone thought you were real cute." And he blushed to his roots.

You are smiling, and this is the man who has more effect on your future than anyone else, and he is not spending that $47 million—*which was given to him specifically to test AIDS drugs*—and you are smiling!

Everybody likes Dr. Fauci and everybody thinks Dr. Fauci is real cute and every scientific person I spoke to whispers off to the side, "Yes, he's real cute, but he's in way over his head."

Dr. Fauci is an ambitious bureaucrat who is the recipient of all the buck-passing and dumping-on from all of the above. He staggers, without complaint, under his heavy load. No loudmouth Dr. Koop he.

Dr. Fauci, with his devoted staff of several dozen—that's right, folks, no more than a couple dozen doctors and scientists are fighting against AIDS at NIAID; I guess $47 million doesn't buy what it used to—is chief administrator of the nineteen AIDS-designated treatment units around the country, called ATEUs, and of all AIDS research and testing for the entire country, and no major decision can be made without him. He works eighteen-hour days, his wife is an AIDS nurse in his hospital, he must summon committees, preside over meetings, supervise the selection of drugs to test, monitor their results, deal with pharmaceutical companies, keep up on all the latest information, attend conferences all over the world, and put up with complaints from absolutely everyone.

Dr. Fauci, of all the names in this article, is certainly not the enemy. Because he is not, and because I think he does care, I am even more angry at him for what he is not doing—no matter what his excuses, and he has many.

Instead of screaming and yelling for help as loudly as he can, he tries to make do, to make nice, to negotiate quietly, to assuage. An ambitious bureaucrat doesn't make waves. Yes, Dr. Fauci reports to Dr. Wyngaarden who reports to Dr. Windom who reports to Dr. Bowen who reports to the President.

Dr. Fauci has had this $47 million for a year, and worse—the beds in his AIDS wards are empty! A whole floor in America's state-of-the-art hospital, $47 million given him to test new treatments, and his beds are empty, just as the majority of places on the treatment protocols at those nineteen ATEUs around the country are empty.

What the fuck is going on here? Are they actually afraid they might learn something that might save us?

Research at NIH? I have not space to go into the gory details. Let me just say that the research rivalries in and among *all* the institutes at NIH could make a TV series to rival "Dynasty" and "Falcon Crest" in competitiveness, hostility, selfishness, and greed. (Why doesn't the press write about these scandals as they do about all others? Why doesn't the press ever investigate NIH? Is it so holy—like the Vatican?)

Now you know why NIH stands for Not Interested in Homosexuals.

What the fuck is going on here, and what the fuck are you doing about it?

If I use gross language—go ahead, be offended—I don't know how else to reach you, how to reach everybody. I tried starting an organization: I cofounded GMHC, which becomes more timid as it becomes richer day by day. I tried writing a play. I tried writing endless articles in the *Native* and *The New York Times* and *Newsday* and screaming on "Donahue" and at every TV camera put in front of me. I helped start ACT UP, a small bunch of too few very courageous people willing to make rude noises. I don't know what else to do to wake you up!

I will tell you something else to try to wake you up: If AIDS does not spread out widely into the white, non-drug-using, heterosexual population, as it may or may not do, then the white, non-drug-using population is going to hate us even more—for scaring them, for costing them a fucking fortune, for our "lifestyle," which they will say caused this. AIDS will stay a disease of blacks and Hispanics and gays, and it will continue to be ignored, it will be ignored even more.

The straight world is scared now because they're worried it's going to happen to them. What if it doesn't? Think about that for a while. If all this lethargy is going on now, think what will happen then—just as you are coming down with it and facing death.

Who is fighting back in any and all of this? Twenty-four million gay men and lesbians in this country, and who is fighting back? We have a demonstration at the White House and we have three hundred people and we think we're lucky! We get our pictures in all the magazines and newspapers for one or two days and we feel real proud. Sixty thousand Catholics march in Albany. Two hundred fifty thousand Jews march in New York against the treatment of Soviet Jews. One million people march for nuclear disarmament.

What does it take to get you off your fucking asses?

"You want to die, Felix? Die!" That's a line from *The Normal Heart.* In his immense frustration, Ned Weeks yells it at his dying lover. That's how I feel about all of you.

What does it take to make people hate? I hate Ed Koch because he is the one person in this entire world who could have done something in the beginning and didn't and it took us almost two years even to get a meeting with him (we must always remember that, as Dr. Mathilde Krim tell us, "this is an epidemic that could have been contained"), and he has put yet another powerless wimp in place as his Commissioner of Health, and gay men and women in New York still kiss Koch's ass, as gay men and women still think Ronald Reagan is peachy wonderful, and gay people in Massachusetts think that Ted Kennedy is wonderful, and he is in charge of health issues in the Senate and he has been silent and cowardly about AIDS for six long years, and how many dead brothers have to be piled up in a heap in front of your faces before you learn to fight back and scream and yell and demand and take some responsibility for your own lives?

I am telling you they are killing us and we are letting them!

Yes, I am screaming like an hysteric. I know that. I look and sound like an asshole. I told you this was going to be my last tirade and I am going to go out screaming so fucking rudely that you will hear this coarse, crude voice of mine in your nightmares. You are going to die and you are going to die very, very soon unless you get up off your fucking tushies and fight back!

Unless you do—you will forgive me—you deserve to die.

I never thought I would come to say anything like that. Nobody *deserves* to die.

I recently spoke at a *Village Voice* AIDS Forum in New York on a panel with Dr. Ron Grossman, who has one of the largest gay practices in New York. "Larry," he said to me, "our most outrageous early pronouncements are short of the mark. And so have been our efforts. We are so *behind.*"

AIDS is our holocaust. Tens of thousands of our precious men are dying. Soon it will be hundreds of thousands. AIDS is our holocaust and Reagan is our Hitler. New York City is our Auschwitz.

"Holocaust" is another word for "genocide."

"Genocide" is a word I hear myself and others using more and more frequently. You don't hear it as much as you hear words like "mandatory testing" or "no sex education in the schools" or "no condom ads on TV."

Why doesn't everybody realize that all the screaming and yelling going on about "education" and "mandatory testing" is one whale of a red herring?

Why doesn't everyone realize that while all the hatred and fury from the right wing, from the fundamentalists, Mormons, Southern Baptists, born-agains, Charismatics, Orthodox Jews, Hasidic Jews, Phyllis Schlafly, Paul Cameron, Governor Deukmejian, Representative Dannemeyer, Jesse Helms, Jerry Falwell—and all their equally as vocal supporters—goes on, that while they are screaming and yelling about the naughtiness of condoms and sex education and homosexuality, the killing culprit virus continues to spread and spread and spread and kill and kill and kill. While Rome burns, the Falwells fiddle, fanning their fundamentalists into fury against the faggots—and the junkies and the niggers and the spics and the whores and . . .

And they *know* it!

It is perfectly clear to me—no matter what Ronald Reagan and his henchmen say—that no substantial battle for a cure will be mounted while he is in office and that we must endure, at the least, another eighteen months of untended, *intended* death.

Very consciously they *know* that the more noise they can make, the more stalling tactics they can put into action, with the aid of their President, who supports them, and with the aid of his staff and his Cabinet and his Vice-President and his Attorney General and his Justice Department and his Supreme Court and his Secretary of Education and his various Secretaries and Assistant Secretaries of Health and Human Services and his director of the National Institutes of Health and his Centers for Disease Control—the more gays and blacks and Hispanics will die.

They *know* this! I believe it is a conscious act.

And we are allowing it!

We have fallen into their trap!

Our leaders—such as they are—their energies are consumed fighting these battles against mandatory testing and for better education—and no one is fighting the NIH for drugs and increased protocol testing and faster research. I am telling you that there are drugs and treatments out there that can prolong the quality of our lives and you are not getting them and no one is fighting for them and these drugs and treatments are caught up in so much red tape that they are strangled in the pipeline and the Reagan administration knows this, knows all this, and does nothing about untangling the red tape and half the gay men here can die because of it.

Yes, by our own passivity we are actively colluding with, and participating in, our own genocide.

We are allowing ourselves to be knocked off one by one. Half the gay men here could be dead in five years.

Our gay organizations are weak and *still* don't work with each other and our AIDS organizations have *all* been co-opted by the very systems they were formed to make accountable and you all sit by and allow it to happen when it's your lives that are going down the tubes.

Politicians understand only one thing: PRESSURE. You don't apply it—you don't get anything. Simple as that.

And it must be applied day by week by month by year. You simply can't let up for one single second. Or you don't get anything. Which is what is happening to us.

For six years I have been trying to get the gay world angry enough to exert this pressure. I have failed and I am ashamed of my failure. I blame myself—somehow I wasn't convincing enough or clever enough or cute enough to break through your denial or self-pity or death wish or self-destruction or whatever the fuck is going on. I'm very tired of trying to make you hear me.

I'm shutting up and going away. The vast majority of the gay world will not listen to what is so simple and plain. That there are so few voices as strident as mine around this country is our tragedy. That there is not one single gay leader who has any national recognition like Gloria Steinem or Cardinal O'Connor or Jerry Falwell or Jesse Jackson is also our tragedy. Why is that? Why does every gay spokesperson finally just collapse under the apathy of trying to make you listen—and failing, failing utterly.

Don't you ask yourselves quite often the Big Question: Why am I still alive? Untouched? At some point I did something the others did. How have I escaped?

Don't you think that obligates you to repay God or fate or whomever or whatever, if only your conscience, for this miraculous fact: I am still alive. I must put back something into this world for my own life, which is worth a tremendous amount. By not putting back, you are saying that your lives are worth shit, and that we deserve to die, and that the deaths of all our friends and lovers have amounted to nothing.

I can't believe that in your heart of hearts you feel this way. I can't believe you want to die.

Do you?

I guess this is the angriest speech I have ever delivered. I was pretty fed up and tired. Boston was an unlikely city to deliver it—they're a quiet, polite bunch up there, and the local gay papers had never been very kind to me. But this group kept calling me up, offering me a thousand bucks (I'd never been paid to speak before), and I decided I was going to diva-out and make my farewell appearance. And what better place than historic Faneuil Hall?

And for a while, I really meant it. Even though, much to my surprise, because as I'd harangued them they'd sat there stone-faced, I received a standing ovation; even though, much to my surprise, I got letters from as far away as France and places like Utah and Nevada, from strangers begging me not to quit. I'd had it.

I don't know why I can't confess to burnout when it happens to me, but I can't. I told everyone that I was quitting activism. I'd devote my energy to writing my plays and trying to get them on and writing another novel and trying again to get *The Normal Heart* made into a movie. You'll see, you'll see, I said. Larry's never going to make another speech again.

None of my friends believed me.

Whose Constitution Is It, Anyway?

I never knew what it felt like to be a nigger or a spic. Now I know. I'm a fag. Fags and niggers and spics aren't protected by the Constitution. Nor are junkies, whores, and broads.

Discrimination—consciously allowing some people to be treated as inferiors—is on the verge of totally bankrupting this country: financially, creatively, and morally.

This is not a good time in history to be a gay man or a lesbian, but particularly a gay man. I don't know if there ever was a completely good time to be gay, but for a little while there we were making some headway toward equality and acceptance. Until Ronald Reagan and AIDS came along, unfortunately at the same time.

I know you're celebrating the Constitution today. I don't feel very much like celebrating. The Constitution, as it is being administered today, doesn't protect me in the ways I need protection. In fact, I'm ashamed to be an American today— ashamed of how this precious document is being hypocritically

---

* Remarks made to a symposium sponsored by the New York Civil Liberties Union on Thursday, September 7, 1987, to celebrate the two-hundredth anniversary of the United States Constitution.

177

misread and misapplied to suit those who would wish me and all like me dead. I personally think that conscious genocide is going on. This administration's determination—which has persisted for a very long seven years—not to do anything sufficient to fight the AIDS epidemic can only be construed as an attempt to see that minority populations they do not favor will die. Seven years, 25,000 dead, over 50,000 cases, a quarter-million predicted in a few years' time, soon after that to be a million— and still there is no one in charge of combating AIDS, and still this city and this country do not provide adequate essential services, and still this government will not release the many life-saving drugs available in other countries, or educate the public so that a poor Florida family is not burned out of everything they have in this world.

I am going to tell you something you've never heard before. I am going to tell you that the AIDS pandemic is the fault of the white, middle-class, male majority. AIDS is here because the straight world would not grant equal rights to gay people. If we had been allowed to get married, to have legal rights, there would be no AIDS cannonballing through America.

The concept of making a virtue out of sexual freedom, i.e., promiscuity, to use that loaded word, came about because gay men had nothing to call their own *but* their sexuality. The heterosexual majority has for centuries denied us every possible right of human dignity that the Constitution was framed to provide to all. The right to marry. The right to own property jointly without fear that the law will disinherit the surviving partner. The right to hold a job as an openly gay person. The right to have children. The right not to be discriminated against in just about every area and avenue and byway and nook and cranny that can be found in which hatred is stored. Indeed—the right to walk down the street holding hands, as you do when you are freely in love. Yes, the right to love. We are denied the right to love. Can you imagine being denied the right to love?

So, rightly or wrongly—wrongly as it turned out—we decided we would make a virtue of the only thing you didn't have control over: our sexuality. Had we possessed these rights you denied us, had we been allowed to live respectably in a community as equals, there would never have been an AIDS. Had we been allowed to marry, we would not have felt the obligation to be promiscuous.

The poor, black, and Hispanic have also been forced into AIDS by your oppression. The awfulness of their destitution and deprivation, the absolutely zero chance they face to better their status in the world, forces them to seek peaceful respite and brief relief in the only oblivion available to them—the never-never land of drugs—which drugs, I might add, this country, for all the "Just Say No" mentality of an imbecilic First Lady, makes remarkably available through inept law enforcement and just plain looking the other way.

AIDS, having thus been caused to seed and sprout, is allowed to grow and fester and increase a millionfold. Yes, indeed, the white man made AIDS—the heterosexual white man. The heterosexual white man with money. The greedy heterosexual white man with money, who, two thousand years into the so-called Christian era, is still boss and master.

I am not going to speak in legalese, or cite the wretched decisions of the Supreme Court against us, or quote you lines from the Constitution or its Fourteenth Amendment or from the Bill of Rights. I am only going to say that some 25 million people constitute a sizable minority who are entitled to the same rights as everyone else. We do not practice behavior that can be changed, despite what that horrible monster, Robert Bork, or that equally horrible monster, the dogma of the Catholic Church, maintains as one reason for denying us these rights—that homosexuality can be changed. For decades, the psychiatric couches of the world sagged under the weight of gay people trying to change. At last, enlightened knowledge is finally beginning to concede the battle. We are born just as heterosexuals are born, just as people with blue eyes or people who are left-handed are born. Twenty-five million people cannot all be the result of any neurotic maladjustment or anything mothers or fathers do or don't do. Twenty-five million people are too many, too high a figure, to be anything but born, just as everyone else is born.

For our institutions—the Church, the Pope, the State, the Supreme Court—to pretend otherwise is, quite simply, immoral. How dare they presume to speak for God and for

Everyman? Because of these immoral institutions and their immoral pronouncements, we have been estranged from our families, and we have been forced to create a ghetto. We have been forced to suffer. We were forced into AIDS.

Would that 25 million people were not so frightened and not so invisible and had more courage to say out loud, all and at once: We are equal, whether you like it or not.

But we are frightened of you, with good reason, because of what you have done to us and continue to do to us, which is yet another tragedy, this fear of ours. I do not think the Constitution had fear, as well as enforced suffering, in mind as a prerequisite for minorities living under it. But so it has turned out.

I have learned, during these past seven years, to hate. I hate everyone who is higher in the pecking order and in being so placed, like some incontinent pigeon, shits all over all of those below. And, sadly, tragically, as more and more of my friends die—the number is way over two hundred by now—I hate this country I once loved so much. And as each day Ronald Reagan and the Catholic Church and various self-styled spokespeople for God—the Right Wing, the Moral Majority, fundamentalists, Mormons, Southern Baptists, born-agains, Orthodox Jews, Hasidic Jews, La Rouchies, Jesse Helms, Representative Dannemeyer, Governor Deukmejian, Phyllis Schlafly, Jerry Falwell, enemies all—take the law into their own hands, a law that neither the framers of the Constitution nor Christ himself, if indeed there ever was a Christ, ever envisioned would be so used to cause the deaths of fellow men, I not only hate, but I know there will never be freedom, or peace on earth, or America the Beautiful, or Oh, Beautiful for Spacious Skies.

Oh, say, can you see? our national anthem asks. Yes, I can see. I see a country more and more divided by hate. I see a country where the rich ignore the poor. I see a country where selfishness exceeds all other character traits. I see a country where education is no longer valued as the necessary force to give us strength and knowledge and compassion. I see a country where the media is controlled by and prepared for the privileged. I see a country where those less privileged have a voice that diminishes day by day until our cries are only heard as whispers. I see a country—and, I might add, a city—where crime and corruption and political chicanery and thefts of every conceivable sort are such a daily occurrence that we no longer protest and can no longer imagine a world otherwise. I see a country that the framers of the Constitution would be ashamed of. I know I am.

My country 'tis of thee? Oh, beautiful for spacious skies? God bless America? Oh, say, can you see by the dawn's early light? Our hymns have all turned into horseshit.

So go ahead and celebrate the anniversary of this once-precious document. I cannot do so.

The audience for this symposium appeared to be composed mostly of elderly men and women, with nothing else to do, who filled their days attending activities like this one, costing nothing. The first time the word "gay" was mentioned, a number of them got up and walked out. While I spoke, I saw only stony faces and icy stares. When I finished the applause was scattered. When questions were asked for, a handsome and well-dressed elderly woman stood up and told me, with a huge, positive smile, and a forceful, positive tone in her voice, that I must not talk about black people the way I had done, that it was possible for all people with the right attitude to improve their lot and better their lives, that she had seen, during her lifetime, the huge amount of progress in the black community, and that she thanked the Lord God for this and knew that He would carry on doing such a Fine Job for black people everywhere, everyone, every day.

Before the President's Commission

I'm a cofounder of Gay Men's Health Crisis, this country's first and largest community self-help AIDS organization, and founder of ACT UP—the AIDS Coalition To Unleash Power, a gay and straight group that's picketed, among others, the White House, *The Saturday Evening Post,* St. Patrick's Cathedral, and is at this moment picketing outside this meeting itself.

The fastest way this horrible epidemic can be stopped is to find a cure. Dr. Burton Lee, of your Commission, has been quoted as saying that you will not concern yourself with the basic science of AIDS. But the field of AIDS research is a huge mess. It's strangled in bureaucratic red tape, inefficiency, and a lack of cooperation among people, agencies, and countries.

We fought so hard for money. Congress has finally appropriated money. Now we find this money is either not being spent at all—hard as that may be to believe—or is being spent foolishly. The system set up by Dr. Anthony Fauci of NIH, of designated hospitals called ATEUs—AIDS Treatment Evaluation Units—is still, *after two years,* not functioning tolerably.

* Testimony before Hearings of the Presidential AIDS Commission, Washington, D.C., September 9, 1987.

Money for testing twelve thousand patients with promising drugs has been available for over a year. As of July, less than one thousand of these slots were filled. AZT—already approved by the FDA and effective for only half of those taking it—is still the main drug being tested. Other promising treatments are ignored. Dr. Fauci—who's been described by many AIDS experts as "in way over his head"—takes up to two years to make decisions that an organization like the American Foundation for AIDS Research can make in three months. The situation at NIH is now so bad that some drug companies and hospitals would prefer not to work with them at all. Couldn't some system be devised by which more *direct* funding is available, bypassing the NIH quagmire? Why must NIH get *all* the money? We in New York think we've found such a way. We've set up our own Community Research Initiative, with its own Institutional Review Board. The manufacturers of Ampligen—tired of waiting for NIH—are so excited about our CRI they're preparing a $4-million protocol. We'll provide two hundred patients—they'll provide this most promising drug, personnel, and money.

From the very beginning, we in the gay community have begged to do such as this. Let us help! Let us be your guinea pigs. You must remember that time is not on our side. Rules and laws that were formulated for slower fatal illnesses, or accidents such as those from thalidomide, simply don't apply with AIDS when patients have only two years to live, and something infectious is going around.

Our desperate circumstances often make us better informed than most doctors. Our grapevine often tells us about effective new treatments first. We pass this information to NIH and we're ignored. Anecdotal evidence is dismissed with holier-than-thou hauteur. AL 721 remains largely untested, even after a glowing report two years ago in the *New England Journal of Medicine,* as does Colony Stimulating Factors, which received similar praise. We've now learned, by sheer accident, that antabuse—the harmless medication given to help alcoholics—has an ability to raise T-cells. Antabuse, it turns out, is made up of the same molecules as Imuthiol. We've been begging for the testing of Imuthiol for a year. Why is there no mechanism available to *immediately* begin pilot studies with harmless antabuse? Must we wait two years while Dr. Meyers at NIH develops her protocols and Dr. Fauci's drug-selection committee has meeting after meeting, only to arrive—as they often do because they are so big and unwieldy and so timid—at no conclusion.

The FDA is a *passive* organization; you must go to them and prove everything *to* them. But often valuable drugs are controlled by inexperienced, poor, or inept companies that don't know how to maneuver the treacherous FDA waters. Why is there no mechanism in place to *actively* help these companies?

Now we face the growing difficulty of finding and keeping experienced personnel. The head of New York's Mt. Sinai ATEU gave as his excuse for his abysmal record that he couldn't find doctors or nurses willing to work on AIDS. NYU can't find data-base *computer operators* who aren't frightened. Soon we're going to find that not only is all the money there, the drugs and patients ready—but there's no staff to administer.

Indeed, the best scientists and researchers seem to be too scared to come anywhere near AIDS at all. Thus we're at the mercy of Drs. Broder and Gallo of NIH, who use their positions of power to intimidate. Indeed, Gallo is known at NIH as "the Godfather."

We implore you to investigate these areas. The epidemic will be in its *eighth* year by the time you report. Yet another precious year lost! The federal government's own General Accounting Office has proclaimed that there is a "perceived lack of leadership which is preventing a quick response."

You begin with many strikes against you in the eyes of the world. Much has appeared in the media about your credibility— and the fact that a *majority* of your membership is *on record* as saying something offensive about gay people. Right now, we don't expect you to either accomplish much or put aside your personal prejudices. Quite frankly, we think many of you would as soon see us dead.

But sometimes the challenge makes the man or woman. There are many instances in history where the most unlikely heroes have emerged and triumphed over their perceived images. We pray this will be one of those rare and precious and God-inspired occasions.

In closing, I would like to remind you of a few gay people who are a part of your history, too. Leonardo da Vinci, who painted *The Last Supper.* Michelangelo, who painted the Sistine Chapel and sculpted the most beloved *Pietà.* King James I, who undertook the most famous translation of the Bible. St. Augustine. Cardinal Newman. Cardinal Spellman. Pope Julius II. Pope Paul VI. Pope Benedict IX. Pope Sixtus IV. Pope John XXII. Pope Alexander VI. Pope Julius III. Joan of Arc.

Thank you.

I delivered this list while staring Cardinal O'Connor right in the eye.

Oh, My People

In reading over my collected diatribes of the past years, I realized I still am unable to resolve this fundamental problem—how to inspire you without punishing you.

We must live with facts that become more horrible with every passing minute. And no sooner do we fight one engagement than another one pops up in yet a completely different theatre of war. And we are losing to AIDS, at a rate that accelerates with every single minute.

I know we are all so tired of mourning. Because, as Mart Crowley said in *Boys in the Band,* "it takes a fairy to make something pretty"—we have managed to turn mourning into some kind of art form. I simply cannot attend another funeral or memorial service, although I know I shall. I often think I don't have any tears left.

I turned on the TV last night, and there, on "ABC World News Tonight," the Person of the Week was our own Cleve

---

* Acceptance speech delivered upon receiving the Arts and Communication Award at the Sixth Annual Human Rights Campaign Fund Dinner, Grand Ballroom, Waldorf Astoria, October 17, 1987.

Jones and there was that quilt—*that quilt!*—and I started crying again. And I couldn't stop crying.

I pray so much that our magnificent March on Washington is a mandate for us all. I pray it's a beginning, and not a last dying gasp, because we're so exhausted. Will every man and woman who danced down the middle of Pennsylvania Avenue return home to reinforce that energy and commitment in their lives and to their friends and families and jobs? Or was it, for them, just a dance down the middle of the road?

But what happened in Washington was, as Nelson Mandela would say, just another link in a long, long struggle.

They didn't give us very much time to feel good. This past week, after our return, came the Jesse Helms hate bill. Ninety-four senators voted *for* that bill. With the exception of Senators Weicker and, surprisingly, Moynihan, every single friend we thought we had suddenly turned against us. Then came the Dannemeyer hate bill. It's almost as if we're being immediately punished for our March. Slap them down quickly before they get too uppity. Even though the stingy media coverage robbed us, once again, of the accurate report of our true numbers, Washington saw that 650,000 of us were there, and now they're going to show us how powerful they are.

I'm afraid.

I've never said that out loud to you before. I think the torrents of hate are really just beginning. I don't think we've begun to see the horrors of what they're going to do to us. And we're crying "Genocide" now.

Oh, my people, I beg you to hear me. We are woefully unprepared:

We still have no leaders with national recognition.

We still have not learned how to broker our power.

We still don't know how to deliver votes in blocks to politicians.

We still have no national publication that is worthy of respect.

We still have no national organizations that are strong.

We have many small organizations that don't cooperate, many duplicating the same efforts and budgets and responsibilities and fighting for the same turf. We have too many Boards

of Directors and Task Forces and Defense Funds and Advocates and Action Councils and AIDS Networks and Coalitions
and Alliances for this and that. Each fights for the same dollars
and, hence, none of them receives enough to be truly effective.
The AMA has over 100 lobbyists. The tobacco industry has over
250. Twenty-five million gay people have—five.

The time has come when we must consolidate. We need one
or two powerhouse organizations, as blacks and women and
Jews have learned. Numbers, numbers, numbers, that's what
scares them, numbers, and we have to ram our numbers down
their fucking throats!

In my writing, I make a lot of comparisons between gays
now and the Jewish community before the war. The Jews
thought of themselves as good Germans first and good Jews
second. When the horror started, they couldn't believe what
their own fellow Germans were doing to them.

After the war, the Jewish leaders, those who were still alive,
came together in one room and determined that what had happened must never happen again. They vowed they would speak
with only one voice, and they would keep their arguments in the
confines of that one room, and the world would never see their
divisiveness in public again. And they've pretty much operated
successfully in that fashion ever since.

Somehow we've got to sit down in one room. From across
the nation, we've got to summon our boards of directors and
our executive directors and our rich and powerful. Our prominent professionals. Our well-connected. Our closeted presidents
of corporations and banks and the partners in law and accounting firms. In this room alone tonight is an assortment of talent,
brains, and money that should be enough to move mountains.

We are prioritizing our battles in the wrong order. There is
only one thing that is going to save us. The battle is, first and
foremost, for a cure. And we're not fighting this battle.

Definitive studies in San Francisco now prove beyond any
doubt that after six and a half years, 76 percent of those with
the virus will definitely come down with ARC or AIDS if they
have no treatment at all. This percentage gradually increases
in the following years to almost 100 percent. Even if my current
candidate for Public Enemy Number One, Dr. Anthony Fauci

of NIH, were to be on top of the situation today, 76 percent of those with the virus would still come down with ARC or AIDS.

We all now know there are many potentially life-saving drugs, almost all of which are available somewhere else in the world, that are simply not being tested here with speed and urgency, and there is not one single humanitarian reason why they aren't available to us. We all know the system of treatment centers that Fauci has set up isn't working. We know he's been given $141,349,398 to use for testing promising new drugs and that he's had this money for two years and five months and *still* he isn't spending it or testing anything much beyond AZT, which half of all AIDS patients cannot tolerate. So half of all AIDS patients are being told to just lie down and die. And AZT only works for about eighteen months. I've seen the list of all NIH protocols planned for the next five years. Eighty-seven percent of these are still for AZT. Not one of the drugs we've been begging for for three years is on this list. Until these are tested, how dare NIH tell us what won't work! We know the NIH receives $8.2 billion each and every year.

We are being murdered.

Oh, my people, why don't you hear me when I use this word "murdered?" Why don't you believe me when I tell you that Dr. Fauci and his boss, Dr. Wyngaarden, and our President, Ronald Reagan, and our mayor, Edward I. Koch—all megalomaniacs playing God—are murdering us?

When even one of our enemies, Cardinal O'Connor, starts talking about the need for a Manhattan Project to deal with AIDS—as he did on Thursday—is this not impetus enough at last for our leaders to meet in one room and consolidate our power toward demanding the very same and mobilizing all our energies to bringing such a Manhattan Project about?

I want to tell you about the Community Research Initiative: CRI. This is an offshoot of the PWA Coalition that is desperately seeking endowment. Its intention is to test drugs directly on patients in our own community, bypassing all government red tape. Results would be faster, cheaper, and we'd know very quickly if these drugs were working. Easily half of all gay men in San Francisco and New York are now infected with the virus. We are told *half of all gay men in San Francisco and New*

York are now infected with the virus! We are walking time
bombs. We have guns to our heads. Seventy-six percent of
those of us infected will come down with ARC or AIDS if we
receive no treatment at all. Latest CDC figures are worse than
ever: 95 to 98 percent of patients die within three years. We
simply can't wait for Dr. Fauci or Ronald Reagan or Edward
Koch. We can't wait for HRA and HHS and FDA and CDC and
PHS and NIH, the alphabet soup that is our government. Ron-
nie is senile and Nancy now is sick and cabinet members and
top officials are now resigning in droves and we face fifteen
more months of a sinking ship and we can't sink with it, we
must act! A number of prominent New York doctors are connected with CRI: Dr. Donald Armstrong of Sloan-Kettering,
Dr. Joseph Sonnabend, and our devoted friend and ally, Dr.
Mathilde Krim. We must fund CRI and put it into operation as
swiftly as is humanly possible. I beg you to be generous to it.
We must, repeat, *must* make the CRI work. Tom Hannan and
Michael Callen are here tonight, should any of you want to give
them checks or ask questions. Tom and Michael—stand up so
we can see two men of courage and vision.

I find it upsetting that the American Foundation for AIDS
Research, which CRI begged for funds, refused them, despite
appeals from Dr. Krim. Quite frankly, the less the wonderful
Dr. Krim is allowed to speak for AmFar, the less I like AmFar.
Slowly, she appears to be becoming a victim of and silenced by
a board of directors composed of many NIH monsters, or doctors funded by NIH monsters, so that AmFar, which is now
receiving millions and millions of dollars in charitable contributions, is unable to pressure the very NIH, which is not doing the
job it should be doing in the first place. Oh, the nooses tighten
and strangle us all to death.

I am ashamed of AmFar, as I now begin, once again, to
become proud of GMHC. Under Nathan Kolodner, GMHC is
moving forward in directions so many of us have begged it to
take for so long. But GMHC cannot take care of the world,
which is what it is being asked to do.

With pride, I close by acknowledging ACT UP. The AIDS
Coalition to Unleash Power—now almost one thousand very
energetic men and women who glory in nothing more than
protesting in the streets. I cannot tell you how infinitely moving

this organization is—this new generation that has no political agenda other than fighting against AIDS—many of them young men who never knew gay life free from fear, a life that I and many of you were, oh, so privileged to know. Their commitment is astounding. They have picketed and yelled and screamed and been arrested on some dozens of occasions—outside the White House, before the President's AIDS Commission, they totally destroyed Pat Robertson's presidential launch—and we will protest this coming Monday at twelve-thirty at City Hall at an AIDS Conference of Mayors and on Tuesday from three to seven at the United Nations, at their emergency plenary session on AIDS. I beg all of you to come and join us at both of these and at our Monday-night meetings at seven-thirty at the Community Center.

In a desperate struggle to secure their new homeland, the Jewish people in Palestine fighting to establish Israel had an organization called the Irgun. It was an underground guerrilla army, and its members were extremely disciplined and daring. They started fires. They threw bombs. They kidnapped. They assassinated. They executed their enemies. They won. Dr. Mathilde Krim belonged to the Irgun. So did Dr. Ruth.

We are such passive people, we gay people. We take all the shit they lay on us and then we lie down and take some more. And then we lie down some more and take even more. And more and more and more and more and more.

Oh, my people, I beg you to listen to me. I say all of this because I love you and I don't want to leave you or lose you.

And I thank the Human Rights Campaign Fund very much for my Arts and Communication award.

The award was presented to me by Nathan Kolodner, the president of GMHC. It was his idea to do so. It was the first time in four years that a public gesture of reconciliation was made by GMHC, and we hugged each other.

I was able, at the beginning of my remarks, to acknowledge my brother and sister-in-law, Arthur and Alice Kramer, Joseph Papp and his wife, Gail Merrifield, and Dr. Lawrence Mass, the only cofounder of GMHC still living, along with me, in America (Ed White is in Paris; Paul and Paul and Nathan are dead)—all of whom were in the audience. I was particularly happy to make Larry stand up and hear the huge applause for him; he is one of the true heroes of these years of horror; his impeccable medical reporting during those first years was the only information most of us had, and he has not been remembered for it or honored for it nearly sufficiently.

A wise friend urged me not to be so over-rhetorical in my choice of "Oh, My People" for my running refrain. I guess it looks corny in print, but it sounded good in the Waldorf. If it does seem too much (Wise Friend had recommended "Oh, My Friends")—well, it won't be the first time I've erred in that direction. Anyway, I like it.

An Open Letter to Dr. Anthony Fauci

I have been screaming at the National Institutes of Health since I first visited your Animal House of Horrors in 1984. I called you monsters then and I called you idiots in my play *The Normal Heart* and now I call you murderers.

You are responsible for supervising all government-funded AIDS-treatment research programs. In the name of right, you make decisions that cost the lives of others. I call the decisions you are making acts of murder.

At hearings on April 29th before Representative Ted Weiss (D.-N.Y.) and his House Subcommittee on Human Resources, after almost eight years of the worst epidemic in modern history, perhaps to be the worst in all history, you were pummeled into admitting publicly what some have been claiming since you took over some three years ago.

You have admitted that you are an incompetent idiot.

Over the past four years, $374 million has been allocated for AIDS treatment research. You were in charge of spending much of that money.

It doesn't take a genius to set up a nationwide network of

---

* *Village Voice*, May 31, 1988, and *San Francisco Examiner*, June 26, 1988.

193

testing sites, commence a small number of moderately sized treatment efficacy tests on a population desperate to participate in them, import any and all interesting drugs (now numbering approximately two hundred) from around the world for inclusion in these tests at these sites, and swiftly get into circulation anything that *remotely* passes muster. Yet, after three years, you have established only a system of waste, chaos, and uselessness.

It doesn't take a genius to announce that you have elected to personally supervise the study of a broad range of new drugs. Yet, two years later, you are forced to admit you've barely begun.

It doesn't take a genius to request, as you did, 126 new staff persons, receive only eleven, *and then keep your mouth shut about it.*

It takes an incompetent idiot!

To quote Representative Henry Waxman (D.-Calif.) at the above hearings: "Dr. Fauci, your own drug selection committee has named twenty-four drugs as high priority for development and trials. As best I can tell, eleven of these twenty-four are not in trials yet. Six of these drugs have been waiting for six months to more than a year. Why the delays? I understand the need to do what you call 'setting priorities' but it appears even with your own scientists' choices, the trials are not going on."

Your defense? "There are just confounding delays that no one can help. . . . We are responsible as investigators to make sure that in our zeal to go quickly, we do the clinical study correctly, that it's planned correctly and executed correctly, rather than just having the drug distributed. . . ."

Now you come bawling to Congress that you don't have enough staff, office space, lab space, secretaries, computer operators, lab technicians, file clerks, janitors, toilet paper; and that's why the drugs aren't being tested and the network of treatment centers isn't working and the drug protocols aren't in place. You expect us to buy this bullshit and feel sorry for you? YOU FUCKING SON OF A BITCH OF A DUMB IDIOT, YOU HAVE HAD $374 MILLION AND YOU EXPECT US TO BUY THIS GARBAGE BAG OF EXCUSES!

The gay community has been on your ass for three years.

For thirty-six agonizing months, you refused to go public with what was happening (correction: *not* happening), and because you wouldn't speak up until you were asked pointedly and under oath by a congressional committee, we lie down and die and our bodies pile up higher and higher in hospitals and homes and hospices and streets and doorways.

Meanwhile, drugs we have been *begging* that you test remain untested. The list of promising untested drugs is now so endless, and the pipeline is so clogged with NIH and FDA bureaucratic lies, that there is no Roto-Rooter service in this shitty country that will ever muck it out.

You whine to Congress that you are short of staff. You don't need staff to set up hospital treatment centers around the country. The hospitals are already there. They hire their own staff. They only need money. You have money. YOU HAVE 374 MILLION FUCKING DOLLARS, FOR CHRIST'S SAKE!

The gay community has, *for five years,* told the NIH what drugs to test because we know and hear first what is working on some of us somewhere. You couldn't care less about what we say. You won't answer our phone calls or letters, or listen to anyone in our stricken community. What tragic pomposity!

The gay community has consistently told you that unless you move quickly your studies will be worthless because we are already taking drugs into our bodies that in desperation we locate all over the world (who can wait for you?!!), and all your "scientific" protocols are stupidly based on utilizing guinea-pig bodies that are "clean." You wouldn't listen, and now you wonder why so few sign up for your meager assortment of "scientific" protocols, which make such rigid demands for "purity" that no one can fulfill them, unless they lie. And why should those who can obtain the drugs themselves take the chance of receiving a placebo in one of your "scientific" studies?

To quote Representative Waxman again: "Aerosolized pentamidine was named High Priority *fourteen* months ago and there are still no people in trials. Everyone is now taking bootleg versions. Will you ever be able to get enough volunteers for placebo studies when it is now in routine use?"

How many years ago did we tell you about aerosol pentamidine, Tony? That this stuff saves lives. And we discovered it ourselves. We came to you, bearing this great news on a silver platter as a gift, begging you: Can we get it officially tested, can we get it approved by you so that insurance companies and Medicaid will pay for it (as well as other drugs we beg you to test) as a routine treatment, and our patients going broke paying for medicine can get it cheaper? You monster.

"Assume that you have AIDS, and that you've had pneumonia once," Representative Nancy Pelosi (D.-Calif.) said. "You know that aerosolized pentamidine was evaluated by NIH as highly promising. . . . You know as of today that the delays in NIH trials . . . may not be solved this year. Would you wait for [an NIH] study?"

You replied: "I probably would go with what would be available to me, be it available in the street or what have you. . . ."

We tell you what the good drugs are, you don't test them, then YOU TELL US TO GET THEM ON THE STREETS! You continue to pass down word from On High that you don't like this drug or that drug—WHEN YOU HAVEN'T EVEN TESTED THEM! You pass down word from On High that you don't want "to endanger the life of the patient." THERE ARE MORE AIDS VICTIMS DEAD BECAUSE YOU DIDN'T TEST DRUGS ON THEM THAN BECAUSE YOU DID!

You've yet to test Imuthiol, AS 101, dextran sulfate, DHEA, Imreg-1, Erythropoietin—all drugs that Gay Men's Health Crisis considers top priority. You *do* like AZT, which consumes 80 percent of your studies, even though Dr. Barry Gingell, GMHC's medical director, now describes AZT as a "a cumulative poison . . . foisted on the public." Soon there will be more AIDS victims dead because you did test drugs on them—the wrong drugs.

ACT UP was formed over a year ago to get experimental drugs into the bodies of patients. For one year ACT UP has tried every kind of protest known to man (short of putting bombs in your toilet or flames up your Institute) to get some movement in this area. One year later, ACT UP is still screaming for the same drugs they begged and implored you and your world to release. One year of screaming, protesting, crying, cajoling, lobbying, threatening, imprecating, marching, testifying, hoping, wishing, praying has brought nothing. You don't listen. No one listens. No one has ears. Or hearts.

Whose ass are you covering, Tony? (Besides your own.) Is it the head of your Animal House, the invisible Dr. James Wyngaarden, director of the National Institutes of Health (and may a Democratic President get him out of office *fast*)? Is it Dr. Vincent Devita, head of the National Cancer Institute, another invisible murderer who lets you be his fallguy? Or Dr. Otis Bowen, secretary of the Department of Health and Human Services, no doubt the biggest murderer on this list; George Schultz and Caspar Weinberger would never take the constricting bullshit from the Office of Management and Budget that Bowen wallows in. All you "doctors" have, continuously, told the world that All Is Being Done That Can Be Done. Now you admit that isn't so.

WHY DID YOU KEEP QUIET FOR SO LONG?!

I don't know (though it wouldn't surprise me) if you kept quiet intentionally. I don't know (though it wouldn't surprise me) if you were ordered to keep quiet by Higher Ups Somewhere and you are a good lieutenant, like Adolf Eichmann.

I do know that anyone who knows what you have known for three years—that, to quote Representative Weiss, "the dimension of the shortfall is such that you can't possibly meet your needs," and, to quote *The New York Times* and their grossly incompetent AIDS reporter, Philip Boffey (whose articles read like recycled NIH press releases; who doesn't know how to get The Other Side of any story; who refuses to investigate anything he christens A Fact), "Official Blames Shortage of Staff for Delay in Testing AIDS Drugs"—I repeat, anyone who has known all this and denied it for the past three years is a murderer, not dissimilar to the "good Germans" who claimed they didn't know what was happening.

I will also tell you two things I have learned in the last few weeks. New York doctors are now seeing AIDS patients who are not testing HIV-positive during the course of their illness. What does that say about your AIDS test? What does that say about the safety of the nation's blood supply? What does that say to the millions of people who have been tested and think they're fine when in fact they could still be carriers? As more and more cases of AIDS appear, there are going to be more and more bizarre phenomena like this. Everything is not going to fit neatly into your little, simpleminded, HIV-only package.

The New York Blood Center is discovering AIDS happening in people with no known risk behavior (translated: white heterosexuals who've never had contact with drugs or engaged in homosexual acts). But their funding sources (translated: Centers for Disease Control; New York City Department of Health; New York State Department of Health; U.S. Department of Health and Human Services) are suddenly uninterested in funding research that provides this kind of information. So the New York Blood Center has discontinued cataloging these cases. So the world can go on thinking AIDS only happens to gays, blacks, Hispanics, and junkies.

But then, I guess this kind of information is really not your problem. Your problem is to learn how to spend your own $374 million.

With each day I realize a little more that the gay community has lost the battle. And that we haven't even begun to experience the horrors that still await us—horrors even worse than those you represent. We have lost. No one important enough has ears. Or hearts.

You care, I'm told (although I no longer believe it). I've even heard you called a saint. You are in essence a scientist who's expected to be Lee Iacocca. But saints, miracle workers, good administrators, and brilliant scientists have imaginations vivid enough to know how to spend $374 million in a time of dire emergency. You have no imagination. You are banal (a word used so accurately to describe Eichmann).

Do I want you to leave? (Yes.) Could your replacement be more pea-brained than you? (Yes, it is possible.) Will this raving do any good at all? Will it make Congress shape you up? Will it make my own community's bureaucratically mired AIDS organizations finally ask the right questions? (Judy Peabody of GMHC, please take note.) Will Dr. Mathilde Krim ever—as she indicated she would—get the American Foundation for AIDS Research to fund the desperately needed and desperately needy Community Research Initiative, which is valiantly attempting to do what you should be doing, so tired are we of waiting for you to do it. (Leonard Bernstein and Harry Kraut, please take note.)

I have no answer to most of these questions. You may (God help us all) be the best that will be given us. You may, like John Erlichman, once accused, desire redemption and forgiveness by rethinking, retooling, and, like Avis, trying harder. Even more miraculous, those Supreme Murderers in the White House might tomorrow acknowledge that families simply everywhere have gay sons and daughters.

But I fear these are only pipe dreams and you'll continue to carry on with your spare equipment. The cries of genocide from this Cassandra will continue to remain unheard. And my noble but enfeebled community of the weak, the dying, and the dead will continue to grow and grow—until we are diminished.

The level of rhetoric gets higher, the pitch more shrill. The separation between gay readers of this diatribe, for whom it reads with the utmost sane clarity, and straight readers, who think I've now gone round the bend, increases.

How do you finally get the system to work? How do you get important people to listen? And act?

After seven years, I no longer know.

I remember, while writing my earliest pieces, thinking they sounded very angry indeed. Rereading them now, they seem almost calm. Will this attack on Fauci, in a few years' time, sound calm? I think so.

After we had attacked each other in print for several years, it was gratifying that Richard Goldstein, the openly gay editor of the *Village Voice*, welcomed this piece into that publication, whose record on AIDS reporting, while better, is still pretty awful. But it's a strange publication—purchased, I think, mostly by yuppies who want the *Voice*'s encyclopedic listings of weekly Village events, and edited, for the most part, by heterosexual left-wing liberals, who have never been gays' best friends.

Indeed, where have been the voices of Norman Mailer, Saul Bellow, Irving Howe, Alfred Kazin, George Steiner, Victor Navasky, Philip Roth, Arthur Miller, Michael Harrington, Naomi Bliven—to name only a few I used to admire but have yet to hear from on the most crucial issue now facing modern man?

Dear Max

16 June 88

Mr. Max Frankel
The New York Times
229 West 43rd Street
New York, NY 10036

Dear Mr. Frankel,

Thank you very much for your letter of 8 June. I am pleased you thought my *Voice* "polemic" "brilliant." It's been picked up by about twenty newspapers across the country.

I feel your letter requires an answer, and a long one. You say that you "reject the paranoid theories about our suppression of news and I'm satisfied that after a slow start we're doing quite well on the AIDS story."

I must somehow prove to you that my "theories" about your "suppression of news" are not "paranoid" and that, indeed, the *Times* is still not doing a very good job of covering AIDS.

I thought the best way I might accomplish this was by simply taking your recent AIDS articles, day by day, and pointing out to you some facts about them.

■ ■ ■

Friday, June 3, page 1: Philip Boffey's lead article on Admiral James Watkins and his Presidential AIDS Commission Report. Boffey focuses almost exclusively on the report's antidiscrimination recommendation. For a report of many hundreds of pages, containing 578 other recommendations, seven-eighths of Boffey's prose is about one point only. Nowhere in the entire article, or in the excerpts from the report itself you chose to run, is any of its biting criticism of the FDA and NIH for their tragic intransigence. So far as I can see, you were the only major American newspaper to overlook this. As far as coping with AIDS is concerned, there is no more important subject today than getting experimental drugs into research protocols. This is the one subject that the *Times* has been exceedingly bad on, and, as you know, it's the one subject I feel is the most important subject out there. Research.

[I had written Frankel on May 29th: "Boffey's articles read like recycled press releases from NIH, or pharmaceutical companies, or various government agencies. He rarely bothers to get the other side of any story, or opinions from dissenters. And when he does, the way he uses them, writes them in, so obviously conveys his bias that these dissenters appear as crazies. Well, as happens so often in science, in discovery, in anything on the cutting edge, I submit to you that it is often the crazies who make the discoveries. NIH, NCI, NIAID—none of these has such a hot record on major cancer stuff."]

■ ■ ■

Sunday, June 5, page 1: Gina Kolata's article on the ability of "the AIDS virus" to remain undetected. This story, about macrophages, is one year old. Macrophages have been written about in the gay press for fully one year. Indeed, when I saw Boffey at the Presidential Commission's meeting on September 9th, 1987, I asked him why he wasn't writing this story. He knew nothing about it and didn't seem particularly interested in finding out anything further. I offered him names of New York doctors who were noting patients with AIDS testing negative for "the AIDS virus" over a long period of time.

[In my earlier letter, I'd said: "Boffey isn't the only one. Gina

Kolata, who wrote so well when she was at *Science* magazine, now appears to write most vapidly—her heart just doesn't seem to be in it, and a number of her stories appear to go against the grain of what she in fact thinks."]

■ ■ ■

Sunday, June 5, editorial: Nick Wade (if he indeed wrote this) has, in general, been one of your most effective observers of AIDS. He is accessible to outsiders, which Boffey, Kolata, and Dr. Lawrence Altman are not. This particular editorial is fine, but, again, there is absolutely no mention of Watkins's steaming criticism of FDA and NIH.

■ ■ ■

Thursday, June 9, page A-32: Boffey's article on the *Nature* magazine report warning on heterosexual spread. Why is this buried at the bottom of the back page? This is one of the most important issues today, and an extremely respectable magazine is saying something terrifying, and you not only bury it on the back page, but everything in Boffey's contorted prose is geared to refuting the *Nature* warning, calming the waters. Surely this article should have been on page one, and should have been longer and filled with fewer caveats, and Boffey should have sought supporting opinions from other experts who feel the same.

■ ■ ■

Monday, June 13, page A-13: Lawrence Altman's first report from the International AIDS Conference in Stockholm. I don't know what conference you sent this man to cover, but he's not at the same conference as reporters from the *Washington Post*, the *San Francisco Chronicle*, and the *Los Angeles Times*. Each report Altman has filed deals with only one issue. Every other reporter has filed stories containing four, five, or six major announcements. "AIDS outlook bleak." "Aren't we fortunate AIDS wasn't called GRID?" What kind of stupid article is this? Filled with filler, verbiage that doesn't say anything. On this day, Dr. Jonathan Mann of the World Health Organization presented frightening and comprehensive *detailed* figures and projections that even every major network excerpted on the national evening news. Dr. Robert Gallo made some specific predictions about vaccines, including the astonishing statement that there might never even be one that was any good.

■ ■ ■

Tuesday, June 14, page B-4: Bruce Lambert's article on New York State medical societies seeking to force State Health Department officials to deal with AIDS as a communicable disease. There are two huge holes left open in this article. One is that nowhere is mentioned any statement to refute the medical societies' spokesmen, to the effect that "the AIDS test" as presently available is not sufficiently useful a tool to do what the societies want. The other is that you simply cannot use a statement like "He accused the state of bowing to homosexuals," without getting a statement from a homosexual source to balance it. And, boy, I wish we were that powerful in reality! I hear so many remarks about "the tough tactics of gay lobbyists," which is just absurd. We have, in total, six full-time lobbyists working for AIDS and are they not tough! To Bruce's credit, he is your only reporter who, quite rightly, qualifies the putative cause by saying "the virus believed to cause AIDS." Everyone else has bought HIV hook, line, and sinker. There simply is no agreement that HIV is the *only* cause.

[In my May 29th letter to Frankel, I'd written: "Bruce Lambert took me out to dinner to pick my brains. I thought this was very enterprising of him, and I liked him, not only for that. I gave him—it must have been a dozen or more story ideas, which he wrote down greedily. I've called him several times since to pass on a few more. Not one of these ideas has ever made it into a story in the *Times*. When I asked him why, he said they'd all been submitted, but had not been approved by those Higher Ups to whom these decisions evidently fall." I've since learned that all *Times* AIDS reporting falls under one of three desks: Metro (for New York), National, and Science. Each desk has one or two or three editors. Often AIDS stories aren't clearly local or national or scientific: They're all three, or two of them. Then, evidently, rivalries take over, disputes over turf, or the story falls, by default, to the editor least interested in it, or a story that contains political implications is handed to Science, where all the nonscientific matter is edited out. The *Times*—and why should anyone be surprised—is as bureaucratically mired and inefficient as every other AIDS service provider. And if the story should be for the Sunday *Times,* or for "The Week in Review," or the magazine section, then there are yet *further* editors involved in the tussle.]

■ ■ ■

Tuesday, June 14, page B-4: Altman from Stockholm again. On the day when vital new evidence was presented about additional possibly causative viruses, Altman chooses to report on results of the experimental drug Imreg. Fine. As far as it goes. Nowhere does he mention that we have known about these results for about six months, that we have been clamoring for Imreg for over a year. Nowhere does he raise the troubling question: Why were the Imreg studies so small, when it has been known to be so promising for so long? He mentions that the company that produces it is "small." He doesn't tell us how hard it is for "small" companies to get cooperation from the FDA. He includes the most pathetic quote from "a spokesman from the Federal Food and Drug Administration," to whit, "We look forward to receiving the clinical data that would substantiate the claims being made for this drug." This breaks my heart. Neither *The New York Times* nor any other paper, except *The Wall Street Journal,* has done an exposé of the subtext of this FDA spokesman's response: The FDA is a *passive* organization. You have to present everything *to* them. Nowhere in this entire government is there any mechanism for *actively* helping a "small" company that doesn't have the savvy skills of a Burroughs Wellcome, the manufacturers of AZT, in maneuvering through the treacherous FDA (and NIH) waters. Here comes a promising drug, Imreg; why isn't the FDA spokesperson saying, "We look forward to doing everything in our power to helping Imreg gain approval and get out into the world." I beg of you—please get someone to write about the FDA not working at all, as Watkins's report so bravely pointed out.

■ ■ ■

Wednesday, June 15, page A-21: Altman, still from Stockholm, writing about the great efficacy of aerosol pentamidine. This story, too, is over one year old. Dr. Donald Armstrong at Sloan-Kettering ran his original study over a year ago, and the results of this study are widely known (not, certainly, from the *Times*), so much so that this drug is in widespread and general use just about everywhere in the world. I and many others have tried innumerable times to get various *Times* reporters (not Altman, who doesn't return phone calls, and has behaved like this since 1981) to write about this over this past year. No one was interested. Altman writes: "The National Institutes of Health is now sponsoring a large trial that is being conducted in several hospitals." This is a huge distortion of reality. You read my *Voice* "polemic." In it I quoted testimony from the Ted Weiss hearing in which Fauci was raked over the coals for *not* testing aerosol pentamidine a long time ago, and Fauci admitted that the trials were planned but still in the future, and that he, under pressure, admitted that if he had *Pneumocystis,* he'd go out in the streets to get this drug.

In this same issue of the *Times* there is an important letter to the editor from Arthur Leonard, a professor of law and an exceptionally able writer about AIDS legal concerns, in which he also takes issue with Philip Boffey for omitting vital facts from his June 3, page-one article on Admiral Watkins's recommendations—the heinous tactics Representative William Dannemeyer and Senator Jesse Helms have used to kill any possible legislative vehicle for achieving the protection against discrimination that the Watkins report makes top priority. How could you not be writing about these two murderous dumbbells?

■ ■ ■

Thursday, June 16, page A-25: My least favorite (edging out Boffey by a nose), Altman, again from Stockholm, reporting on the slowdown of AIDS in the addict population. (Would that it were so!) He must have gone home early. On this day, exceedingly important information was presented concerning the promising efficacy of *four* experimental treatments, including dextran sulfate and naltrexone. Indeed, the naltrexone results were reported by a New York doctor, Dr. Bernard Bihari, of SUNY-Brooklyn. Additionally, there was a vitally important report on the promising CD-4 (even the networks reported on this one), as well as promising reports from Israel on AL 721, and mixed results on Peptide-T. The *San Francisco Chronicle* ran *four* separate articles about AIDS and about this conference on this date. (The *Times*'s coverage of the entire conference, which was a very important conference, has been so sparse and piddling as to be tragic. It is a sad commentary when all three networks—particularly George Straight on ABC—do a better job covering a major happening than *The New York Times*.)

Information about these drugs is information this city should and must have, and you are not reporting it. How dare you overlook this? People are desperate for this kind of news above all other.

And you think I am "paranoid" about your suppression of the news!

■ ■ ■

Now some further thoughts: Your reporters just write the same stories everyone else writes. Mostly, when something "new" is reported in a medical journal, they just rewrite it and put it out. That's not reporting. That's really just a form of plagiarism. It doesn't take much talent to rewrite a medical journal article. Most of them contain news, as I've shown above, that's old news anyway, which we knew about a long time ago, and, in many instances, tried to get your people to write about a long time ago. No one does much "reporting" up there. What are you paying them for? To thumb through the medical journals as soon as they arrive on their desks?

Dextran sulfate: This is a terrific story. I've told Boffey and Lambert, as have others. It comes from Japan. It seems to raise T-cells. Doctors in New York have been sending couriers over for about six months to get it. As soon as the FDA heard about this, they clamped down, made it illegal to import it into this country, so that it's now seized at the borders if you try to bring it in. Further, the FDA instructed Japan not to sell it to Americans. The Japanese therefore made it a prescription drug—it had been available there over the counter *for twenty years*, with no reported bad effects. So now AIDS sufferers can't get it. Why aren't you writing stories like this? It puts the FDA to shame. Talk to Dr. Barbara Starrett about the tests she's doing with dextran sulfate. She is, by the way, one of the "AIDS

Heroes" profiled in the current issue of *7 Days*. Here is a local doctor, sick and tired of waiting for the NIH and FDA to study and release promising drugs, who is doing the damned (and expensive and tedious) testing on her own. With her own patients. With her own money. She sent her own lover, Ann Silver (who is hearing-impaired), over to Japan to courier supplies back. Why aren't you writing human-interest stories like this? Barbara's story has certainly been pitched to your boys and girls.

Every single drug or treatment that is promising and that we can't get hold of has a story of chicanery or slipups of some sort. Susan Spencer said on "CBS News" the other night that there are now *two hundred* drugs that are promising, and that aren't available here. That's awful. Where are your reporters? Isn't this suppression of vital news? Am I paranoid? I can't tell you how many times many of us have tried to get your reporters to write these stories.

The stupid (if it weren't so tragic) story behind the unavailability of AL 721, for instance. It comes from the Weizmann Institute, certainly a distinguished place. They licensed the patent, it seems, not to one of the international drug companies that were after it, but to one of the members of the Weizmann Institute's American board, a New York attorney, Leslie Jacobson, whose nephew had a tiny drug company with little track record or, as it turned out, experience or ability to manufacture the stuff in sufficient quality or quantity to supply the NIH for their planned protocols. That's a tragic story, Mr. Frankel. You haven't written it. The *New England Journal of Medicine* described AL 721 as promising and worthy of study *three years ago!* And it still remains improperly tested. And here are reports from Stockholm that it's still promising, three years later.

One of the problems is that your reporters are very haughty. They aren't interested in putting their ears to the ground. They're only interested in listening to establishment doctors, most of whom don't know very much about AIDS treatments because these treatments aren't recognized by the FDA or the NIH. Why don't your reporters listen to the gay community, which knows more about what's going on than most doctors? Dr. Barry Gingell, the medical director of GMHC, is now so frustrated that he puts out a GMHC treatment newsletter that prints all of the stuff you should be printing. If the power of the *Times* isn't available to get the system to move forward on malfeasances, what good is the *Times* in a time of dire emergency?

Another story you refuse to track is the Community Research Initiative. This is an historic attempt by the gay community to test drugs on ourselves. Indeed, they did the aerosol pentamidine study with Dr. Armstrong of Sloan-Kettering, which, over a year ago, discovered the same thing that Altman is just now "reporting" from Stockholm. Your reporters are invited to all CRI press conferences, but they never show up. Dr. Mathilde Krim is on CRI's board. So is Dr. Armstrong. It is not a fly-by-night group. They desperately need media attention so they can raise money. They just got a small grant from Du Pont to test Ampligen—from Du Pont! A tiny community group that was sick and tired of waiting for NIH and FDA to test important drugs found, somehow, a way to legally set up their own protocols, and is doing invaluable work on a shoestring. Talk about a continuing human-interest story! But is the *Times* there? No.

Every time a black or Jewish group holds a protest or performs some act of civil disobedience, it's reported in the *Times*. Every time ACT UP protests, the *Times* never shows. This group of several thousand (which has even finally been profiled in *Newsweek*) has done monumental acts of civil disobedience in this town and in this country, and the *Times* never notices. They held a four-day, around-the-clock picketing of Sloan-Kettering last summer, and where were you? It's pretty hard to ignore a four-day, around-the-clock event, but you managed to do so. A very angry zap of Mayor Koch last week, which made the local TV news and the *Post* and the *Daily News*, but not the *Times*, prevented Koch from speaking for a full half hour, until he left in a huff. Why can't *our* activism be reported?

Did you know about the mess at the New York Blood Center? I tipped Bruce Lambert off to this many months ago. The *New York Observer* just ran a long article on part of the mess, but no one else has. It goes even further than they reported. Rather than be forced into admitting that a heterosexual rise is occurring in non-drug or non-gay-contact persons, which they are discovering, the Blood Center has discontinued tallying these results. That's a scandal! The *San Francisco Chronicle* ran an article yesterday on another aspect of this: "AIDS Suspected Behind Rise in Female Deaths." Evidently women diagnosed with other illnesses are now thought to have died from AIDS. Where are your reporters? I even think this one was on the wire service.

I could go on endlessly about other stories you're not reporting, or are reporting badly. I do hope you can concede that I've made a bit of a point in disputing your letter. I'd like to close with querying your last sentence. "Please don't make them [your reporters] hostile with unfounded and unsubstantiated accusations." (I hope I have more than substantiated my accusations!) I query your notion of what happens if and when my criticisms turn your folks hostile. Are you saying that criticism will turn them against writing about AIDS in a responsible fashion? (Not that they're doing so now.) That is what it *seems* you are saying. If that is so, and I can't believe you mean this, then your reporters are not any reporters I should like to have on the staff of any newspaper I want to read.

I hope you realize that I write this, and keep after you and yours, because, like so many others, I care deeply not only about AIDS, but about the *Times*. We all want it to be perfect, which nothing can be. But on AIDS, for some reason, you have been, from the very beginning, very poor indeed. Yes, you are better than you were under your hated and hateful predecessor, Abe Rosenthal. But you are just not yet good enough.

[I closed my May 29th letter with: "So, once again, after a short spurt of recovery, the *Times*, the supposed paper of record, has reverted to its earlier Rosenthalian blind lethargy. More and more books are being written about your awful showing—to go along with Randy Shilts's *And the Band Played On*. I have been interviewed for several of them, including ones written by academics, who seem to be very interested these days in the role, or lack of it, of proper media attention to the AIDS epidemic. No one has a very good word to say about the *Times*, before you or, really, during you."]

We have been writing to each other for so long that I feel we are somehow almost friends. Would it be permissible at this stage to deal with each other on a first-name basis?

I received a short note in return, which began with "Dear Larry" and was signed "Sincerely, Max," and which said, "Yes, first names help. So would more staff. Without agreeing on all your points, we would like to do yet more and are looking to find a way to get it done along with everything else."

I understand that both these letters of mine were circulated to all the desk editors and all the reporters I criticized. This both pleases me and surprises me, happily so. In the week following, Dr. Barry Gingell was taken out to lunch by Deputy Science Editor Erik Eckholm and reporter Gina Kolata, and asked to provide them with a list of important stories. *Times* metropolitan reporter Tom Morgan was assigned a feature article on ACT UP. Bruce Lambert was assigned to covering AIDS full time. And Washington AIDS reporter Philip Boffey is still there.

Max and I write to each other several times a month now. It's almost impossible for me to believe that the editor-in-chief of the world's most powerful newspaper actually answers my letters, and with occasional sympathy, but always politely and quickly. For the first six years of AIDS, the *Times* was edited by a monster. Abe Rosenthal would not only never respond to a letter, but he rarely allowed acknowledgment that gay people even existed. May he go down in history as the culpable villain he is. Along with his henchman, Dr. Lawrence Altman, the principal AIDS "reporter" for those long, silent years at the *Times*.

Max appears a kind man, certainly a liberal one. One of his first acts in office was to allow use of the word "gay" instead of "homosexual" as Rosenthal had demanded. But I don't think Max really comprehends that there are one million gay people in New York, and that a goodly number of us are his readers and his advertisers. His response to AIDS is that of a decent heterosexual responding to a few cries from the wilderness, rather than that of a pragmatic editor cognizant of the necessity that this million is entitled to have its history written about with the depth, frequency, and integrity granted to other minorities like blacks and Jews.

While most *Times* coverage has improved, the main AIDS reporter is still the incompetent Phil Boffey. I do not know what the specific problem with this man is. Is it a lack of compassion, a lack of energy, a lack of reportorial skills, or is he just plain dumb? Article after article finds him completely missing the main point of discussion. He always defers to the same few people for information or quotes of attribution. He does not understand AIDS, and yet he is the the principal *Times* spokesperson on it.

I think history will eventually record that it is one of the truly great tragedies—of an epidemic not lacking in them—that it fell to Altman and Boffey to be the principal AIDS investigators for *The New York Times.*

And so, I notice, I end as I began—with the *Times*. I suppose it's not a bad symbolic symmetry, the *Times*.

The times.

To relive these years, as I have done in preparing this book, has been to relive a lifetime. I've been plagued with mixed emotions: Dare I include this? Did I really write that? This makes me sound so self-serving. Or too self-righteous. Or too righteous, period. Or an ass. What a megalomaniac.

What are the main lessons I've learned? One is this: I no longer believe America is a country where one voice can make any difference.

I started out, in 1981, believing it could. Oh, I can see where certain things I raged against were now and then affected. But it shouldn't take so long when so many people are dying. And something infectious is going around. And everything's going to get much, *much* worse.

I also learned, after an earlier life of comparative privileges, what it's like not to have them anymore. I have learned—in a more tangible and visible way than I ever thought or was taught I would encounter in a "free" and "democratic" society—how gay people are hated and expendable.

I believe I said everything I said in the only way I knew how to say it at that moment. In so doing, I became the "activist" I never wanted to be. The angry kid I was found a way to use that anger. I'm no less angry now that I've grown up. But I'm much more tired.

Well, whatever I wrote, it's all here. The ups and downs of antagonisms and of friendships. The loss from death. The death of hope.

The making of an AIDS activist.

Part Two

Report from the holocaust

I

I don't think any heterosexual can understand what it's like to be a homosexual man in New York today—or in any other major American city: Los Angeles, San Francisco, Houston, Dallas, Miami, Boston, Chicago, but particularly in New York, which, with some one million gay men and women, is the largest gay city in the world.

I don't understand much of it myself, and writing this essay has been yet another attempt to do just that. I've been asked, though rarely, by heterosexual friends: "How do you stand it? How do you live?" And I can't really answer, except to say something annoyingly clichéd like: "We all take it one day at a time," or, more often, "I try not to think about it," which is a lie but serves to cut off further discussion. It's not that I mind talking about it; it's just that I've come to find heterosexual inquiry just that, and only that: inquiry. More like checking to see what my opinion is of the latest movie. I've come to be very angry about this heterosexual attitude, and less tolerant of the perfectly valid (to them), reasonable excuses heterosexuals use

217

to support it, as voiced by my brother, Arthur, a lawyer: "We have our own lives and our own set of problems; I don't ask you to fight my battles, don't expect and demand that I fight yours." So, rather than destroy what few straight friendships I have left, I've found myself changing the subject or, more often of late, withdrawing more and more from my straight friends and even my family.

Most gay men don't know how we're enduring it. If we're still healthy, we clutch that fact to our hearts and minds, and attempt to take strength from it: I am here, I am alive, I don't know *why* I'm alive, or how, but I am alive. I have never before, in my fifty-three years of living, been particularly grateful to be alive. It's just something I never thought about. It's a notion that always seemed to accompany facing old age and death. There'd always been good days and bad days then, mixed together.

I hesitate to state that over the past seven years I have lost some five hundred acquaintances and friends to AIDS. I realize that putting a figure to this loss is both gruesomely macabre and too Madison Avenue. It makes me sound weird: that I have for over seven years kept a record of these names. It also sounds vaguely opportunistic: trafficking in dead bodies to make a morbid point. Further, I think it makes me sound a bit—I don't know—self-serving? How could anyone *know* five hundred men? It sounds like I'm scouring to make a point, which, of course, I am. Nobody *knows* five hundred people, straight friends tell me disbelievingly, proving to me that this isn't the right approach for argument or pleas for help.

Because gays live in a ghetto, we know personally and generally recognize most of the people in it. We live together in this world-within-a-world: certain neighborhoods in Manhattan, Fire Island, the Hamptons; the discos we once danced in; the organizations we belong to, from religious congregations (gay synagogues, Catholic worship groups) to social ones like gay alumni from one's college, Men of All Colors Together, choruses and marching bands, to athletic teams: soccer and baseball and football (now even a Gay Games, which would be called the Gay Olympics, were it not for the Supreme Court disallowing it) to AA meetings, affiliations of gay physicians, social workers, men in advertising, the law, even the police, to charitable endeavors, and, now, AIDS organizations in which we attempt to take care of our own; or just walking down city streets everywhere. But even in rural areas of New York State and New Jersey and Staten Island, gays know where other gays are. It's like the old American idea of life in a small town. We know everybody.

We know who we are. When the first man who ever loved me, a professor of mine at Yale, told me during my freshman year in 1953 that, yes, we could all pretty much recognize each other passing on the streets, I didn't believe him. How could one tell? Well, one can mostly tell.

If an infectious illness were happening to Jews, in which *over 50 percent* of their population was thought to be infected—one out of every two Jews—how many people would a socially active Jew in, say, Rego Park, or Boro Park, or Woodmere, or Great Neck, or the upper West Side know? How many Jews would a person like Cynthia Ozick or Laurence Tisch or Bella Abzug or Edward Koch know? Such an occurrence would seem devastating not only to their community, but to the world. Happening to gay men, it doesn't seem to register very high on the devastation scale. That's the problem.

Because I have helped to start two AIDS organizations, one, Gay Men's Health Crisis, for self-help (though it was originally founded to fight to make the world pay attention and help us) and one, ACT UP—the AIDS Coalition to Unleash Power—for political activism, and because I have written extensively about the gay world, beginning with my novel, *Faggots*, which I wrote between 1975 and 1978, and continuing with many pieces of political journalism, I guess I know more gay people than most, and more dead gay men than many. Too, because I am a writer fascinated by everyone's story, I tend to recognize many people who might not know me, but whom I know about. When I was an unhappy and exceedingly lonely student at Yale, I could identify almost everyone in my class of over one thousand men because I had memorized our Class Directory from poring over it so much, or from listening and observing so much from the sidelines: This guy is from Shaker Heights and this one's from La Jolla and that one went to Groton and that one grew up in Switzerland and that one's father is a barber and that tall guy's mother is a Du Pont. Few of them knew me. I didn't know

then that I would become a writer, and that this almost pathological interest in everybody's history would pursue me. Except
now it *is* pathological—"pertaining to or caused by disease."

Oh, how I, as a homosexual, have always loathed that word
"disease," and, worse, "caused by disease." I have fought so
hard—even to the point of not speaking to my sister-in-law,
Alice, for many months when, years ago, she said emphatically
that she knew homosexuality was an illness. "I just know it in
my heart of hearts," she said, looking me straight in the eye,
as I stood there speechless and fuming, having no ammunition
to fight back with, beyond the same argument: I knew, and
know, in *my* heart of hearts, that she's wrong. I was born just
as she was born.

And also—because AIDS has brought gay men much closer,
so that friendships that would ordinarily take years to develop
are now quickly made and cemented—those of us fighting this
epidemic find ourselves with many new friends very quickly
indeed. (It's not unusual to go to a funeral and find that most
of the mourners are men and women the deceased became
friendly with after his AIDS diagnosis.)

I believe most gay men now know more dead gay men than
they realize, or allow themselves to think about.

I only recently discovered that the number of dead I knew
was so great. For the first several years of this epidemic, I
dutifully kept a list in a little green notebook. When the number
reached two hundred, sometime in 1985, I stopped. I'm not quite
certain why. Even then it seemed hyperbolic to discuss such a
large number; or perhaps I was going through one of my periodic bouts of burnout, deciding enough was enough. But I
didn't really stop. When I came across an obituary anywhere of
someone I knew, I'd clip it out and toss it into a box. When I
heard another name in conversations, on the phone, walking
down the street, at dinners or other social gatherings, I'd make
a note of the name on a piece of paper and toss that into the box
too. (Listening to conversations of gay men at social gatherings
recently, I've realized how completely we've come to absorb the
morbidity of our lives; men pass along information of deaths
casually interspersed in the flow of whatever else they're talking about, as in "He's got a new Volvo, Peter must have left
him some money, he says it's the best car he's ever had," or

"Frank got the house when Terry died, and Frank and Tom, his lover died . . . was it in August . . . are going to Europe, I got them into the Connaught in August, you know how hard it is to get anyone into the Connaught in August. . . ." These quotes come from men still in their twenties and thirties.)

When I started to write this essay, I pulled out the box and dumped the pieces of paper on the floor. I transferred the names and taped the obituaries onto three-by-five file cards, and then copied all the names from the green notebook onto file cards, too. I began to be aware that the task was taking me longer than I thought it would. Then I alphabetized them all, as best I could, because a number of the dead men were identi-fied not with names, which I couldn't remember, but with de-scriptive phrases: "Alice's hairdresser"; "the guy I had a date with after the opening night of *No, No, Nanette*"; "Bruce Kaye's lover"; "the brother of the *Newsweek* reporter, they both came here to talk"; "the short doctor with the Italian name who was a friend of DW's [a man I was desperately in love with in 1975]"; "Coconut Grove—the guy with the Spanish first name and the Jewish last name"; "the kid who became an Or-thodox Jew when he got sick, and then got married." I can still see most of their faces, even though I'm no longer as good with names as I was at Yale. After completing this task, I began asking friends to list for me names they remembered, and when I recognized one I didn't have, I added it to my own list. It was only when I counted the cards after I'd done all of this that I was startled to discover I had about five hundred. Just as star-tling is the knowledge that there are always more to be added. I continue to hear new names of acquaintances and friends I hadn't included. And *The New York Times* comes out every day.

(I used to encourage friends who were dating to settle down into relationships. I wasn't a matchmaker—just a romantic egg-ing-on from the sidelines, hoping others would find what I hadn't. While filing my index cards, it upset me to note several couples I'd encouraged who had perhaps then infected each other.)

The publication that the Centers for Disease Control, the government agency responsible for monitoring this epidem-ic, puts out with the latest numbers, the latest physical manifestations and permutations—for there are many illnesses and diseases all under the category AIDS—is called the *Morbidity and Mortality Weekly Report*. The *MMWR*. On last (1988) June 5th (the date, in 1981, that the *MMWR* first listed cases of what was eventually to be named AIDS and, by this inclusion, officially designated it an "epidemic"), this country entered the eighth year of the AIDS epidemic. There is no cure. There is still marked uncertainty about what is going on inside our bodies. There is, among some of us, a growing conviction that what we're told *is* going on may perhaps not be accurate. Despite congressional appropriations—at last—of hundreds of millions of dollars that would seem to dispute this, there is still monumental indifference on the part of the straight world to addressing this catastrophe, and predictions for the future are even more grotesque than the numbers I live with now.

Figures, which all Americans, myself evidently included, wallow in, from TV ratings to increased sales of gourmet take-out, aren't really meaningful to me any longer. The figure "five hundred" seems unreal. Death as a profound philosophical subject is currently ridiculous. Even now, in its non-philosophical form, it's impossible to grasp, to get hold of, this unreality, just somehow to live with it. With an average of several deaths a week (there is a new American case diagnosed every fourteen minutes), how could anyone? There's no time for grief or mourning, certainly not for contemplation. I can't cry easily anymore anyway. Phone calls advising me of another departure from this world are too routine. As is finding familiar names in the obits of the *Times*. I read the latest overall tallies. They're awful. Everything's awful. And it's been awful for so long.

Over a year ago, I set out to write something—I wasn't quite certain what. I'd submitted a proposal to several publications. I wanted to write regularly about AIDS, stories that weren't being written and that I felt demanded to be written. The AIDS epidemic is enormously complicated. It's so complicated that few reporters appear to understand what's going on. I consider all AIDS reporting everywhere, without exception, to be imprecise and superficial. The latest news, be it a medical or scientific discovery or a proposed legislative action—each and all tied in knotted strands of potential controversy (usually including either the word "discriminatory" or "mandatory")—

cannot be encapsulated in one-minute segments on the evening news or even in 1,400 words, which newspapers occasionally, at the limits of their generosity, allocate. And I think something very grim has happened to American journalism: It has become bland and increasingly conservative. The sort of deep, investigative reporting that I grew up with and took for granted has apparently disappeared. I was tired of calling my reporter contacts, pointing out the AIDS scandals they weren't writing about, and watching them still not write about them. Or reading their articles and calling them up to say they'd missed the point. Or writing them lengthy letters critiquing their articles in detail. Or berating them for not bothering to get a statement from someone representing another point of view. Most AIDS reporters seem to think there is only one point of view: that promulgated by the United States government and its many agencies dealing with the epidemic (but not with each other). I thought I'd better stop complaining about this and do it myself—that, as a writer and someone well acquainted with this awful drama and its huge cast of characters, I could be most effective in this way.

My proposal was accepted by a large newspaper and its syndicate. I went to Washington for a month, to research my first article. I decided I wanted to write about the total lack of any AIDS chain of command, the fact that nobody was really in charge, and the complete disarray among those who were meant to be involved—to try to make readers understand that, in these circumstances, little would get done. I wrote the article, which appeared in the "home" newspaper I was attached to by the syndicate, and then I became despondent as I silently watched it not picked up at all when it was wired—two times— in full to some 300 newspapers across the country, wired in summary to some 1,200 newspapers across the country, and even when the syndicate salesman personally made an appeal to his twelve leading newspapers.

But that is not the point of *this* essay, beyond demonstrating how hard it is for the gay community to get our story out to the straight world. All writers are familiar with rejection. The point that *is* applicable, that I do want to make, is that in my discouragement I quit. Instead of persevering and hoping that the forthcoming articles, as sometimes happens, would begin to accrue additional syndicated outlets, I absorbed my rejection and frustration and took my marbles and went home.

As with the mounting tallies of lost friends, those of us who have been trying to confront this losing battle seem to have an infinite capacity not only to absorb the worst, but to be defeated by it. So many deaths have not turned very many of us into fighters. We are all, naturally, infinitely tired ("AIDSed-out" is the expression). Whatever energy can be summoned to fight perceived wrongs has, for many, long since dribbled away.

That it's taken over a year for me to sit down and tackle this project again is less a token of my energy or commitment, or my ability to overcome my conviction that whatever I write will again fall on deaf ears, or my renewed energy after a period of burnout, than it is of my realizing again that there's nothing else to do. There's nothing else important enough to write about. I should be making a living writing something that might produce for me the income I need like everyone else (my brother, Arthur, only half-jokingly remarks that I'm using AIDS as an excuse *not* to work and write), but I don't have the interest or energy for that kind of writing. What actually gets me started again is not the inspiration (I am sorry to say that the loss of five hundred no longer works, as it once did, as the more-than-sufficient inspiration), but the realization that over a year has passed. Where did that year go? How many three-by-fives? (About ninety.) How many more of us became infected? What dynamite will ever ignite experimental drug-testing at the Food and Drug Administration and at the National Institutes of Health, of the more than two hundred promising treatments that "CBS Evening News" casually mentioned recently were available somewhere else in the world but not here? What did I do with my life for one whole year? Oh, I know what I did—but what did I *do?*

In other words, I became frightened again. If, as I fear, my days are probably numbered, how can I afford to be so wasteful of time? I was brought up a Jew, by two intelligent parents, both professionals (my father a lawyer and my mother a social worker), and fifty-three years of the instilled necessity to achieve does not disappear, especially, it would seem, in the face of death.

Why do I feel I have to offer these excuses? Excuses for

what? For my year of inactivity or for my decision, once again, to try to write about this? I haven't been completely honest with you. I did not waste a year doing nothing. I wrote two plays. I put together a book of my political writings of these AIDS years. I rewrote a screenplay of my play *The Normal Heart,* about the early years of the epidemic. That is certainly a good year's work, by any standards, Jewish or otherwise. Why do I discount it so?

Because none of it has any meaning for today, now, this minute? How can that be? I ache for *The Normal Heart* to be a film, because there have been no motion pictures, yet and still, documenting these years of horror. One of the new plays is a farce "inspired by" some of those I consider monstrously responsible for the AIDS predicament—the First Family and the Mayor of A Large City. The other play, a companion piece to *The Normal Heart,* which I call *The Furniture of Home,* is about growing up with my parents and my brother, covering some forty years; its theme, which evidently provided enough energetic fuel for me to write it, can be stated simply: You spend so many years fighting to come to terms with being homosexual, you finally not only accept yourself but like yourself, and then the fucking plague comes along.

All of this work contains ideas I want people to hear. So why do I disparage it? Do I feel guilty because I'm not fighting this fight twenty-four hours a day? Do I feel guilty I'm alive?

I come back to my opening sentence: I don't think any heterosexual can understand what it's like to be a homosexual man today. I somehow want every heterosexual to understand that. I want my brother and sister-in-law to understand that.

I am presently, as I write this sentence, in various stages of estrangement from both of them because of a recent example of my "gay activist" behavior. I wrote a strong and threatening letter to a large corporate client of Arthur's firm to protest their unjust firing of a gay employee; Arthur and Alice took great offense at my involving Arthur in this way. You must know that my brother has always been the most important person in my life and that our devotion to each other has been total; like the only two members of a fraternity, we have prided ourselves, in our adult lives, on our closeness, in the eyes of the world as well as our own. We would have lunch regularly once a week; then—

with the arrival of AIDS and my increasing political activism—
this became less regular, supplanted by weekly phone calls
back and forth. Both calls and lunches have now become sporadic and suffused with forced casualness. Before I wrote the
letter, I had asked him for advice on how to write it. Homosexuality is the only subject between us that, even after some thirty-
five years of knowing about mine, he cannot talk about
comfortably. An edge of upset comes into his voice, which rises
a pitch or two, an edge that I recognize as not only discomfort
but anger—that I've brought the subject up or that he doesn't
want to talk about it, I don't know which. Probably both. And
the rejection that I instantly feel evokes my own hardly sup-
pressed anger: Even after some thirty-five years of knowing
this does that to him, I slam down the phone. And wait for him
to call back. Which he always has done, so far. It is exceedingly
painful for me to confront the possibility that my very own
brother might have to be included in that "straight" world for
which I find myself having less and less tolerance.

Recently, before this episode, in the course of chatting
about many things, including AIDS—for I make a determined
effort to force the subject down his and Alice's and our mother's
throats—he casually asked me, "You're worried about your
health?"

That he could have asked me such a question, eight years
into an epidemic that has taken many of my friends whom he
knew, and despite his cognizance of my political involvement,
and my writings which I've seen to it he's had copies of, and the
organizations I helped to start, to one of which I finagled him
into becoming pro bono legal adviser, and the massive media
coverage (even if I don't think they're the right stories, at last
now there are plenty of stories) has, as our mother puts it when
she stews about something that upsets her, "stuck in my craw."

What does he think I worry about? To watch friend after
friend be taken from me to die after ghastly and punishing
illnesses and not be frightened? To see dread spots erupt over-
night on previously unblemished skins and limbs of still-living
other friends and not be frightened? To hear incipient coughs
transmute from hacking barks into sudden silence and not be
frightened? I guess this sounds melodramatic. And my prose

has turned purple too. Am I begging for sympathy? Yes. Am I begging for help? Yes. Am I frightened? You bet your life.

In the end, I realize I can't write about anything else. Every story is the same story. What I have written this past year is the only thing I can write now. Primo Levi, the survivor of Auschwitz who somehow managed to write magnificently of his horrible memories, said in *If This Is a Man* (reprinted as *Survival in Auschwitz*): "The need to tell our story to 'the rest,' to make 'the rest' participate in it, had taken on for us . . . the character of an immediate violent impulse, to the point of competing with other elementary needs."

Several months ago I met the first man I have allowed myself to make love with, and be (safely) intimate with, and consider having a relationship with—in five years. Luke. I have not made love in five years. One of the last men I loved died from AIDS in 1983. Men who have been romantically important in my life in earlier, pre-AIDS years (there's no margin of safety in thinking like this: the putative causal virus might have an incubation period of twenty years) have also died. It is very difficult for me to make love, even "safely," when the very act is now so inextricably bound up with death. I don't mean the memory of my dead lover, though that, too, of course, is there. (I have undergone periodic satisfactory tests on my body's immune system—though not for HIV, because I consider this test, perhaps irrationally, unconvincing. It's not that I disbelieve its probable efficacy, it's just that I still don't believe *enough* to subject myself to living under such a sword of Damocles. To be fair, I must say that I have many friends whose opinions I respect who consider my refusal to be tested for HIV a state of denial.) I mean the very act itself—of kissing, of gently masturbating each other, of sweating bodies lying side by side. All the educational material in the world proclaiming that "safe sex" is possible does not reduce the fear that some slipup might occur. Is it fatal if his semen on my hand enters the tiny exposed cuticle under a minuscule hangnail on my thumb? Or my sweat into his scraped knee (he belongs to a gay wrestling team)? Is kissing really safe? I know they say it is, that no cases have been discovered that result from kissing, but do they really know? How do you define "kissing"?

How do you draw distinctions between kisses and kisses? There are reported cases of single-contact infection. Contact with what, exactly, and where? Anal intercourse is considered to be the most dangerous activity. But I know dead men who never engaged in it. So many hard-and-fast dicta have been issued at some time during these years of scientific and epidemiological investigation, only to be refuted, contradicted, contravened days, weeks, months, or years later. And so many of the men and women making these pronouncements I know to be, from personal encounters, truly second-rate (many first-rate minds have refused to participate), or corseted by ironclad requirements of a bureaucracy determined, at any cost, not to create panic in "the general population." (Before 1981, I'd always considered myself a part of "the general population." But before 1981, I also believed in democracy.) So it's difficult for me to believe anything.

And yet I found myself falling in love. Like other human beings, I desire the experience. I wanted to hold this man and to kiss him. Is this wanting too much? Is this wanting too much *now?* Can any straight person understand what it is like to want to make love but to be terrified that to do so means possible death? Even breaking the most stringent and necessary diet for one's health doesn't kill you; you have a binge and go back on the diet tomorrow, plagued only with guilt. It took me many years of psychoanalysis to rid myself of guilts—over being homosexual, over not being as financially successful as my brother, over . . . oh, the endless agenda of what we think the world expects of us that we're not fulfilling; now guilt creeps back in yet another door. I feel guilty falling in love. I should have more control over my emotions. I don't want to die. I have important work to try to do quickly, before I die. I don't want to die.

I want to live and I want to love and I want, in the universal as well as the specific sense, all my brothers to try to understand why this epidemic is here—because I think there are reasons why it is here—and, with your understanding, to help us, for we, and I, desperately need help. That's why I'm writing this. For Arthur and Alice and for every heterosexual friend I find myself hating, when I don't want to hate.

And in so writing, perhaps I can also try to offer thoughts on some questions:

■   Why are homosexuals not allowed to state that many of us *know* we are born homosexual, as straight men are born heterosexual, as bisexual men are born bisexual, without such staunch opposition from so many others, on so many fronts? Why is it so important to *them* that this cannot be so? What is their vested interest in keeping us sick? And illegal?

■   Why has the straight world, by and large, been unable to face or cope with the realities of what is happening to us—to such a degree that I now believe some form of intentional genocide is going on?

■   Why have not more gay men fought against the world's intolerance of us, the way we are treated, in just about every way? Why do gay men accept the decisions of others so passively?

■   Are gay men, cooperating with the System, being the "good little boys" we were brought up to be, helping to kill our own? Are organizations like GMHC *in any way* like the Jewish councils set up during World War II to help the Germans exterminate them?

II

In May 1987, prior to my trip to Washington to research my article, I made these notes, using information published in *The New Internationalist,* a British magazine published in Oxford:

The World Health Organization estimates that some 50,000 people around the world have so far died as a result of AIDS, with a further 50,000 terminally ill. To many experts, this figure of 100,000 cases in all is a conservative figure. What we do know, from statistics compiled over five years in many different countries, is that for every full-blown case of AIDS there are *at least* one hundred carriers of the infection who have not as yet developed the disease. Of these one hundred, at least ten already have come down with ARC—AIDS-Related Complex. If we accept the World Health Organization's figure of 100,000 AIDS cases, then this implies that there are a million people in the world with ARC, and 10 million carrying the putative virus. The World Health Organization's 100,000 dead or dying from AIDS today becomes 10 million dead or dying by the year 2000.

And, again, WHO's figure is conservative. Research in Africa strongly suggests that 10 percent of the 100-million population of the worst-affected central zone are now carriers of the putative virus: In other words, there are, at this minute, 10 million infected *in Central Africa alone.* Add to this the infection in the rest of the world, including the United States, with an estimated 2.6 million carriers—also thought to be a very conservative estimate (Dr. Robert Gallo, of the National Cancer Institute, claimed, in the London *Observer* in April *1985,* that two million were already infected)—and we obtain, according to WHO, a current global figure of 15 million or more people infected with the putative virus. All these people are infectious as well as infected, capable of passing on a virus to others with whom they have sexual contact. So 15 million infected today implies a great many more infected a year from now and the year after that. Indeed, the World Health Organization estimates a world total of *100 million* infected within five to ten years.

One year later, at the Fourth International AIDS Conference in Stockholm, these figures have been more than generously confirmed.

I won't dwell on the possibility that troubles me and a few others: that HIV is not the *only* cause of AIDS, that it's possible it isn't, that there's a cofactor, or an additional cause, or additional causes, or that HIV might be only a marker (and a marker not 100-percent present), or not the cause at all. Though many scientists everywhere claim HIV is the only cause, there are a few distinguished ones who now maintain otherwise.

And I won't dwell on this either: That, for reasons I find incomprehensible, the non-African world and the straight white population in America and elsewhere seem to put enormous confidence in an unproved theory: that AIDS cannot happen to them. That something "different" is going on in Africa and gay (and now parts of black and Hispanic) America. That viruses discriminate. (Heterosexual Americans, both white and black, prefer to ignore what's happening in Africa, setting up yet another prejudice.)

And they ignore a proved theory: that this putative virus appears to have an incubating latency of, so far as is known at present, up to twenty years. If this is so, it would not be inconceivable that someone with whom one had sex twenty years ago might have passed along the virus.

Why doesn't it make sense to them that what's happening now in Central Africa began much earlier in time? Why doesn't it make sense to them that gay men's AIDS and drug-related AIDS are just another stage, as Central Africa is an earlier one?

For every "expert" public official who has proclaimed that "the general population" need not be concerned, there's a medical or epidemiological or scientific "expert" (who, more often than not, is not interviewed or on television) who just as emphatically proclaims that a virus has no way of knowing who's black or white or straight or gay.

I don't want this essay to be a compilation of damning statistical predictions. Surely we've learned by now that just about any argument, no matter how extreme, can be supported by "statistics." (I consider most epidemiologists to be, along with insider traders, major gonifs.) At the worst, even providing mountains of horrible evidence, as Jonathan Kozol recently did in preparing his moving and cogent exposé of the homeless in New York City, appears to result in nothing beyond a blizzard of numbers and facts and details falling on an uncaring world. The ability of exposés to ignite action seems to have diminished substantially in recent years. It's almost as if we have not only seen the worst, but we now expect it. It (whatever "it" stands for) is not going to change. There's been a little spurt of a reaction of disgust recently to this Age of Greed we live in, particularly in New York, where the two extremes are extraordinarily noticeable; but it seems only a spurt, and a long way from being revolutionary enough to turn the landowners off their land. The downtrodden are weak, not angry. There doesn't seem to be very much anger around these days, but there is a lot of exhaustion or, worse, acceptance. I watch too many PBS documentaries about those who "fall through the cracks." These documentaries all seem to wind up with someone saying something like, "The future will judge what kind of people we were by how we took care of_____." Fill in the blank with your own favorite set of problems.

In a letter defending herself against an attack "on my political views and my personal motives," the philosopher Hannah Arendt responded: "What Mr. Halpern, like many of our politically interested intellectuals, does not understand is that we deal in politics with warnings and not with prophecies. If I were foolish and resigned enough to play the role of prophet, I certainly should also be content to share his eternal fate, which is to be proved wrong time and again, except at the decisive moment, when it is too late."

The figures I have cited are not prophecies of doom, "only" warnings. Why do people refuse to hear warnings?

Why is it that white heterosexuals prefer not to think about or deal with AIDS? For the African and the black and Hispanic American cases, it's because of racism. For the gay male cases, it's because of homophobia.

III

I wonder why so many gays demand that our lives and experiences be viewed "positively," when in fact we have lived through such horrors to get here. Jews demand, of themselves and the world, constant remembrance of their tortured history. Homosexuals have been hated by religion, state, country, world, and history, by parents and families and peers. (This is a horrible singularity of the gay situation: Can Jews imagine being hated *by their parents* for their Jewishness?) If a writer, gay or straight, attempts to detail the fallout from these experiences in his work, accusations of "self-hate," "negativism," or the worst offense, of course, "homophobia"—which, when leveled by one gay against another, brings the charge full circle back to "self-hate"—are the automatic, knee-jerk responses. Why are we so insistent on wringing only joy and laughter out of our painful history—to such an extreme degree that we now pride ourselves in naming ourselves and what we are "gay"?

Perhaps because I am both, I find it remarkable how many similarities I notice between homosexuals and Jews. I turn for support for these convictions of mine to Hannah Arendt. History recently made a pretty good attempt to destroy the Jewish people, and as I think history now has an opportunity to do (and is already doing) pretty much the same to homosexuals, there are obvious lessons to be learned in a study of her work.

It would be interesting to know what Hannah Arendt (who died in 1975) thought of the Italian chemist and writer, Primo Levi. "Anyone who has been tortured remains tortured," Levi quotes a friend tortured by the Gestapo who committed suicide some thirty years later. Levi, in his last book, *The Drowned and the Saved,* published in 1986, before his own apparent suicide in 1987, attempts to establish hierarchies of innocence and guilt among both the victims and the victimizers. Levi concluded it was possible to be "less guilty." I doubt Arendt would allow this.

It is fascinating how harsh Arendt is in her etiology of modern anti-Semitism. She looks no further than her own front door. As the Princeton professor George Kateb writes in his book, *Hannah Arendt—Politics, Conscience, Evil:* "She argues that antisemitism could not have become the elemental force that it became . . . unless the Jews themselves had something to do with it."

She asks, as I ask of gay people: Why are we so hated? Why are we disliked? Why do we make so many uncomfortable? Why do we particularly offend the "good family man" Arendt describes so disparagingly as the great modern criminal, who would do anything to save his family, up to and including murder (Adolf Eichmann)?

In our case, I can understand some of the reasons for the repugnance felt by the "good family man": to start with, we gays are perceived to have what he doesn't and fantasizes he desires—freedom, sexual choice without commitment, continued unlimited sexual choice (until eight years ago). We are perceived to be utterly and totally promiscuous, even though for most of us this description has always been far from accurate. But again, particularly during and after the "swinging sixties" (and seventies), into which the heterosexual populations were also released with abandon, this stereotype took hold, in full disregard of that overwhelming majority of us who were either in monogamous relationships or just as inept or frightened of sex as everyone else. But it seemed to serve the straight world's purpose, and perhaps our own, to be seen as so sexually athletic. It's certainly more manly than being seen as a sissy.

For reasons as incomprehensible to me as the ancient "reasons" for hating Jews (that they drank the blood of Christian children), I don't understand the irrational fear that apparently grips so many parents of school-age children, that we will "recruit" these children. (And why is there never fear that straight male teachers will seduce little girls?) Study after study has proved that gays are not child molesters, that child molesters are overwhelmingly heterosexual, and yet the belief persists. (Although curiously no one goes after the Catholic Church, where so much of the priesthood *is* gay; I have few Catholic friends who weren't aware of this when they were young. As Dr. Robert J. Stoller remarks in his generally inadequate entry on homosexuality in the *Encyclopaedia Britannica:* "To the church's discomfort, those most able to abstain from heterosexuality may lean toward homosexuality.") I know of no gay people who enjoy seeking sexual relations with someone who is not gay; it simply isn't a gay characteristic. So this myth of recruitment, like the belief that all gay men are promiscuous, must serve some purpose for the straight world—to keep us different and dangerous—and the dangerous must always be watched and rallied against, to the extent of law.

(In those instances where children do have sex with their homosexual elders, be they teachers or anyone else, I submit that often, very often, the child desires the activity, and perhaps even solicits it, either because of a natural curiosity that will or will not develop along these lines, or because he or she is homosexual and innately knows it. This is far from "recruitment." Obviously, there are instances in which the child is unwilling, and is a victim of sexual abuse, homo- or heterosexual. But, as with straight children anxious for the experience with someone of the opposite sex, there are kids who seek, solicit, and consent willingly to sex with someone of the same sex. And, unlike girls or women forced into rape and traumatized, most gay men have warm memories of their earliest and early sexual encounters; when we share these stories with each other, they are invariably positive ones. What has not been positive is our knowledge, from that early date, of the world's disapproval. I realize that this is a very volatile issue, and that this in no way absolves the adult participant of responsibility in colluding in such acts, be it with boys or girls. Nor am I sanctioning sex with children, most of which I personally find as abhorrent as if I was a parent of a child myself. I am just saying that the issue is not so cut-and-dried as many laws and many parents and many righteous moralists maintain.)

As with all kinds of sex, attempts at prevention aren't going to stop them. They only increase the quotient of guilt and self-loathing—results exceptionally costly, both in economic terms and those of mental health. Most gay people knew they were gay from a very early age, whether they acted on it or not. Not only have we always known it, but we also know what many don't wish to hear: that we can't change and, more important, most of us don't want to change—just as heterosexuals can't change and, more important, don't want to change. Why can't society accept what we've known for so long, that sexuality is a *given?* I know I am stating a blasphemous heresy to too many when I say this. I'll be coming back to it later.

Many gay kids are now discovering their homosexuality earlier, accepting it earlier, acting on it earlier, and, mercifully, becoming more comfortable with it earlier. It's now possible for gay kids to know other gay kids (something I never experienced) or, if not actually to know them, at least to see them portrayed on television or read about them in newspapers or novels. It's no longer necessary to think you're the only person in the world with these feelings. Of course, not all of these experiences are going to be positive; there is always going to be peer rejection, for instance. Yet, gradually, there are places for the young to go: youth organizations in cities like New York, and gay high school and college groups. The recent brouhaha that erupted among Yale alumni when an article in *The Wall Street Journal* correctly identified that university as having a large gay student population no doubt will be repeated in a growing number of other centers of higher learning. The still-continuing legal battle between the administration of Georgetown University and the city of Washington, D.C. (which has an antidiscrimination ordinance that protects homosexuals), over whether a gay student organization should be allowed on campus and funded like other student groups, will also no doubt be repeated elsewhere. What is also going to continue is the growing visibility of this young gay population. It becomes increasingly evident that many of them are not going to hide in the closet for most of their lives, as so many of their predecessors have done.

The concept of "manliness" is the stereotypical straight expectation for all males; somehow, all gay men are therefore "sissies." (How gay men hate this word!) As with all stereotypes, there are many examples to prove them true. But there are larger numbers that do not. (In a 1957 study, Dr. Evelyn Hooker demonstrated that less than 10 percent of gay men fulfill any stereotypical category.) Many effeminate men are totally heterosexual, and many gay men are indistinguishable from their straight brothers. But it is the stereotypes which are seen, photographed, televised. When Gay Pride parades are photographed across the country in late June, it's always the few gays in outlandish costumes who catch the eye of the media. The hundreds of thousands who look just like everybody's son or daughter or husband or wife are not so visually titillating.

If all gay men are sissies, the stereotypical reasoning follows, then all gay men wear dresses. This makes little sense. As Brian McNaught, a gay counselor and teacher, points out, why would a *man* who is attracted to *men* and wants to be attractive to *men* wear a dress?

Over the last fifteen years, gay men have worked very hard to change their perceived image. The 1970s were years of "clonedom." Levi 501 jeans (the kind with the button flies), work boots, flannel shirts, mustaches, beards, and bodies heavily muscled from constant gymnasium workouts were all requirements for this look; we *were* the Marlboro men. (Indeed we were the model, the prototype, for the Marlboro man—straight men across the country were soon copying *us,* and now television and movies are filled with the mustached, work-booted, flannel-shirted, muscled "straight" man we made popular. As with the discos and disco music of this era that we also popularized, the gay contribution to popular culture is an area that sociologists have conveniently overlooked.) But, ironically, this new look came to be just as stereotypical as the former swish, limp-wristed model we were so anxious to replace—and the very sight of a group of men wearing work boots, 501's, and mustaches became just as gay-identifying, and just as likely to produce the homophobic response of "look at those faggots." (The standard shot used ad nauseum on television and in photojournalism, when homosexuality or anything about the gay community is discussed, is that of two men, shot from behind, with their arms around each other, their hands on each other's Levied asses.)

Non-Jews also embrace stereotypes when hating Jews: Jews are moneylenders; Jews are criminals; Jews are greedy; Jews are more loyal to each other than to the outside world; Jews, through secret cabals, control the world. All Jews are dark and hirsute. All Jews are Shylock or Fagin. All Jews are smarter, more ambitious. All of these stereotypes could be perceived as being somehow interconnected, pollen from the same plant. They all involve money, greed, power. Even that favorite Christian slander hurled at Jews—that they killed Christ—can be conceived as an attempt to maintain power.

On the surface, gay stereotypes don't seem to blend so well. For instance, at the same time that we are perceived as amusing, decorative, effeminate, and creative (I often think that the entire gay population is considered to be composed of nothing but hairdressers and interior decorators), we are perceived as being sexually threatening to children, or to husbands and wives. It doesn't seem to occur to many that foppishness and sexual prowess are an unlikely combination. And our sexual "threats" seem to provoke peculiar, contrary reactions: I've heard of wives who are far more upset when they lose their husbands to another man than to another woman, when she should be less so—it has little to do with her, or what she might have been or done. But, instead, she often sees this rejection as some sort of challenge: She will "change" him. Indeed, I know straight women who pursue gay men for just this reason (when in actuality this pursuit might reflect the woman's desire not to have a sexual relationship at all). Too, the woman who enjoys the company of the amusing gay man because he is amusing is usually less interested in the straight man because he isn't. (It was Proust who pointed out that the homosexual was one of the few members of society not bored to death and still capable of passions.) The pool of available, eligible, interesting and interested straight men, for some women, is often limited, and they turn to gay male friends for companionship; such women, unkindly termed "fag hags," are seen quite often in large cities like New York. So gay men would seem to serve as less of a threat than a convenience.

Here is a short compilation of responses I've received when I've asked people, both gay and straight, why they think homosexuals are hated. Invariably the first thought is that people hate *difference.* Anything that veers from the norm. Anything that veers from the rigid family way. (It seems slightly ludicrous that gays not procreating should be considered—in this age of woeful overpopulation—as a reason for disapproval.) An inability to perceive differences: They're frightened because they *can't* see us, they can only sense our threat. People aren't flexible in general. (Look at how many churches have boundaries on what is acceptable sex.) They don't see multiple points of view as being an option. They see black and white without many shades of gray in between. We're hitting people where they live their most secret terrors. My niece, Liza, a graduate student in English literature, said, "It's just too threatening: People can't deal with that part of themselves, because I think everybody has homosexual as well as heterosexual feelings." Straights are shackled to their families and family values, which we flagrantly disavow. It's not unlike racism and anti-Semitism or sexism. (Gay women are not nearly so ostracized as gay men. Here is a bit of perverse sexism: women's sexuality is considered unimportant, therefore not a threat.) We go against the theory of capitalism (say some on the gay left): We produce no children to become workers. (But capitalism breaks up the family, sending women and children away from their homes.) Everyone has a *need* for a scapegoat—a way of not facing their own problems and responsibilities. The heterosexual majority must be in control; they're going to oppress all who, in any way, threaten their power (their beliefs).

While each of these reasons could no doubt serve as the basis for an entire book, I think they don't get to the root cause, but are rather manifestations, perhaps even rationalizations, of it.

Hannah Arendt believed quite simply, as Professor Kateb puts it, that "modern antisemitism depends on the character of modern Jews." Arendt talks about the two main Jewish responses to anti-Semitism, the parvenu and the pariah. The parvenu tried to become assimilated at all costs, and the pariah was an outcast, who accepted his position as an outcast. Either way aggravated anti-Semitism.

Arendt begins *Antisemitism,* the first part of her monumental trilogy *The Origins of Totalitarianism,* with a thought so simple as to be shocking. Who has ever thought of this?: "There is hardly an aspect of contemporary history more irritating and mystifying than the fact that of all the great unsolved political questions of our century, it should have been this seemingly small and unimportant Jewish problem that had the dubious honor of setting the whole infernal machine in motion." The "infernal machine" obviously is World War II. By then European Jews had long since lost what power they had accumulated, despite the Nazis' claim that it was Jewish world political power that must serve as the pretext for killing them off. Arendt goes all the way back to "Tocqueville's great discovery" that "wealth without visible function is much more intolerable because nobody can understand why it should be tolerated." Translated to the situation prior to World War II, this meant: "Antisemitism reached its climax when Jews had similarly lost their public functions and their influence, and were left with nothing but their wealth."

Arendt makes a clear distinction between anti-Semitism and Jew-hating, which always existed but, in those years of Jewish power, only on an unofficial, behind-the-back basis. When Jews lost this power, it was all right for Jew-hating to be officially codified as anti-Semitism. So long as any group has power, it's not in the majority's interest to crucify or cremate its members. But "wealth without power or aloofness without a policy are felt to be parasitical, useless, revolting, because such conditions cut all the threads which tie men together."

For a moment, Arendt turns aside: "Just as antisemites

understandably desire to escape responsibility for their deeds, so Jews, attacked and on the defensive, even more understandably do not wish under any circumstances to discuss their share of responsibility." Why are Jews responsible? Because they "avoided all political action for two thousand years." They are a people without a government, without a country, without one language. Despite the elements of their faith, which did contain well-defined concepts of history and moral philosophy, they spent two thousand years avoiding anything remotely resembling political action to defend and protect themselves or their beliefs. "The result was that the political history of the Jewish people became even more dependent upon unforeseen, accidental factors than the history of other nations, so that the Jews stumbled from one role to the other and accepted responsibility for none." Since they never fought back, it became increasingly easy to punish, torture, and scapegoat them.

I think it can quite easily be maintained that gay people have been marching around the earth for just as long. We have not been united in the same way as Jews, although, as John Boswell, Professor of History at Yale, writes so cogently in his *Christianity, Social Tolerance, and Homosexuality*, once upon a time homosexuals were a distinct group, before the centuries of going underground. "Few classicists," Boswell writes, "have doubted that homosexuality occupied a prominent and respected position in most Greek and Roman cities at all levels of society and among a substantial portion of the population." Indeed, in ancient Greece, "many . . . writers use homosexual love as an ideal to which heterosexual lovers might aspire." In ancient Rome, "if Gibbon was right, the Roman Empire was ruled for almost two hundred consecutive years by men whose homosexual interests, if not exclusive, were sufficiently noteworthy to be recorded for posterity."

Concerning the "cause" of homosexuality, Professor Boswell has this to say: "There are in fact no explanations in any classical literature for homosexual desire, which everyone apparently considered ubiquitous and entirely ordinary." And this: "It should be noted that what 'causes' homosexuality is an issue of importance only to societies which regard gay people as bizarre or anomalous. Most people do not wonder what 'causes' statistically ordinary characteristics, like heterosexual desire or right-handedness; 'causes' are sought only for personal attributes which are assumed to be outside the ordinary pattern of life. Since very few in the ancient world considered homosexual behavior odd or abnormal, comments about its etiology were quite rare."

Boswell is also interested in comparing Jews and gays. "The fate of Jews and gay people has been almost identical throughout European history, from early Christian hostility to extermination in concentration camps. The same laws which oppressed Jews oppressed gay people; the same groups bent on eliminating Jews tried to wipe out homosexuality; the same periods of European history which could not make room for Jewish distinctiveness reacted violently against sexual nonconformity; the same countries which insisted on religious uniformity imposed majority standards of sexual conduct; and even the same methods of propaganda were used against Jews and gay people—picturing them as animals bent on the destruction of the children of the majority."

Boswell also mentions what he considers significant differences: Judaism is passed on consciously from parents to children, while gay people "suffer oppression individually and alone, without benefit of advice or frequently even emotional support from relatives or friends."

It is this same aloneness that many psychiatrists insist on using for their paradigm in not only repressing comparisons between the development of Jews and gay people, but also in denying gays anything approaching mental health and social equality. Therapists seem to compile identical lists: Gays did not have families to support them through the years of terror; we had no role models; we were rejected by our parents—in the case of gay men particularly by our fathers; we had so many early rejections from all and sundry as to think ourselves "dirty" and, indeed, morally wrong; therefore we have difficulty forming satisfactory relations with either one another or society; therefore we are ashamed of our homosexuality and hide it.

I submit that it's too easy to use this catalogue of possible truths to flog the mental health of homosexuals. There are Jewish families that are ashamed of being Jewish, that do not support each other against the world's intolerance of their differences, and instead try in every way to be accepted by those in majority. This is Arendt's own point, when she views parvenus with such antagonism: They, too, are denying who they are with misguided determination. Does this send them all to analytic couches? Did this make them sick in the eyes of psychiatry?

No, whatever else they were called, Jews were never thought of as "sick" by the majority, nor Judaism an illness. Where did this notion of homosexuality as an "illness" come from, and why has it persisted for so long? Boswell traces many centuries of "reasons." Most of them emanated from established religions, or from the seats of ruling power (which could, of course, be one and the same) and most of them had to do, not with the fear of "difference" cited by those I questioned, but with a determination on the part of an established interest to cement absolute power. But I am less interested in those early tyrants than in modern ones.

Freud himself considered homosexuality more an inconvenience than anything else. In an often-quoted letter to a worried mother, he said it would be easier, the world being the way it is, if one did not have to be homosexual. (One of these days, somebody ought to research fully Freud's own exceptionally close attachment to Wilhelm Fliess. It was certainly much more than just a friendship, and perhaps, noting this in himself, Freud passed on to other subjects for his scrutiny.) Dr. Stoller, in his *Encyclopaedia Britannica* article, (my edition is that of 1975), refers to "Freud's statement that all human beings possess undercurrents of homosexuality because they are biologically and thus psychologically bisexual." Why, then, did modern psychoanalysis take it upon itself to metamorphose "inconvenience"—indeed, "bisexual" tendencies—into illness? When did "the medicalization of homosexuality" take such a strong hold? The term "homosexual" appears to date from the late nineteenth century; the supplement (not published until 1976) to the unabridged *Oxford English Dictionary* (the main *OED*, published in 1933, does not include it) cites its first appearance as in *Psychopathia Sexualis* by Dr. Richard von Krafft-Ebing, a German neuropsychiatrist and early student of sexual psychopathology. That "ground-breaking examination of sexual aberrations" *(Encyclopaedia Britannica)*—in which just about everything except heterosexual intercourse in the missionary position is made to sound sufficient to ensure incarceration in the local nuthouse—was published in 1886.

It is my opinion that matters took a distinct turn for the worse with the arrival on these shores, from about 1930 on, of Freud's "children," mostly German analysts and mostly Jewish, in need of scapegoats of their own, and finding no others (particularly no others in numbers able to afford their services), they slowly institutionalized us homosexuals, in one way if not another. These German doctors were refugees themselves, and their own insecurities forged a great need to prove to the New World that they would fit in completely. It is perversely interesting to record that, of all the branches of modern therapy, most of which have come to accept the existence of so many gay people as sufficient evidence that nothing sick or abnormal is going on, the entrenched Freudians, in their network of Psychoanalytic Institutes located in each major American geographical area, are still the aggressive purveyors of this homosexuality-as-illness theme. (Boswell, in an unpublished paper, makes a very convincing comparison between today's psychiatrists and yesterday's priests; both have looked upon themselves as the only authorized keepers of the world's "morality.") How truly perverse: The persecuted now turned into persecutors.

That we gays don't pass on our "religion" from generation to generation is also, like aloneness, not a sufficient reason for preventing comparison with Jews. It is more than balanced by the fact that—no matter what methods are utilized to deny or expunge us—10 percent of any and every population will fall into Kinsey's homosexual category. So we are, in essence, self-perpetuating in a way even more reliable than the Jews' religious instruction of their young, which is not always so automatically self-perpetuating as Jewish elders like to think.

Most psychiatric literature, it seems to me, is written by men and women based only on their observations of those who come for treatment. There are many heterosexuals who had poor role models, were rejected by one or both parents, were rejected by many, all, or sundry, and who thought themselves "dirty" for one reason or another. Some become neurotic; many don't. The continued insistence by those who should now know

better, like my brother and sister-in-law (for at last the psychiatric literature now has a growing number of works to refute
it), that homosexuality is "caused" by an over-possessive
mother and a rejecting or absent father, is no longer tolerable.
Some 24 million gay men and women cannot all be here because
of bad parenting: The number is simply too huge. I know too
many gay men who loved their fathers and were loved by them
in return. Or who had no mothers. Or who rejected the mothers
they had. I know too many gay men and women who had and
continue to have warm and loving families. I know plenty who
haven't, but I know plenty of heterosexuals who haven't either.
Homosexuality is not, in and of itself, the problem that causes
gay people to seek treatment. It is the world's response to
homosexuality. That and that alone is the "trouble" with homosexuality.

This response continues to be inhumanly perplexing in the
light of so many scientific studies by notable academics, studies
that have been generally accepted as valid. Dr. Alfred Kinsey,
in 1948, startled the world with figures that have yet to be
attacked or disproved. He said that 10 percent of American men
were pretty much homosexual, that 4 percent of American men
were exclusively homosexual, that 37 percent of American men
had had a homosexual experience leading to orgasm post-pu-
berty, and that 50 percent of American men have homosexual
fantasies. Studies by Clellan S. Ford and Frank A. Beach, an
anthropologist and a psychologist, found, in 1951, that homosexuality was accepted as normal in 64 percent of primitive
societies, and in 1957, that homosexuality exists in every species of every mammal and that as the cortex of the brain develops, i.e., as creatures get smarter, the percentage of
homosexuals increases. (This latter study is cited by Brian
McNaught in *On Being Gay.*)

Surely it makes sense that if all mammals can be homosexual so naturally, these acts must be innate rather than learned.
At least it does to me. Why is heterosexuality considered innate, an existential given, and not homosexuality? Or, if homosexuality is *learned,* why isn't heterosexuality *learned?*
Homosexuality's attackers can't have their cake and eat it too.
Even some gay people are unwilling to concede that they were
born gay. One friend of mine says, "Your sexuality is deter-

mined by your third year." But another friend rebuts: "I know some three-year-olds who sure know how to dress."

Homosexuals are born, just as heterosexuals are born. This is what I think, feel, know, and there has been no evidence to prove otherwise.

I offer this rephrasing of Arendt's notion: There is hardly an aspect of contemporary history more irritating and mystifying than the fact that of all the great unsolved political questions of our century, it should have been this seemingly small and unimportant problem of homosexuality that had the dubious honor of setting the whole infernal machine in motion. Only this time the "infernal machine" is the AIDS holocaust.

People hate victims, because they see in them something they're terrified of becoming: themselves as victims. People hate others for not doing what they themselves also feel powerless to do. All of this is embedded in the nineteenth-century origins of anti-Semitism. European society and Western Jewry disintegrated and declined pretty much together; there was no balance of power between nations; there was no cooperation between countries; and "the non-national, inter-European Jewish element became an object of universal hatred because of its useless wealth, and of contempt because of its lack of power," both of which were now "atomized into a herd of wealthy individuals." Powerless non-Jews came to look upon wealthy Jews not exercising the power commensurate with their wealth as parasites.

I think that many heterosexuals look upon today's homosexuals in much the same way. Compared to most people, we appear to have large disposable incomes, we appear to exercise few family or community responsibilities, we appear to be entirely frivolous and, until recently, utterly hedonistic, and this hedonism has resulted in AIDS, which we are now expecting the straight world to take care of immediately. Is it any wonder that there is little sympathy for gay people and their plight? This is Arendt's very point about the Jewish situation prior to World War II.

For gays, this might appear in many ways a double-edged sword, a situation of damned if you do, damned if you don't. We hide because we know "they" don't like us; by our hiding, "they" hate us even more. And the more we try to emerge from our cocoon and into full view, the stronger are the forces prepared to slap us down and into hiding again. (I think it no coincidence that the Jesse Helms amendment, refusing AIDS funding to any organization that "advocated" or "promoted" homosexuality, came immediately following the October 1987 March on Washington of some 650,000 gay men and lesbians.) It's at this crucial juncture that we must realize that only by capitalizing, in the many meanings of this word, on our coming forth, can we save ourselves: When we capitalize on the power inherent in our numbers, when we demand recognition in return for this power, only then will we not be murdered.

One of the richest men in America is gay; he is president of one of the largest and wealthiest financial institutions in the world; he is not known to be gay and shudders at the thought that he'll be identified and revealed. This situation is repeated across the country; in corporations, in banks, in businesses, in family fortunes. If these gay men could unite, surely their voices would be heard and answered in the corridors of power.

It is now a truism that every gay man who stays in the closet is helping to kill the rest of his fellow gay men. Yet, instead of provoking anger and hatred on the part of those who are "out" against those still hiding within, it has fostered protection. We all have our oppression in common and, like Vietnam veterans, we've all been through various versions of the same war. We'll take care of each other—even if, now, we are taking care of those who help kill us. Their secret is safe with us.

I know there is historical reason for this—that the rite of coming out is a precious and individual one, and that, in memory of the pain it often entailed for so many, we honor each person's privacy. But for a growing number of gay people, the maintenance of this protection is becoming increasingly more difficult to sanction, either philosophically or pragmatically.

I offer as an example the late Terry Dolan, founder of the National Conservative Political Action Committee, a PAC devoted exclusively to raising money for the conservative agenda and right-wing congresspersons in league with fundamentalist religions and Reverend Jerry Falwell. Terry was gay, he lived with a lover, he even had an affair with one of my friends; he was a frequent visitor to the New York disco, bathhouse, and Fire Island scenes; he moved comfortably in the Washington gay political community because he knew they would not expose his homosexuality—even as he raised millions of dollars for the enemies of gay people. When a book came out, *God's Bullies* by Perry Deane Young, in which Dolan's homosexuality was revealed, his "heterosexuality" was defended by no less a voice than William Safire, who, in his regular column in *The New York Times*, sharply criticized Young, or anyone, for using such "lies" to discredit Dolan, or any prominent person, and his work. When gays attempted to get a rebuttal to Safire printed in the *Times,* and, when the *Times* refused, in the *Washington Post,* it was not possible to do so. At a gay cocktail party in Washington, I confronted Terry and condemned him for taking so much from our community and repaying us in such a monstrous fashion. I did not expect to be congratulated by the others in attendance, but I certainly did not expect to be condemned by them, which is just what happened. In Washington, one does not criticize one's enemies, even if they are one's own. When Dolan died, from AIDS, his brother, who is a speechwriter in the Reagan White House, attempted to suppress an article that appeared in *Regardies* magazine by *Wall Street Journal* staff writer Ellen Hume, which contained the truth about both his brother's homosexuality and his death from AIDS.

Eight years into an epidemic that has gone largely untended because it is perceived as happening to gays, *and* because gays have not sufficiently demanded the attention it deserves, we witness the tragic spectacle of many tens of thousands dead and many millions infected. It is hard to escape the fact that we gays are helping to kill off our future by protecting this rule of silence. It becomes increasingly difficult, and morally impossible, to sit by silently and watch elected officials (not to mention prominent church leaders) across the nation, whom we know to be closeted gay men or lesbians, as they not only deny their heritage but bend over backwards *not* to help in gay emergencies, lest this very aid, by extension, identify them.

The closeted are also protected by the media and the press, even though it is not against any law to name anyone as gay if that person is gay, if that person has disclosed it publicly, or, as is most important in the case of public officials, if their work in the public arena is compromised by their denying their homosexuality. Terry Dolan would have been a particularly good example of this, should any reporter (other than Young) have had the courage to write his story honestly while Dolan was still alive. But reporters don't discuss a person's homosexuality, not because they or their papers are afraid of lawsuits (which are rarely brought), but because they are worried about offending sources or making themselves personae non gratae.

Representative Barney Frank of Massachusetts, before he came out publicly, had for some time acknowledged privately to many reporters that he was gay; but reporters didn't report it because they thought that he would be offended. If they had reported it, they could not have been sued because (1) it was true, and (2) he regularly debated gay issues publicly. Therefore his sexuality would have been relevant to public understanding of his participation in the debate. As I said, it is no secret to many gays that many of the most important politicians and government bureaucrats forced into dealing with AIDS are doing their work badly, if at all, because they are in the closet, and we cannot get the press to help us expose them.

The battle days of libel cases just for naming a person homosexual are largely gone. That was the legal world that destroyed Oscar Wilde, and it existed until about 1970, when the first mainstream debates in society about homosexuality and the gay rights movement also commenced. Saying someone is gay who *is* gay no longer constitutes defamation or slander or libel. You cannot defame someone by telling the truth. But the press has not caught on or caught up.

So it still comes back to the point that homosexuality is considered something negative. The many of us who are so proud of homosexuality are at the mercy of the many more who aren't. And the law still does protect closeted gays who aren't in the position of politicians or church leaders dealing with gay issues. To name a movie star as gay, even if he or she is (unless he or she debated gay issues), is considered an invasion of privacy. The law doesn't protect Jews denying their Jewishness. Could one imagine the gay actor-playwright Harvey Fierstein getting away with suing someone because he was called a heterosexual?

Homosexuals always seem to be considered entirely as artistic. It comes as a surprise to find Arendt writing, in her essay,

"The Jew as Pariah": "When it comes to claiming its own in the field of European arts and letters, the attitude of the Jewish people may best be described as one of reckless magnanimity. With a grand gesture and without a murmur of protest it has calmly allowed the credit for its great writers and artists to go to other peoples, itself receiving in return (in punctilious regular payments) the doubtful privilege of being acclaimed father of every notorious swindler and mountebank."

It is presently no different for gays. Roy Cohn is identified as gay; John Maynard Keynes is not. Burgess and Maclean are identified as gay; J. Edgar Hoover is not. Boy George is identified as gay; Cole Porter and Lorenz Hart are not.

It appears impossible for homosexuals to claim our own. We "honor" the closetedness of the living. Or we identify our renowned dead, and no journalist, historian, or academic will publish our identification. In the case of the famous dead, like Whitman or Leonardo da Vinci or Michelangelo, some "proof" is required—for everyone since time began is declared heterosexual unless *proved* otherwise. It is not sufficient for us to respond to such questions as "Can you prove he was homosexual?" with our own, "Can you prove he wasn't?" So we are denied our heritage. We are denied the most potent weapons to prove our own worth both to ourselves and to the world.

At the end of his life, Christopher Isherwood urged every homosexual of some authority to reveal his homosexuality. Of all the major widely published poets over fifty, only Allen Ginsberg, Richard Howard, and James Merrill have done so. There can't be just three major gay poets over fifty.

IV

Homosexuals are at an historic moment in our own emergence, and we have been so placed, I would estimate, for ten to fifteen years. When I was a child, I thought I was the only homosexual in the world. When I was a student at Yale, I thought I was one of only a few. Now I have concrete and visible confirmation that I am one of tens of millions, one in eight, one in ten, one of twenty-four million—whichever estimate, they are all comforting. We are here, and seen to be here, and known to be here, more than ever. Beginning with the mid-1970s, much to our surprise and gratification, mental, spiritual, and sexual, we began to take full note of this.

As gays become more visible, we provoke more hatred. As I said, we have, in many cases, comfortable disposable incomes that allow us to live well and deny ourselves little in the way of consumer goods. (Of course, there are poor gays, but, whatever our income, we often have little to spend it on but ourselves.) We have, in most cases, no responsibilities raising children. If we find old houses in marginal neighborhoods and remodel them, thus revitalizing that neighborhood, we're a threat to those living there already. We appear as leeches: taking much from the world but putting little back into it (always excepting our taxes, conveniently overlooked by our critics; and we have historically asked little in return for these annual contributions), though when we try to do so, we are hated even more for our very attempts and visibility. Or our perceived "freedom." My sister-in-law, Alice, once said to me that she was jealous of my life in many ways: I could do what I wanted to do, while her life is circumscribed by a large suburban estate, partnering a successful lawyer in his social and professional endeavors (which are more than a little intertwined), raising and instructing three children in the ways of their world, with little time for herself, while I have nothing but time for myself.

Like Jews, homosexuals historically have had little interest in power. We never think of exercising it, or indeed that we possess it. Of course, this comes from centuries of having no political experience, even though these centuries were eons of tension, ostracism, and, quite often, extermination because we were what we are. We have failed to notice that these centuries also allowed us, as they still do, great possibilities for the use of power, so large are our numbers, as they have always been.

If a reporter wished a quote on women's rights, or the black reaction to anything, the reporter would have at his fingertips a list of many prominent respondents, most of whom have national recognition. One thinks immediately of Gloria Steinem or Betty Friedan, or Jesse Jackson or Barbara Jordan. In all of gay history, there has never been a gay name with national recognition, not at least while he or she was alive.

Why has it been impossible for the huge numbers of homosexuals, in this country and this world, to foster, nurture, and produce such visible leadership?

There are practical reasons: There's no money to be made as a gay leader—it doesn't lead to election to political office anywhere; it doesn't provide a substantial living, because few are the organizations to run and even lower their budgets to pay anyone; nor is it necessarily good for business, unlike, say, being a politician in New York, which has recently enabled so many to make so much. It only leads to aggravation, and eventually to desperation and futility—not only for these reasons, but also because the gay population itself has thus far evinced little interest in participating in what few gay political organizations there are.

The few gay men and lesbians actively involved in the political process, in their so far unsuccessful attempts to make their words heard, thus find themselves scrambling for the few constituents and meager territory available. This has given rise not to cooperation among themselves, but to distrust, anger, and backbiting. Few are able to withstand the toil and anguish of this fighting; the frustrating disillusionment, when realization finally dawns that their inspiration has not been sufficient to attract a crowd and exhaustion sets in, has robbed us of many important voices. The average length of time a person is able to step forth with the best of intentions before being struck down by lassitude or fury seems to be a few years at the most. (San Francisco Supervisor Harvey Milk, the first openly gay person ever elected to public office, was assassinated.)

Any leader not only has to have a message—certainly not hard to come up with—but he or she has to have the ability to raise funds and attract enough supporters. No openly gay leader working for a gay organization has been successful at these tasks, nationally, or for very long.

The National Gay and Lesbian Task Force has a mailing list of 13,000 members. The Human Rights Campaign Fund mails to 22,000. National Gay Rights Advocates mails to 18,000. Lambda Legal Defense and Education fund has 15,000. And a large proportion of these members are the same—i.e., many of us belong to two or more of these organizations. With a potential 24 million joiners, plus supportive friends and families, and with the AIDS crisis threatening us more each day, these are our *largest* political organizations. (We seem able only to summon large numbers to march in parades, which, of course, provide protection for anonymity.) The gay community has nothing like a National Organization of Women, a B'nai B'rith, an NAACP. Even Gay Men's Health Crisis, headquartered in the city worst afflicted with AIDS, and with an estimated one million gay people to draw from, has been able to attract only 1,800 volunteers, a number of them heterosexual women. Sixty-eight percent of GMHC's charitable donations come from heterosexual donors. This is an even more remarkable fact to contemplate when it is realized that 80 percent of GMHC's $12 million total annual budget comes from charitable donations. So much for the perception of successful AIDS fundraising from gays.

Though we lack charismatic leaders with national recognition, we have a superabundance of part-time leaders, dropping in and out of running organizations, depending on their energy and the organization's health. Unfortunately, as in any community where there are many scrambling for the same dollar and the same constituents, there is much territorial infighting—with little realization that there's enough for all if only cooperation and alliances could be forged. Gay organizations in every major city seem eventually to fall victim to endemic bitchiness and bitterness. The very sarcasm that makes gay humor so amusing is also the potent weapon that stabs us to death. And people who should plug into these organizations don't: lawyers, accountants, teachers, doctors; at a time of national emergency it's the professional skills that are needed most.

The backbiting and backstabbing are horrendous, and perhaps typical of most marginal political groups, particularly those on the left—all fighting each other and not the issue, and all being politically ineffective.

When a population cannot even prevent scurrilous attacks on it from appearing in the press, how could it ever mobilize against something like AIDS? A recent issue of *New York Woman* contained comments from the columnist Jimmy Breslin about *Burn This,* a Broadway play by the gay writer Lanford Wilson. "I thought the play was written by a faggot, it's a fag play written for fags. . . . Faggoty—oh, they love fag plays. Anything with latent homosexuality scores big, because that's the strain in this city. You have little unmarried guys building big buildings." That a major New York columnist, late of the *News* and now of *Newsday,* would say anything like this in print, and that a publication would then publish it, shows the extent of our weakness. What paper would publish a description of *Fences* as "a nigger play written for niggers"? Or of *A Shayna Maidel* as "a kike play written for kikes"? Or what newspaper would ask anti-Semites their opinions of a Jewish parade down Fifth Avenue, or note the words on placards racists were holding on the sidelines of a black march, as the *Times* felt compelled to include vicious anti-gay slogans purveyed by no more than twelve along a parade of over 100,000 on Gay Pride Day?

I recently spoke with Vivian Shapiro, the former co-chair of Human Rights Campaign Fund, which, in an era of the declining importance of PACs, is now America's ninth largest one. (HRCF made contributions to the campaigns of politicians they deemed helpful and friendly toward gay issues; unfortunately, a number of the candidates found it embarrassing to receive this money, so concentration has now been turned toward funding several full-time lobbyists in Washington. The entire gay population supports only six lobbyists.) Vivian is popular, an excellent speaker, and an effective fundraiser. After four years of intense political activism, which found her constantly traveling back and forth across the country, to the detriment of her job (she is vice-president of a successful firm that represents major metropolitan newspapers and sells advertising space for them), Shapiro suddenly quit gay politics. "You've got to be a lunatic to volunteer to do this. You lose your personal life. You're exhausted. If you care, you're worried all the time. You don't sleep. You wake up in the middle of the night—until one day you wake up and ask yourself, 'Why am I one of only so few doing this?' And you finally quit in guilt and grief."

This situation repeated that of an earlier promising gay leader, Virginia Apuzzo, who headed the National Gay and Lesbian Task Force for three years. One of the most inspirational speakers in the memories of many, she was unable either to build her membership or to attract donations substantial enough to retire an ever-increasing debt. Finally, one day she left to take a position working in Consumer Affairs for Governor Cuomo.

"Nobody knows what to do anymore," Shapiro says. "I used to think I knew. I just don't know now. I can't personally force 24 million people to come out of the closet."

For a while, San Francisco was the gays' Israel. For decades, gays migrated there, and in time they attained great power in the political structure of that city. No mayor there would consider *not* consulting with gay leaders. And this gay power was sufficient to keep most local heterosexual opposition in check. Tragically, with the devastation of AIDS, gay power in San Francisco has waned considerably: Many of the leaders have died.

Where do we go? We don't have Zionism as a hopeful haven from the world's hatred of us. And, as Arendt pointed out, Zionism's solution was not one of fighting anti-Semitism on its own ground, that is, wherever it existed, but to escape it, "denying the Jewish part of responsibility for existing conditions" in the first place, and sinking "to the assumption, as arbitrary as it is absurd, that every Gentile living with Jews must become a conscious or subconscious Jew-hater." "The upbuilding of Palestine has little to do with answering the anti-Semites; at most it has 'answered' the secret self-hatred and lack of self-confidence on the part of those Jews who have themselves consciously or unconsciously succumbed to some parts of anti-Semitic propaganda." Perhaps homosexuals should be grateful that we're relieved from setting up our own nation-state, though the relief from such an affiliation obliges us to an even sterner battle.

It is, of course, this battle that I think we are losing.

"Every pariah," Arendt declares, "who refused to be a rebel was partly responsible for his own position and therewith for the blot on mankind which it represented. From such shame there was no escape. . . . For insofar as man is more than a mere creature of nature, more than a mere product of Divine creativity, insofar will he be called to account for the things which men do to men in the world which they themselves condition."

Are we at just such a juncture in the development of homosexual emergence into political stability and power? As I mentioned, this notion that every closeted gay person is the single most important hindrance to the achievement of this goal by those out of the closet is something said so often that it has become meaningless. The words, the plea, continue to remain insufficiently inspiring. The gay writer Edmund White, in mock despair, once announced that of the 24 million gays that are supposed to inhabit America, no more than 100,000 were openly so and no more than five thousand of these were politically active.

My friend Robert Prager wrote me from San Diego: "But what is the correct course of action in the world where the worst has happened and is happening?" This is not such a peculiar question as it sounds when one is asking gays to engage in civil disobedience *against* someone. That "someone" quite often receives sympathy for the "persecution" he's receiving at the hands of the hated homos. A candidate who might in fact be sympathetic to gay causes will arrange to be picketed by gays so that he will appeal to the homophobic vote. Rumors of just this sort of strategy on the part of Governor Michael Dukakis have been reported in the gay press. "Oh, I can't vote for homosexuals, a homosexual issue. I'll get killed at home if I vote for those homosexuals": These are the words that liberal Senator Tom Harkin (D.-Iowa) used to chide his fellow senators for their bigotry, hoping to get them to vote against an amendment that would remove an antidiscrimination (against gays) clause from a D.C. ordinance (the Georgetown University case mentioned earlier). The amendment passed overwhelmingly.

In his book, Professor Kateb describes what Hannah Arendt most prized: "Freedom exists only when citizens engage in political action. . . . Arendt's mission as a philosopher is to attempt the recovery of the idea of political action in a culture that she thinks has (except episodically) lost the practice of it and in which almost all philosophy is united, if in nothing else, in denying intrinsic value to it."

The word "political" has, for most gay people, uncomfortable innuendos and repercussions. It suggests we must be obstreperous, obnoxious, rebellious—and visible. We must confront a system that does not want to accept us. For most gay people, the recent decades, even the present one—providing we are not ill with AIDS ourselves; and most gay people mercifully still fall within this category—have been good ones. There appears to be a margin of acceptance, and tolerance enough; no one is yet coming to haul us, as a group, into the streets or march us off to camps. This is comfort enough for most. For those with financial capital, the Reagan years have been generous, and gays, like most people, vote their pocketbooks. Better to accept this existence, most feel, than to make waves and endanger it.

It is overwhelmingly difficult, almost impossible, to change this way of thinking. It is useless constantly to cite references to the dangers into which this attitude led the European Jews. Gays do not identify with Jews, any more than Jews identify with gays. And most Americans, certainly, believe that we've all arrived at a more tolerant time in history, that Santayana's lesson has been learned, and that we can't go back again. To suggest that we most assuredly can is considered, by many gays, ridiculous hyperbole.

In the same way that the creation of Israel was an attempt by the Jews to take control of their lives—and by so doing actually withdrawing themselves from those geographical-political areas where they were most hated, while still thinking that they were doing no such thing, so the institution, growth, and proliferation of myriad AIDS organizations has been considered by many gays as a conscious, positive, creative political response, indeed a historic one, to fight against oppression. Only now do we realize, too late, as did the Jews, that the powerlessness remains. I don't know how many of the hundreds of volunteers to GMHC and its fellow satellites across the country actually thought, when signing up, that they could help change the course of this epidemic "politically," a word as much anathema to them as it was to millions of Jews before the war, but I'm certain they considered this contribution of their time and energy as a step in this direction—certainly a more "political" act than most of them had ever participated in for any gay cause in their pasts. I believe that for most of them there was some sort of inchoate, unverbalized, perhaps even unconscious, but nevertheless existing notion inside them that, somewhere, there were leaders, there was leadership—somewhere in the hierarchy of the organization, with its board of directors and honorary directors and numerous well-known contributors and supporters—which would be on the front lines, in Washington, or New York City, or Albany, or Sacramento, petitioning for all the requisite materiel for winning the war.

I doubt that it occurred to any of these volunteers that GMHC (and its fellow AIDS organizations across the country) has actually made it easier for the system to ignore gays and AIDS. (Theodor Herzl, the founder of Zionism, once described Jewish charity as "a mechanism for keeping the needy in subjection." This is cited by Ron H. Feldman in his excellent collection of Arendt's miscellaneous writings, *The Jew as Pariah.*) These community self-help organizations have removed a huge burden of responsibility from the local, state, and federal governments. The services they are diligently providing are services these governments *should be providing.* Indeed, contributors are paying twice for these services, the first time in their taxes.

But, people protest, if GMHC et al. didn't provide these services, no one would be providing them. Perhaps. But not providing such services—including crisis counseling; legal, welfare, and ombudsman advisers; group therapies of many sorts; and community education—would long since have shamed an administration into its duty. Obviously some people aren't going to sit by and uncomplainingly let their friends die. But it doesn't seem to register that if you're going to do something yourself to alleviate the problem because your government refuses to, you have to protest *twice* as much against that government inaction. Not complain less, but complain more. As Arendt wrote to support her thesis: "The simple truth is that Jews will have to fight anti-Semitism everywhere or else be exterminated everywhere."

Even with AIDS, where there is an emergency that far surpasses such other gay problems as immigration, adoption, discrimination, anti-gay violence (although these also are endemic to AIDS), the organizations that have been founded discover in very short order that a conservative attitude is the first thing to arrive in the board room as soon as minimal success in numbers and dollars has been achieved. Gone immediately are all the original intentions to fight to make the system accountable. As organizations such as GMHC attract prominent closeted lawyers or wealthy heterosexual socialites, conservatism becomes even more entrenched than when the organization was run by inexperienced, naïve, young gay volunteers, who, at least, had fury on their side and anger as their original agenda.

What has happened, of course, and this applies to all governmental agencies as well, is that energy is being converted to *managing* the crisis, turning the crisis into a condition, something that is a part of the way things are, something that happens like a flood or hurricanes or poverty—to be managed, thus creating new bureaucracies. The very source of the problem is ignored and negated. As Randy Shilts, author of *And the Band Played On*—a book filled with as much damning evidence on AIDS being ignored as Jonathan Kozol's *Rachel and Her Children* is filled with facts on the ignoring of the homeless—said, "AIDS didn't just happen. It was allowed to happen."

All these AIDS organizations are *managing* AIDS. No one is trying to *stop* it. It is impossible now, and has been impossible from the very beginning, to get the ear of our President, our mayor, our governor, any of the Presidential candidates (with the honorable exception of Jesse Jackson), or indeed that of the two most important government officials in charge: Dr. Otis Bowen, the director of the Department of Health and Human Resources, and Dr. James Wyngaarden, the director of the National Institutes of Health, both of whom have been singularly silent on the issue. What Dr. Mathilde Krim, the founding co-chair of the American Foundation for AIDS Research, said from the very beginning must not be forgotten: "This is an epidemic that could have been contained. Everything about this epidemic has been utterly predictable, from the very beginning, from the very first day. But no one would listen. There are many people who knew exactly what was happening, what would happen and has happened, but no one of any importance would listen. They still won't listen. We definitely could have contained it."

It seems not to occur to an organization that has placed the wife of one of New York's wealthiest men, with connections at the White House itself, on its board—as GMHC has so placed Joan Tisch, wife of Preston Tisch, Reagan's former Postmaster General—that the thing to do would be to have this wife or, even better, her husband, deliver a plea to the President. If they are thinking of this possibility, they are not acting on it. I have been unable to understand why Elizabeth Taylor, AmFar's other co-chair, for all her considerable devotion to the AIDS fight, never achieved a personal meeting with Ronald Reagan, certainly someone she knows or has access to as a fellow performer, if nothing else. Such a meeting—scheduled as it would be with a list of requests, and publicized as it should be to let the world know whether it was granted or not—would do far greater good than hours of fundraising in Miami Beach.

Gays are certainly not alone in disdaining political action. Arendt, in *The Human Condition,* traces this disparagement all the way back to an early and continuing fundamental doctrine of the Christian faith—a faith that insists on the possibility of eternal life, which "brought hope to those who knew that their world was doomed, indeed a hope beyond hope, since the new message promised an immortality they never had dared to hope for. This reversal could not but be disastrous for the esteem and the dignity of politics." Kateb says, "The desire to substitute the inner life for a worldly life is understandable, but for Arendt unforgivable." This same desire is no doubt partly responsible for many of the noble deeds of sacrifice offered up by countless volunteers. (It is also no doubt partly responsible for the fatalistic attitude of so many: "If I'm going to go, I'm going to go.")

I don't know if gay people are "more religious" than non-gays. I do think there is such an amazing compliance with the rules of the world, and how it is run, and such an extreme avoidance of upsetting apple carts, as to be traced, less to centuries of religion, than to childhoods of being raised as good little boys and girls, obedient to parents and school and church. We knew we were different, and we knew we were hateful to institutions, and this resulted only in our denying our naturalness, not in our confronting the institutions that hated us. Gay children will often attempt suicide rather than tell their parents about their homosexuality; "I don't want to hurt them" is the unvarying answer in response to "Why don't you tell them you're gay?" The response that is never made is, "Haven't my parents hurt me by hating homosexuality?" "I love you, dear, even if you're gay" seems to be the most supportive parental acknowledgment most honest gay children can hope for. For too many gays with AIDS, their parents would rather have them *die* than admit they're gay. (There are too many cases of gay sons going home to die, to be with parents and family who haven't known these sons were gay or had AIDS; and, when confronted with both these facts, these parents and these families turned these sons out.)

For Arendt, there is no higher calling than the political. "The *raison d'être* of politics is freedom, and its field of experience is action." *(Between Past and Future.)* Arendt drew her inspiration from ancient Greece (for gay people, also that last page in history when we were free and accepted), where all citizens were willing to participate in the political process. For Arendt political action was a moral imperative. She even thought that civil disobedience was permissible, and that any democracy must allow it. She was very much in favor of the civil rights and antiwar movements, so anchored in demonstrations. Professor Kateb collects her thoughts: "In modern times the civil disobedients are precisely those who guard the limits on the conduct of office-holders. . . . When those in authority attack the Constitution, *and* when judicial review is denied [both certainly applicable in the gay community, particularly since the recent *Bowers v. Hardwick* case in which the Supreme Court ruled against the legality of consenting homosexual acts in the privacy of one's own home], citizens may apply irregular pressures, including lawbreaking, to defend it." The important thing is to get the government not to welch on its constitutional promises.

V

Perhaps this is a good place to say why Hannah Arendt interests me so. I'm old enough to remember vividly the deafening roars of outrage that greeted her "Eichmann in Jerusalem: A Report on the Banality of Evil," which she wrote in 1963 on assignment for *The New Yorker,* and which has remained in print, and blanketed in imbroglio, ever since. Most of the outrage, it would appear, erupted, and continues to fester, because of an imprecise reading of her intentions, even though, as Arendt's biographer, Elisabeth Young-Bruehl (in *Hannah Arendt: For Love of the World*) says, "Arendt's book did lend itself to misinterpretation more than any other she wrote: its conclusions were shocking, it contained numerous small errors of fact, it was often ironic in style and imperious in tone, and some of its most controversial passages were peculiarly insensitive."

The particular "controversy" that upset so many Jews, and which I admire her hugely for having the guts to raise, was the question of the Jews' own complicity in their mass extermination. The imprecision of her antagonists' reading based itself on a belief that she had said Jews let themselves be marched off to death. "I never asked why the Jews 'let themselves be killed,' " Arendt wrote in her defense, in a letter to her old friend Gershom Scholem (included in *The Jew as Pariah*). "On the contrary, I accused Hausner [the prosecuting attorney in the Eichmann case] of having posed this question to witness after witness. There was no people and no group in Europe which reacted differently under the immediate pressure of terror. The question I raised was that of the cooperation of Jewish functionaries during the 'Final Solution' . . . I said that there was no possibility of resistance [at this late date in events], but there existed the possibility of *doing nothing.*"

Arendt felt it was these functionaries—prominent members of Jewish communities—who, under the supremely misguided notion that they were staving off Jewish deaths by performing, unfortunately superbly, all the necessary administrative duties the Nazis requested of them, actually brought these deaths closer to reality. Had these Jewish functionaries refused to cooperate, had everyone in essence refused to do anything but be passive, the Nazis, with far fewer numbers, would have been unable to kill so *many* millions. But "wherever Jews lived, there were recognized Jewish leaders, and this leadership, almost without exception, cooperated in one way or another, for one reason or another, with the Nazis."

Like Arendt, I believe that my people must answer for a large part of our current predicament. Despite what the Constitution says, one usually has a hard time obtaining one's constitutional rights unless a concerted demand is made for them. If one is poor, black, and uneducated, there are very good reasons why fighting is difficult. If one is economically comfortable, gay, and educated, these reasons evaporate. Like Arendt, "I can admit to you something beyond that, namely, that wrong done by my own people naturally grieves me more than wrong done by other peoples." Twenty-four million men and women sitting silently by as the AIDS epidemic continues to gobble up their own is wrong. The world is what we make of it: This is the cornerstone of Arendtian thinking. I don't believe that we made AIDS, but I believe, by our not rising up in any coherent, cohesive, visible way, we allow it to continue. Jews aren't less responsible, or, in Arendt's words, don't "cease to be coresponsible," because they're victims "of the world's injustice and cruelty." Too many gay people hide behind the mother's apron of "the world's injustice and cruelty." It's easier that way. It's easier and simpler to be a victim than a fighter. If homosexuals are so politically blind that we don't understand the implications of our own actions (and inactions), then we must pay yet a further price. One is responsible for the human world, Arendt said, even if one is a victim.

In her essay, "Organized Guilt and Universal Responsibility," written in 1945, Arendt wrote: "It is many years now that we meet Germans who declare that they are ashamed of being Germans. I have often felt tempted to answer that I am ashamed of being human."

The lessons the Jews eventually learned when their own numbers were threatened and destroyed are the lessons all homosexuals avoid studying at our peril.

VI

"It is no mere accident," Arendt wrote in "The Moral of History," "that the catastrophic defeats of the peoples of Europe began with the catastrophe of the Jewish people, a people in whose destiny all others thought they could remain uninterested."

It's not too early to see AIDS as the homosexuals' holocaust. I have come reluctantly to believe that genocide is occurring: that we are witnessing—or *not* witnessing—the systematic, planned annihilation of some by others with the avowed purpose of eradicating an undesirable portion of the population.

I know that straight Jews, and other heterosexuals, find this comparison of holocausts repugnant.

I certainly don't know what it was like to witness six million die. When I say that I have lost some five hundred acquaintances and friends over the past seven years, I have been told point-blank by straight Jewish people that "their" extermination is the only "holy" one; ours, by contrast, is piddling. Evidently I must not get so upset, because my deaths are less than their deaths.

Does it appear that I am intentionally trying to escalate our horror to that of the Supreme Horror? I am not unfamiliar with charges of hysteria and hyperbole. To read Primo Levi is to know that our suffering, as of this moment, is still small in comparison. But Primo Levi also writes, "A certain dose of rhetoric is perhaps indispensable for memory to persist."

One inadvertent fallout from *the* Holocaust is the growing inability to view any other similar tragedies as awful. Jews themselves are partly responsible for this: memory must in no way be tampered with. But, important as this memory is, the insistence on its primogeniture frustrates efforts to arouse equal public concern when the newest children on the block arrive, demanding immediate succor.

What Hannah Arendt was trying to tell the Jews was that, whether they knew it or not, they have been able to survive thus far because, like it or not, they constituted a political community, and if they wanted to survive they had to break, as Ron H. Feldman puts it in his introduction to *The Jew as Pariah*, "with the past in which accident reigned supreme and take conscious control of their destiny."

The years Arendt writes about were ones in which "being a Jew does not give any legal status in the world." It is hard for young Jews to remember this time, and it is hard for gays to believe Jews were once as unrecognized as gays are now.

Gays remain pretty unconvinced when told that it took World War II to organize the Jewish population finally and effectively—those of them who were left.

(Because I am also Jewish, and find so many similarities in the historic plights of both Jews and gays, I find it painful that my religion is, in most instances, so unkind, uncharitable, and in some instances—that of the Orthodox and Hasidim—downright murderous. People, if they learn lessons at all, learn them, it would appear, only for themselves, and then only if they are lucky. The benefits are evidently neither transferable generally or assignable specifically.)

"The realization that millions of Jews had gone to their deaths without resistance resulted in a change in Jewish consciousness," Feldman writes, then quoting Arendt: "Gone, probably forever, is that chief concern of the Jewish people for centuries: survival at any price. Instead, we find something essentially new among Jews, the desire for dignity at any price."

This longing for dignity at any price has overtaken the gay population in the largest cities. Our holocaust has done that for us. We have learned, if not how to fight, or become "political," how to grieve magnificently. We have established organizations, many of them now huge and rich, to cater to the dying. It is almost as if, rather than bother anyone with our problems, certainly rather than fight to correct what caused them, we shall clutch them possessively to our bosoms and suffer as nobly as we can. It is indeed heroic to witness the amazing devotion that so many, gay and straight, lavish on their dying friends. I do not mean to diminish these sad rituals, though indeed I personally find them slightly ghoulish.

Of course I want to be attended to by those I love when my time comes. I am just slightly stunned when I witness so many electing to give such large amounts of energy, devotion, and caring to these morbid activities, rather than attempting to right the wrongs in a system that's made these activities necessary in the first place. I look at faces at countless memorial services and cannot comprehend why the connection isn't made between these deaths and going out to fight so that more of these deaths, including possibly one's own, can be staved off. Huge numbers regularly show up in cities for Candlelight

Marches, all duly recorded for the television cameras. Where are these same numbers when it comes to joining political organizations, with either their dollars or their skills, or plugging in to the incipient civil disobedience movement represented in ACT UP?

I find in these actions a defeatism that is depressingly negative: Gays are hated, these actions seem to say, and there's nothing to be done about it, gays will always be hated, so let's accept this as we bury our dead.

That an increasingly large number of these saints—and I do think there's also a margin of saintliness inherent here, as well as a yearning for such saintliness—are straight women I find both disturbing and gratifying. But it's as if, not only do we tell ourselves that fighting for our lives is a useless occupation, but now we are joined by heterosexual representatives telling us the same thing and helping us to nail our coffins.

I submit that there are different kinds of holocausts. After all, the word is defined, in my *American Heritage Dictionary*, as "any widespread destruction." Hitler gave it new and grotesque meaning, but despite the Jewish insistence that the word is now totally attached to their own destruction, it is perversely inhuman to deny its attachment to other conflagrations. At this moment in history, it is perhaps thought that such a holocaust as Hitler perpetrated can never happen again, and Jews fight mightily to keep this notion alive, even though there certainly have been mighty holocausts since: Stalin's and Ethiopia's, as well as incomprehensible slaughters in Biafra, Cambodia, and Lebanon, are only the few that come immediately to mind. The Jewish outrage that automatically erupts whenever another endangered minority, under threat of destruction, claims that a holocaust is occurring is selfishly counterproductive to confronting yet another example of man's seemingly innate inhumanity to man.

Certainly, a holocaust does not require a Hitler to be effective. Certainly, a holocaust does not require *deliberate* intentionality on the part of one or several or many or a bureaucracy to be effective. Holocausts can occur, and probably most often do occur, because of *inaction*. This inaction can be unintentional or deliberate. How one defines the line, or level, of intentionality or unintentionality is often a difficult question. How does one accuse a bureaucrat of looking the other way, or of paying no attention, or of paying less attention than he should, when he can counter—as Adolf Eichmann did—with the defense, "I was only doing my job as best I could"?

In all my investigations over these past years into why AIDS has not been attended to with the dispatch it warrants, I have been told at almost every juncture that "all is being done that can be done." Indeed, I'm often accused of being "ungrateful" for this "activity," and that more has been learned about this condition in a shorter time than in any other health emergency. To this hyperbole, I usually add my own: If AIDS were happening to Jews, or to American Legionnaires, or to white tennis players at country clubs, we would be much farther along the road to treatment and cure than we are, which, despite all protestations to the contrary, is not very far at all.

The one facet of the AIDS epidemic that I think almost everyone prefers to overlook is this: *Something infectious is going around.* Whatever the cause (and, as I have said, and it bears repeating, like almost everything connected with this epidemic, I tend to view any statement of definite fact with doubt, so many have been contradicted, contravened, or proved downright wrong since these statements of "fact" started appearing in 1981), it is apparently being transmitted infectiously, and it is not stopping. Nothing has changed since the onset about the most important prediction: There may never be a cure. As Dr. Linda Laubenstein, a hematologist at New York University Medical Center and one of the first doctors to note AIDS in patients and to this day one of the leading doctors treating it, says, "We don't have a very good record of dealing with viruses. There isn't a virus yet that's been cured or eliminated. The best we can hope for, and this is a long way from ever happening, is that there will be some kind of treatment that will be suppressive without being too toxic to use over a lifetime—the way diabetics take insulin."

Opponents of increased AIDS funding use, as one of their excuses, the high fatalities from other horrors, such as lung cancer, various lymphomas, heart disease, even auto accidents. These, they say, are just as much in need of attention. "But they're not infectious," is Dr. Laubenstein's curt response to this kind of thinking.

If I harp on my holocaust comparisons, it is because it is my firm belief that we are in but the early stages of destruction by AIDS of huge swaths of the world's population. And the hideously alarming World Health Organization figures don't seem to do the trick of convincing any powers-that-be. There have been, over these past three years, four damning reports prepared for President Reagan or at his behest: two by the National Academy of Sciences, one by his Surgeon General, Dr. C. Everett Koop, and one, most recently, by his own Presidential Commission on the Human Immunodeficiency Virus Epidemic. Each has said more or less the same thing. The leading editorial in the Sunday *New York Times* of June 5th, 1988, congratulating the commission for its "findings," noted (in words that could as justifiably be applied to the *Times* itself): "The Administration's response to AIDS has from the start been torpid, fitful, fragmented and riven with prejudice against those infected with the virus." The Commission's Report itself says that government leadership "has been inconsistent and not properly coordinated"; the federal response has been "slow, halting, and uneven"; the Food and Drug Administration and the National Institutes of Health were particularly criticized for going *very* slowly indeed.

Amazingly enough, it is no longer even a question of money. Over very long years, Congress has gradually increased its appropriations, so that now there appears to be enough to go around. What Congress is now finding is that this money isn't being spent, or is being spent unwisely, and that no one is in charge of supervising its proper allocation. To cite just one heinous example of malfeasance, Dr. Anthony Fauci, the director of the National Institute for Allergy and Infectious Diseases—that branch of the NIH under which most AIDS treatment research falls—was recently raked over the coals, first at hearings conducted by Representative Ted Weiss and his House Subcommittee on Human Resources, and subsequently by Senator Edward Kennedy, at Senate hearings conducted by his Committee on Labor and Human Resources, who accused Fauci of "doubletalk." Dr. Fauci has had at his disposal some $374 million. He has been unable to set up a network of hospital treatment centers around the country to test, quickly, promising new drugs (calculated, as I mentioned, to be some two hundred by medical reporter Susan Spencer on "CBS Evening News," and most of them unavailable legally in this country until they *are* tested by the NIH and approved by the FDA). After two years, not only is this system not functioning in any coherent way, but 80 percent of the studies Dr. Fauci and one of his many, many committees, and subcommittees, have approved are still only with AZT, a problematic drug that, in any case, has *already* been approved by the FDA. Because of the snail-like pace of Dr. Fauci's work, and because of the equal lethargy of response from the FDA, which must license any treatment that is approved (and certainly because of the lack of effective pressure from gays or AIDS organizations like GMHC), most of these two hundred untested drugs must be obtained by sufferers as best they can. Hence these treatments are unavailable to any but the rich or the most persistently cagy. Dr. Fauci has been described as "a bumbler" by one of the members of the President's AIDS Commission. I myself have called him, in print, an incompetent idiot.

It is not possible to condemn the stupidities of the NIH without adding those of the FDA. They are a dog-and-pony show. The system is such that you can't have one without the other. A drug tested at the NIH must still be approved by the FDA. Dr. Fauci's culpabilities are equal in size to those of Dr. Frank Young, the FDA's director. Despite repeated promises, despite pressure from congressional subcommittees, presidential reports, and even from Vice-President Bush himself, Dr. Young has done nothing to lessen the eight to nine years' time required for a drug to wend its way leisurely through the FDA approval process. (The average length of time AIDS patients have to live is five years.) Dr. Young loudly trumpeted some new regulations about a year ago—ones that would allow drugs that showed promising efficacy to be available to American patients; but in practice he and his staff have demanded *proof* of this efficacy, not just promise of it, and the time required for that proof to be proved to the FDA is eight to nine years.

A particularly inhumane example of what *is* going on scientifically involves an NIH-sponsored study to test the effectiveness of intravenous immune globulin (an existing pharmaceutical product that anyone can get) on four hundred babies with AIDS or ARC. These babies have an average age of eighteen months to two years. Almost all of them are black or Hispanic. It takes four to eight hours for each intravenous infusion. An infusion is administered once every twenty-eight days, for a period of two years. Previous research has revealed that a high number of the babies have to be *physically restrained* during the infusion. Half of the babies will receive a useless placebo. Even those babies receiving placebos must be hooked up to an IV and restrained; because it is assumed that many of the babies will pick up typical hospital infections, the NIH wants to make sure these infections are equally distributed among those receiving both placebo and the actual drug. As if this type of enforced experimentalization was not cruel enough, and as if making half the babies receive a placebo under the same circumstances was not cruel enough, it turns out that it was not necessary to use placebos at all. There already are in existence earlier results to utilize for statistical comparisons. When these earlier studies were presented to the NIH, studies that would save two hundred babies from a needless and painful ordeal, the NIH elected to proceed with the study nevertheless.

The Presidential Commission Report, its strong condemnations and recommendations—they are all words gay men have longed to hear. But, as I said, we've heard them all before, in those three earlier reports, which produced as little result as, in our despondency, we expect this new report to duplicate. There is no gay man who believes that anything helpful will actually be accomplished while President Reagan is in office. (Or if George Bush is elected.) His Commission's Report is seen as window dressing, perfectly timed so that he doesn't have to do anything, for he'll be out of office shortly after its receipt. Again, with the exception of Jesse Jackson, not one of the many candidates who recently competed for their party's nomination mentioned AIDS, dealt with AIDS, addressed any AIDS issues, or presented a plan for the future—a future that, without any doubt, is going to burden any administration with mountainous problems far surpassing any of the ones these candidates *are* willing to discuss. They know that AIDS is not a topic the electorate wishes to hear about. And no one ever seems to ask, nor does any of these four reports address the questions: Just why is it so many people take drugs? Just why is it so many gay men were promiscuous? Just why is it so many people are homeless?

If it is not possible to locate one Hitler responsible for allowing this AIDS destruction to multiply so, it is possible to locate a number of junior candidates. "We don't have one Hitler," a friend of mine said; "we have many Mengeles."

Ronald Reagan, Dr. Bowen, Dr. Wyngaarden, doctors at the NIH and FDA, are equal to Hitler and his Nazi doctors performing their murderous experiments in the camps—not because of similar intentions, but because of similar results.

"You either wait while six million again die, which is complicity, or you do something about it. It is just as sinful to let people die as to gas them." This was said by my best friend, Rodger McFarlane, who then went on to recite to me sentences from Christian theology—about sins of commission and omission—from a religion he no longer believes in.

With all due respect, it doesn't appear piddling to me to place my five hundred dead friends on the altar of history, and to posit the possibility that, at the rate we are going, we are now in a situation historically equivalent to, say, the German Jews circa 1938–1940, when the looming danger was, for the most part, also pooh-poohed. And that there will be millions of gay men dead before our holocaust is over. How can everyone avoid seeing this? How can straight and gay people continue to deny the viciousness of the AIDS epidemic? Why do gay men need to be *convinced* that we are being murdered?

Reluctantly, though for some time I denied this, and fought against it, for I know it is hugely counterproductive, I have found myself coming to hate heterosexuals. All heterosexuals. The ones, naturally, who sit by and ignore or simply observe what is happening to us. The ones who offer me condolences for all the awful things happening to us now, as they would in passing along kind words for a sick friend or relief from a cold that won't go away. The ones who invite me for Thanksgiving and Christmas and offer up prayers to God for a surcease to "Larry's friends who are suffering so much" before commencing to consume the turkey. The ones who help us bury so many dead and do not recognize that such deaths need not continue to occur. I hate them for not doing what I am unable to do—change all this. The same reason they hate me.

The greatest criminal of the century was, to Arendt, the "jobholder and the good family man" who did everything out of "kind concern and earnest concentration on the welfare of his family." "In contrast to the earlier units of the SS men and the Gestapo, Himmler's overall organization relied not on fanatics, nor on congenital murderers, nor on sadists; it relied entirely upon the normality of jobholders and family men."

The family. The family. How these words are repeated and repeated in America—from campaign rhetoric to television commercials. This is a country that prides itself on proclaiming family values, as if there were no others, as if every family was homespun and united and loving, as if it is necessary to produce a child—like a product—to justify or countenance a sexual act. AIDS goes against *all* family values: It is perceived as happening mostly to gay men; it is spread sexually (as if heterosexuals did not have sex); it is an embarrassment. Well, I am a member of a family, too. Or I once thought so. Every gay man has two parents, and other relatives, too. How convenient for them all to have disposed of us so expeditiously, just when we need them most. But the ranks are closed, something is happening to gay men, and we are suddenly no longer affiliated with *the* family. Where do they think we came from? The cabbage patch?

Most gay people see little to admire or to emulate in heterosexual life. It seems filled with hypocrisies we have worked hard to avoid. We see few happy straight marriages and many dishonest ones—husbands and wives cheating on each other, children taking more drugs than we ever took, and people ignoring values that we have made important in our lives: taste, style, education, directness, honesty, energy, friendships. We feel particularly blessed by so many and such strong friendships. We have turned to our friends to take the place of families. "Your friends are your family" is something often heard in conversations of gay people gathered together. We look at Ronald and Nancy Reagan, and the books their own children have written about them, and we watch our President and his wife talk constantly about "family values in America," and we laugh. At least our promiscuity was *honest.*

VII

I spoke earlier about Luke, the appealing man who offered me love. After five dates, I decided not to see him anymore. I offer here a reasonable facsimile of the thoughts that crisscrossed my consciousness while he held me in his arms:

I don't want to die, this is killing me, my need to love can't be worth this—he is so nice, I want him so, he is so gentle and he makes me feel good—he takes me for what I am, and he is kind to me, and he is all the things I have always longed for in a relationship, but my work, my work must come first, I have too much yet to say, I cannot abandon my work, and yet why might it not work out?, why might we not be carriers?, why not take the chance?: But the chance is Russian roulette and the risks are too great, the odds are too much against us, and, too, I might kill him, I might be the carrier, and his life is precious, his youth, he has so much he wants to give to the world. . . .

What it amounts to is that I cannot stand the torture that each coupling brings to our lovemaking, and the nightmares that come into my dreams, and the walking dialogue that plagues me every time I think of it. It constantly jams itself into my thoughts: You must be crazy, you must be out of your mind, you are gambling with your life. Suddenly it doesn't seem to be worth it. When he leaves me, I promise myself I won't see him again. I cannot wait for him to leave. He keeps kissing me goodbye, tenderly, as he goes off to take the GMHC volunteer training—he wants to become a Crisis Counselor, like his sister-in-law, helping to tend the dying. But when he is gone, I miss him already, and I wonder if somehow we can't work it out. No. I must hold firm to my decision. But I miss him. Why didn't I ask him to come back tonight? He has no place to stay before returning to the training tomorrow, without going home to his parents in New Jersey. "Check in," I said, noncommittally, when he left. Will he? When? What will I say then? Do a Nancy Reagan and "Just say no"?

Hours later I am still trying not to think of him. But it's there inside me, my desire for him, my sweet memories, the ingestion of him, symbolic, but perhaps, accidentally, actual. I try to deny these feelings and get to work. Work! I must work. Another hour later, I vomit.

I find I've made this note in my diary after he left, after our fifth night together: When we hold each other, there are three people in bed and one of them is Death. I confide in no one, not even Rodger, who was my former lover and with whom I share everything. In one of our many daily phone conversations, he volunteers, "I think Jesus would have to carry me in his arms to Paris for me to put out."

I am going to say a few words about "gay promiscuity," and let it go. Promiscuity is a loaded word and a controversial subject, and what exactly constitutes promiscuity—how many more than one encounter with how many more than one person?—seems to differ depending on whom you ask. In any event, as Professor Boswell of Yale writes: "There does not seem to be any evidence that gay people are more or less sexual than others." Dr. Richard Isay, a practicing psychoanalyst and Clinical Associate Professor of Psychiatry at Cornell Medical College, writes in his forthcoming book, *Being Homosexual:* "Human males in general are more interested in variations of sexual partners than females." To which Dr. Kinsey's words can be added: "This is the history of his anthropoid ancestors, and this is the history of unrestrained males everywhere." Promiscuity is liberating for some people while for others it's dehumanizing, and thus it's hard to come down on one side or the other without taking into account who's being promiscuous. But the gay community, both before and after the arrival of AIDS, has taken a bad rap for it. The entire heterosexual world, it sometimes seems to me, perceives the entire homosexual world as busily involved in doing nothing but performing endless acts of sexual intercourse. Some of us did and most of us didn't (and now pretty much all of us don't). But it's an issue that must be addressed because if AIDS is transmitted sexually in any way, then there's no question that the promiscuity of some gay men was unwittingly responsible for AIDS killing so many of us. And it's this, of course, that we are being blamed for (particularly by religious groups)—spreading AIDS.

The concept of making a virtue out of sexual freedom, i.e., promiscuity, came about because gay men had nothing else to call their own *but* their sexuality. The heterosexual majority has for centuries denied us every possible right of human dignity (which the doctrines of all religions and most "free" countries, as well our own Constitution, are meant to guarantee for all). The right to marry. The right to tax advantages and employee benefits that married couples enjoy. The right to own property jointly without fear that the law will disinherit the surviving partner. The right to hold a job as an openly gay person. The right to have children. The right not to be discriminated against in just about every area. Indeed—the right to walk down the street holding hands, as heterosexual people can do freely when they are in love. The right to love. We are denied the right to love. Can any heterosexual imagine being denied the right to love? I ask you to try to imagine how you might feel if you had to hide from the whole world the fact that you loved your wife or husband.

So, rightly or wrongly—wrongly, as it turned out—many gay men decided to make a virtue of the only thing the straight world didn't have control of: our sexuality. Had we possessed these rights denied us, had we been allowed to live respectably in a community of equals, I think a good case could be made that there would never have been an AIDS epidemic such as we are seeing. Had we been allowed to marry, many of us would not have felt the obligation to be promiscuous. (While we may not see much to emulate in heterosexual marriages, this does not preclude our desire to try it ourselves. It wouldn't be the first time we've demonstrated to the straight world that we can do something better.) Thus I think a good case also can be made that the AIDS pandemic is the fault of the heterosexual white majority.

"Our society does not now want gay men to be in stable, responsible, mutually gratifying relationships," Dr. Isay writes. "The visibility of such couples is too shattering to the sense of masculinity of men in most segments of our culture." Until this change comes—a change that will benefit both gay men and society alike—the destruction of American homosexuals by the heterosexual majority will continue. It is unrealistic to think that, even with AIDS, an entire population will be able to stop having sex. The irony, of course, is that being promiscuous is a characteristic that straight men congratulate each other on achieving, at the same time they condemn us for the same acts.

The leveling of this blame for the AIDS epidemic is perhaps better understood if an extension of this argument is presented: that the poor, black, and Hispanic have also been forced into AIDS by oppression. The awfulness of their destitution and deprivation, the absolutely zero chance so many of them face in bettering their lot in this world, forces them to seek peaceful respite and brief relief in the only oblivion available to them— the never-never land of drugs. And these drugs, for all the Just Say No mentality of an imbecilic First Lady, this society makes remarkably available through inept law enforcement and just plain looking the other way. It's almost as if a conscious deci- sion had been made somewhere in government to let all these people drug themselves to death.

AIDS having thus been caused to seed and sprout, it was *allowed* to grow and fester and increase a millionfold by the inaction of our government. As I noted earlier, everyone is more interested in *managing* this epidemic than in stopping it, than in taking any time to search for and begin to solve the root causes of what is going on.

VIII

I've perhaps relied too heavily on others' words in trying to state my case. I've done it intentionally. I've been criticized so often and attacked so continuously for so much of my rhetoric that I've tried to find support for my feelings in the philosophies of others whose lives have given them little choice but to think about tragedy and attempt to find, if not definitive explanation, rhyme, or reason, at least a few ground rules on how to get to tomorrow.

I go to many memorial services. I've been to too many where the Bible is invoked, and there are many quotations, like this from the Gospel of John, describing the death of Lazarus: "I am the resurrection and the life; he who believes in me, though he die, yet shall he live, and whoever lives and believes in me shall never die." Every priest, minister, rabbi, or lay speaker seems to put forth versions of the same sentiment. It was refreshing, and quite ennobling, to hear refutation at last. At one service— that for the writer Michael Grumley—the critic and novelist Doris Grumbach had this to say: "The Christian in me would believe in a purpose and a design to life and to the natural world, but such teleology is very difficult at moments like this. To wipe out the brightest, most talented, and most beautiful among us does not seem the action of a just and compassionate God, a God of love who permits this suffering and these deaths to happen."

At another service, for my friend Charlie, the minister had been sent up from the South by Charlie's ex-wife, who hadn't seen him in twenty years. This minister of God was a fundamentalist, and he was accompanied by Charlie's two daughters, whom Charlie had supported all their lives, and who somehow loved him and had been allowed, if not to see him, to talk to him regularly on the phone. Charlie hadn't consciously known he was gay when he married and became a father. When he realized he was, he immediately told his wife and she just as immediately divorced him. Now, after all these years, the wife demanded of Charlie's lover—in return for allowing the daughters to attend—that her minister conduct the memorial service, a service she herself would not go to. In front of a congregation composed entirely of Charlie's gay New York friends, this man began his sermon about sin. Charlie had sinned, and God would forgive the sinner. Riverside Church was exceptionally quiet. In nervousness or embarrassment or disgust, men looked at each other but no one walked out. And then a man got up and screamed out at the preacher: "Charlie wasn't a sinner. Charlie was a fine man and as good a father as he was allowed to be. Charlie wasn't a sinner." And then, obviously surprised at his own temerity at screaming in a church, he turned and ran out.

I recently got a letter from my old friend and squash partner Val Cavalier, who now lives in New Orleans. I didn't know he'd been diagnosed with AIDS. He's terrified, though bravely trying not to be. "I'm tired of candlelight vigils," he wrote to me. "I think we need blowtorches. And we don't need these so-called faiths [Val's a Catholic]: beware of priests and suchlike bearing gifts; they are one of our chief natural enemies. Oh, Larry, it's so scary, this ineffable Fiend I'm dealing with. One of my fellow PWA's [Persons With AIDS] said at a funeral, 'There but for the grace of Gawd.' I said fuck your fuckin' twisted gawd—we/I didn't do *nothin'* to deserve *this.*"

My dear and precious friend, the film historian Vito Russo, sick now three years, gets his energy from being a constant scrapper. He pounds out articles filled with fury, and delivers speeches wherever he can, and he is a constant letter writer to any and all who dare not to understand what we are going through. He is a very busy man. At a sparsely attended ACT UP rally in Albany, in front of those bleak and passionless government buildings on a gray day, he shouted out to those few who trekked up there with him: "Remember that some day the AIDS crisis will be over. And when that day has come and gone there will be people alive on this earth—gay people and straight people, black people and white people, men and women—who will hear the story that once there was a terrible disease, and that a brave group of people stood up and fought and in some cases died so that others might live and be free. I'm proud to be out here today with the people I love, and see the faces of those heroes who are fighting this war, and to be a part of that fight."

There were few there to hear him. And, as I have written, there are few fighting with him. And today the *Times* announced the death of three more friends.

Since I started writing this, I've had a reconciliation with both my brother and sister-in-law. I tried to tell them that I didn't think I'd done anything wrong in writing a blistering letter to one of Arthur's clients for firing a man for his homosexuality. I tried to tell them that I had no other purpose left in my life but fighting for the healthy life of every gay man. They tried to tell me that I didn't understand that my tactics had endangered Arthur's law firm by attacking one of its most important and lucrative clients. I said I found it hard to believe that a letter from Larry would be enough reason for a client to move to another firm after being so ably represented for some dozen years. I said I thought both Arthur and Alice had reacted—it seemed automatically—out of all proportion: sending

me letters threatening me that our relationship might be sev-
ered, and Arthur writing his client that I was "off the wall" and
he would "muzzle" me if he could.

It was after a month of silence that Arthur called and was
the first to apologize. We have all those historical reasons for
not wanting to rupture our ties. Our mother has drummed into
us from the beginning that we must love each other. And we
do. Yes, he finally called, as he always does, after my long
silence. I sometimes think it's easier for him to apologize than
to talk about the issue.

We've had a couple of lunches since he called. The first was
strained, he trying to move on and I insisting on my pound of
flesh. The second lunch was better. Governor Dukakis had
made his acceptance speech and he'd mentioned the word
"AIDS." He'd done even more than that. He'd actually said to
all the world, "I want our young scientists to dedicate their
great gifts not to the destruction of life, but to its preservation.
. . . I want them to work with us to win the war against AIDS,
the greatest public health emergency of our lifetime, and a
disease that must be conquered." I told my brother that when
I heard Dukakis say that, I found myself sobbing uncontrollably. It was as if some great weight had been lifted from my
body. And I realized that if only Ronald Reagan had said these
words in June of 1981, I might have many of my five hundred
dead friends still alive; I wouldn't have had to spend seven
years of my life screaming; I wouldn't have had to write what
I am writing now.

Arthur, who has supported Dukakis from the beginning,
said, "It was a pretty good speech." I had the *Times* with me,
because both he and I were quoted in it that day. (I in an article
about ACT UP and he in an article about his law firm. Our
mother would be proud.) I read to him from the governor's
speech, the part where he quoted John Winthrop, the first governor of Massachusetts, on the idea of community. " 'We must,'
said John Winthrop, 'love one another with a pure heart fer-
vently. We must delight in each other, make each other's condition our own, rejoice together, mourn together, and suffer
together. We must,' he said, 'be knit together as one, be knit
together as one.' " My brother is not as visibly sentimental as
I am, but he kissed me when I dropped him at his office after

lunch. Then he asked me to please make peace with his wife. And I said I would do no such thing. The ball was in her court.

Alice was a harder person to deal with. She wasn't calling me, and I certainly wasn't going to call her. I'd felt her letter to me to be particularly hateful. I felt I was no longer welcome at her home. I felt I was not wanted at my younger niece Rebecca's high school graduation. I was angry at Alice for even getting involved in something that was between my brother and me. But as his wife, someone instrumental in furthering his career, and in whom he always confided, she thought she had that right, she indicated when we finally had lunch. She didn't accept it as appropriate or comparable when I said that my Rodger, who has been as instrumental in my career and in whom I also confide, didn't take it upon himself to write her a letter, much as he wanted to.

Much to my surprise, it was my older niece, Liza, who had brought this lunch about. I thought it would be my nephew, Andrew, who would be the peacemaker. He's a smart, jolly young man, who has that rare ability to defuse tense situations. (He also gives copies of my novel, *Faggots*, to his gay friends.) Liza is quiet and thoughtful and, like me, has had a difficult time fighting to find out who she is. She'd come into the city for a date and spent the night on my sofa and over breakfast I'd presented my side of the argument. I may have become too melodramatic, but this is what I felt and said: that I had known five hundred men who had died, and that I didn't know why I was still alive, and that I didn't think any of my family had an idea what my life on a daily basis was like, and they should enjoy what little of my life might be left to me, and us, because I might not be around much longer.

Alice called me that same afternoon and we had our lunch. She is a handsome woman, beautiful really. She is tall and slim and dresses exceptionally well. And she is very smart. (She is completing work on her doctorate in Art History.) And, after years of therapy of her own, also quite confrontational. Over the years our relationship has been both good and bad. For all three of us—Arthur and Alice and Larry—my homosexuality has been an issue. Yet even when Alice and I have fought, she's never excluded me from what she always calls "our extended family."

At our lunch (which was before my second lunch with Arthur), I maintained that the subtext of the whole damn mess between us was not my letter to the corporation but that they were still ashamed of my homosexuality. She maintained that this wasn't true, and that they both were proud of me for being such a fighter, and why did I insist on beating them forever over the head for how they'd once felt years ago? She was not in an apologetic mood, and I had determined beforehand that an apology was what I was going to get. And I began to think I wasn't going to get one. And once again to realize that Arthur had apologized on the phone because that's easier for him than having a lunch like this. A couple of times I almost got up and walked out. That's my way of making it easier for myself. Here is this woman leaning across this small table and staring intensely into my eyes and not budging an inch. For a while it looked as if I wouldn't have my family anymore. To make my point, I seem always prepared to take my stand, take it or leave it, and take my leave. Either you do this or I don't love you anymore. She seemed to sense this coming and, instead of avoiding it, she was pounding on like a pile driver. She'd heard my hyperbolic statements about hating all heterosexuals. Did that mean I hated her? And Arthur? And Liza and Andy and Rebecca? She had said she knew my life was enveloped in death, and she had great sympathy and sadness for me. And compassion. (A compassion I hadn't shown to the law firm, she added.) Did I expect them to give up their lives for my cause? She used the argument that her best friend is dying of cancer but she didn't expect Alice to spend her life going out to fight for cancer research. I told her that in all these eight years she hadn't sent a check to an AIDS organization, nor had she or Arthur written a letter to all the important people they knew. Why, Arthur is a big contributor to Dukakis: Had he written to him about AIDS? She said I'd never asked them to do any of this. I said why should I have to ask—they should have done so voluntarily. And months ago Arthur had offered to write to Dukakis, but then had told me to write the letter and he'd send it. So why hadn't I written it, she demanded. Because I'm too busy writing other things, I countered. What could be more important, she retaliated. I don't want to have to *ask* you to do anything, I tried again. (Subtext: You should do it without asking, because you love me, and care.) [Arthur has since written the letter, which closed with: "I would welcome the opportunity to visit with you on the telephone about what role Larry *and I* (italics mine) can play in helping to formulate policy in this area."] We went on and on. I began to realize that Alice was trying to bring the argument to some definite conclusion. She wasn't going to leave this table until she knew something one way or another. I started saying it's not so black and white, it's not so black and white—whether I want to see you again or not. She stared at me and said nothing. Right now I feel estranged, I said, from you, my brother, your kids, your world, and I don't think this is going to go away so quickly, just like that. "Are you saying that you feel nothing for us?" I didn't answer. "Are you saying that you don't have any love for us, or feel our love for you?" She was staring even harder at me across a table in this East Side restaurant where we'd now been talking for so long that all the other customers had long since departed and the staff was now gathered nearby for some sort of lecture from the boss. "Are you saying that all our lives together, and our history, amount to nothing? And that you don't care for us or love us?" "No, I'm not saying that," I said softly. And she started to cry. And I leaned across the table and kissed her. And I started to cry, too.

Part Three

Toward a Definition of Evil: Further Reports

I originally entitled this new and closing section "From anger to fury to rage." In going through what I'd written since the last edition of *Reports*, I was struck by how angry everything appears. And—even given this—how not-angry-enough all of what I wrote now seems.

As my own T-cells have dropped, producing the first irrefutable evidence HIV is alive and well and living inside me, and with so many friends and acquaintances now dead, I guess I should feel it's remarkable I'm still alive, still spewing out such distilled fury. I guess I should wonder why I haven't caved in, thrown in the towel, gone nuts, slit my wrists, or retired to the country to live out my final days in peace. I guess I should ask myself: Where the fuck does all the energy come from that allows me, day after day, to continue to summon up and into action this never-ending rage? Since 1981 until this very moment I've seen no sufficient rewards, no bones less than measly thrown by any President, to shut me up or appease me. Or to inspire a change of tone. Fourteen years is a long time to churn out such bile in the face of such an obdurate and impenetrable stone wall.

Oh, I know the answer. Everything connected to AIDS is *wrong*. AIDS shouldn't have happened. And it drives me to this rage and fury that it's *still* allowed to happen. I shouldn't question how I do it, just be glad I *can*. And attribute it to genes and an ornery personality.

Anger quietly just became a part of my daily life, like going to the toilet—another knee-jerk reaction to the constant slaps in the face gay people endure. After a while, it becomes automatic. As one automatically says, "Have a nice day," I now say to every enemy (now an awfully large group), "How dare you, you fucking son of a bitch."

People ask me: Aren't you grateful you're alive? Well, I don't think about it in quite that fashion. It's hard to think in terms of gratitude when so many just like me have been taken away. Yeah, I'm glad. I'm glad I've still got a set of lungs.

Am I finally nearing the end of my rope? After the last piece in this book, there doesn't seem any higher pitch I can reach. Like the tenor who can't hit any higher notes without being castrated, I no longer seem physically capable of raising the pitch. Yet the wrong that made me so angry in the first place is still everywhere I look. It hasn't gone away. AIDS is still here, and the idiots are still minding the store.

As I plowed through all my writings, I noticed another theme—my never-ending struggle to understand, to find some explanation for what we, the living, do and don't do. *This* is the search that comes closer to killing me. I know why AIDS is wrong, but I still don't understand why most people behave the way they do. By the time I get to the last speech, I'm pretty tired of trying to figure out why people don't fight. They just don't. And it breaks my heart that we don't.

As I write this, the plague has been with us for some fourteen years. The number of cases, like the fallout from the clouds over Hiroshima and Nagasaki, has mushroomed from forty-one known dead in 1981 to a projection (by Dr. William Haseltine, formerly of Harvard and now of the National Genome Project) of one billion HIV infections around the world early in the next century. My editor, Michael Denneny, wanted me to elaborate on these numbers—how many dead, how many dying, risk categories, that sort of thing. I used to do that in my speeches and appearances. I stopped. I stopped because reciting statistics doesn't seem to make any difference. The bigger the numbers, the more blank the faces. One case a day, one case a minute—is either changing how this plague is attended to? Most deaths are in vain, and AIDS deaths even more so because so many people *want* us to die. No, I no longer trot out the numbers because they don't work and I don't know why they don't work.

When I make statements like "The research still isn't being done" or "The government still isn't doing anything," there are always people who just as righteously confront me with "That isn't so." Yes, I speak in hyperbole, and yes, I speak the truth. Yes, there's been progress, and no, there's been no progress. Yes, people are living longer because some doctors know how to keep us alive longer; there are drugs that mitigate various infections, for a while, and patients have a better understanding of how to take care of themselves, even to the point of self-medicating when their doctors are too dumb. No, there is still no one in the White House who has cared to take a leadership position and see that this particular war—like Desert Storm and every other war in our, or any, country's history—has a general. No, there still remain so many unanswered questions on the pathogenesis of AIDS (how the virus works inside us) that I have no doubt that bureaucratic lassitude, an intentional lack of interest at the top, is the reason these questions remain unanswered.

In other words: Official genocide is going on.

I say that a lot in the rest of this book.

In retrospect, 1988, where the earlier edition of *Reports* left off, was a turning point. After eight horrible, grotesque, inhuman, tragic years under Ronald Reagan, hope was utterly lost with the election of George Bush and his appointment of his henchman extraordinaire, John Sununu. If we thought we'd had it bad under Reagan (and *his* court monster, Gary Bauer), we soon found out that now we had it worse. I firmly believe being so completely shut out for another four years destroyed whatever hope AIDS activism had so valiantly and courageously and miraculously nurtured. Many simply couldn't find any more energy. Bush, too, was a master of what Reagan had perfected: Ignore that which you don't wish to address. If you don't say anything, the media won't either. It worked as flawlessly for him as for his predecessor. I'm still amazed that, for twelve years, not one reporter ever asked either Reagan or Bush a question about AIDS. Here's incomparable and irrefutable evidence, if you needed any, of the complicity that the successful perpetuation of official genocide commands and requires. Not one White House reporter at any Presidential news conference, not one reporter on any TV news show, ever asked one single question about AIDS. Kind of raises your hackles when you think about it, doesn't it? And people still read the newspapers and watch the nightly news and think they're being exposed to truth.

But there's enough complicity to go around. Most of the gay community, to instance the saddest collaboration, has remained as negligent in speaking out, fighting back, demanding rights, asking questions, as anyone else.

Following the first publication of *Reports*, George Bush was elected President (when asked during one of his Presidential debates with Michael Dukakis to elect a "hero," Bush named Dr. Anthony Fauci); Ed Koch ran for an unprecedented fourth term (and lost, giving us in David Dinkins a mayor as weak as Koch was obnoxious); *The New York Times* (which reviewed this book with extreme dismissiveness) promoted its chief AIDS reporter Philip Boffey to deputy science editor (he's now an editor of the editorial page); my "play about a farce," *Just Say No*, in which I tried to find yet another way to expose our two most active murderers, Reagan and Koch, and hope that people would hear me, was crucified by the *Times* ("Imagine the worst possible taste, then take it several steps further"); and ACT UP, for a few brief shining hours, flourished.

ACT UP wrought a revolution that changed the drug approval bureaucracy forever. Washington is a byzantine place, filled with swamps, labyrinths, shifting sands, tar pits, and mirages. Just when you think you've found the right person to call, the power shifts to another part of the forest. Somehow ACT UP managed to figure this system out and began to pin the faceless no-necked monsters to the mat. We started with dogged, continual, perpetual demonstrations at every possible point of opposition—the FDA, the NIH, HHS, AIDS conferences, and meetings of every description and all over the world; followed this with the identification of promising-sounding treatments, requesting meetings with their manufacturers, threatening boycotts and demonstrations if refused (you'd be surprised how quickly corporations are ready to sit down and talk with you when they find a picket line around their buildings or demonstrators, handcuffed together, chained to desks in their offices, with a couple of newspaper photographers and CNN cameras just happening to be around), and then negotiating with them for the earliest possible "compassionate use" release of these treatments (meaning the drug is provided free until FDA approval is granted); wrapped all this activity in intense, continuing media coverage; capped it all by writing position papers about what must be accomplished, both immediately and in the long run, widely circulating these position papers to all and sundry, then shepherding them into presentation at relevant conferences; and, finally, demanded and obtained seats on whatever committees had been formed to approve whatever it was ACT UP was fighting for in any or all of the above. A complicated process, all of this, and very labor intensive.

It was an impressive sight—so many young men and women devoting so much time and intelligence and energy to mastering and masterminding all of this.

The time it now takes to get a drug approved can be as little as less than a year. Before ACT UP started, the average time was between nine and twelve years. I hope all those right-wing arch-conservatives who hate gays know that even they now benefit from the availability of a host of treatments that have come to them courtesy of the sweat and screams (and arrest records) of thousands of ACT UP members everywhere.

Lo and behold, even Dr. Anthony Fauci, the government's chief point man on AIDS and, up to that moment, just about Number One on all our Public Enemies lists, made a smart and sharp *volta face*. First, he crusaded for the implementation of a notion known as "parallel track"—a plan for making experimental drugs available widely while they were still in Phase Two efficacy protocols under the FDA (a sort of glorified extension of "compassionate use")—which helped to break the rigid system down even more.

Then he decided that the best way to shut us up was to invite us to sit at his table. One of the truly sad and infinitely tragic developments over these next years would be the metamorphosis of some of the smartest of the treatment activists into bureaucrats, indeed into bureaurats more bureaucratic than the bureaucrats. Had they not sat down at Dr. Fauci's table, I doubt this would have happened.

(Ironically, Fauci's action was to curtail his own power: In a plot right out of *Julius Caesar*, the activists who became bureaucrats turned on their former host and unseated him from his throne, pretty much killing off someone who—again ironically—had become the best friend, and certainly one of the smartest scientists, we'd had.)

The more I came to understand the entire drug delivery system in this country, the more I came to see that more people die on a regular basis because they can't get unapproved drugs than would ever die from receiving them; and that the elaborate machinery our government throws up to protect us from the "unsafe" actually does the reverse—protects us from stuff that's so safe it more than likely doesn't do any good anyway. (If two dozen drugs are to be discussed and a winner chosen from among them, you can bet that any government committee organized on democratic, politically correct principles will choose the safest one, one that won't do any harm and won't do any good either, the one right in the middle.) People who maintain they only want "safe" drugs don't seem to realize people die on "safe" drugs, too. Those who want drugs without any side effects don't seem to realize there's probably never going to be any such thing, or if there is, it'll be too weak to work. People forget that approved forms of chemotherapy, for instance, have many side effects, and kill many people, even though they were—once upon a time, when such approvals were easier to obtain—approved.

I guess what I'm saying—and this is a principle ACT UP originally fought so hard for—is that people should have the right to make up their own minds about what they want to ingest. I believe many sick people feel the same anger toward well-meaning (and usually physically healthy) busybodies that a woman feels when some man orders her not to have an abortion: "Keep your laws off my body!" There's an army of volunteers out there ready and willing to test not-yet-approved drugs on themselves. Yes, they're probably desperate, but isn't participating in trying to ward off your death a hell of a lot more healthy than lying down and submitting to it? Unfortunately, what's left of the treatment activist movement fights less hard for this principle now, often sounding as prim and prissy and negative as the "official" medical advice they once challenged.

As I indicated, in 1988 I tested HIV-positive, as I suspected I would. No amount of suspicion matches the actuality of discovering the truth. Even though there appeared to be nothing different in my body except this new bit of information in my mind, my life changed forever. A new fear now joined my daily repertoire of emotions, and my nighttime ones, too. I didn't want to have the test, but it was discovered that being infected with hepatitis B had given me cirrhosis of the liver and that it was essential to know what my HIV status was before choosing which among several treatments to try to calm my liver down.

Am I glad I had the test? Would I recommend it to everyone now? These are still difficult and puzzling questions. "I don't know" is my cop-out answer—or "It depends on who you are and how your head is and how you live your life." There's no question that knowing you're HIV-positive is a giant bummer; I don't care what any "positive" HIV-positive person maintains. There are still no treatments that are going to really alleviate your basic condition. On the other hand, there are a few things you can take to slow certain declines as well as the onset of some of the opportunistic infections that, if unchecked, can kill. It is possible not to have the test and just to monitor T-cells, which can probably be an accurate-enough indication of health for a while. If and when these start declining, and the decline does not reverse itself, then *the* test can be taken. In my case, if I'd just monitored my T-cells, I'd have had a good five more years during which I didn't have to live with that particular new sword of Damocles in my life, before the falling nature of my T-cells became undeniably a trend. But test or no test, everyone should live as if they're positive—that is, safely in all sexual matters.

I'd like to say a few words about the moment in time when I believe ACT UP got its first real power—the infamous demonstration at St. Patrick's Cathedral on Sunday, December 10, 1989, which sort of got out of hand. Outside many thousands were protesting in a more or less orderly fashion while, unbeknownst to most, a small group of demonstrators entered the Cathedral and disrupted, in many ways, the Mass. These demonstrators (most of whom, interestingly enough, were Catholics) screamed and interrupted the service, lay down in the aisles, received communion wafers only to spit them out—oh, the bevy of sacriligious behaviors was quite long. Cardinal O'Connor was so upset that he retreated to a far throne and sat there holding his head with his hand, looking like nothing so much as a frazzled Whistler's *Mother*.

None of any of what transpired inside had been planned in advance, or sanctioned by any discussion or vote on the floor of ACT UP. It just happened. The kids got inside and something possessed them—that something no doubt having a great deal to do with centuries of their religion's horrific treatment of gay people.

The shit hit the fan. Newspapers and TV and politicians and commentators and editorials and front-page headlines *all* screamed hideous condemnations of us all. Indeed, we condemned us! ACT UP's meetings for the next few weeks were filled with our screaming at each other. No one knew quite how to respond—if indeed we should. There were many who felt we were compelled to apologize publicly and there were many who felt our infiltrators had performed a mighty act. No consensus could be reached, and for a moment or two I wondered if this might be some sort of organizational donnybrook—that the more militant among us would break away to start another group or the group itself might fold.

But a funny thing happened. We discovered the world was afraid of us. We were identified in not a few places as some sort of terrorist army. A few of us realized how enormously useful this could be.

We learned how to play with this fear and use it. I doubt that either Cardinal O'Connor or Ed Koch, both of whom immediately commenced never-ending denunciations of us, realized how mightily they helped to make ACT UP what it became. They created our image of guerrilla warriors to be frightened of. And we caught that ball and ran with it. And the media did the rest. If ever an organization's perception was created, at first, more by the media than by its own members, we were it.

ACT UP was, of course, exceedingly important in the history of both the gay movement and grass roots activism. For a moment, it almost seemed as if we could forge a worldwide army of us—all fighting for the same thing.

■ ■ ■

I'm grateful to my editors, Michael Denneny of St. Martin's Press in New York and Steve Cook of Cassell's in London, for their interest in this expanded edition. Quite frankly, for someone who saves every scrap he's ever jotted anything down on (I'm pleased to note Jane Austen did the same), it's been difficult to make a selection. I'm greedy for it *all* to be on the record, because I still don't see anyone else recording for posterity who all the murderers actually were and are. How they still murder us. How they're still getting away with it. How criminal *The New York Times'* AIDS coverage remains. How puny the activities of yet another President, despite the kind words spewing from his mouth.

In other words, how intentional the genocide of AIDS remains.

In other words, how evil.

Yes, you'll find me—in the rest of this book—grappling, finally and at last, with the issue of evil.

As I also say more than a few times, I don't care who thinks I'm crazy for saying any of this. I know history will bear me out. Nothing has come along to shake that confidence a whit. Just the reverse.

It's been an exceedingly painful job revisiting and revising this book. Everything I'm saying at the end is only another regurgitation of what I said in the beginning. This doesn't help to shore up any complimentary notions one tries so hard to maintain about the importance of the writer or the validity of the witness or, indeed, the quality of our species.

So let's begin Part Three. Toward a definition of evil . . .

June 1994

We Must Make Tomorrow
Happen Today[*]

To the members of ACT UP:

Dr. Samuel Broder has said AIDS can be cured. Yet every impediment imaginable is being placed in the way of our receiving this cure.

I BELIEVE WE ARE SUDDENLY IN MORE TROUBLE THAN WE HAVE BEEN FOR SOME TIME.

Why, after all these years, and after all our protests, and after all the media coverage, and after nine years of a plague, aren't we getting this cure that Dr. Broder says is there?

1. George Bush has shown little interest in AIDS. There is still no one in charge. Enormous budget restrictions are planned that threaten all the progress we have made in obtaining appropriations.

2. The Secretary of Health and Human Services, Dr. Louis Sullivan, is a useless, faceless cipher. Dr. James Mason, his assistant secretary, appears to be less powerful and helpful than we had hoped (and a Mormon who opposes fetal tissue research and abortion).

---

*A letter to the floor of ACT UP, November 27, 1989.

3. There is no director at the Centers for Disease Control. There is no Director at the National Institutes of Health. The director of the FDA, Dr. Frank Young, has been fired, just when he was beginning to be effective for us. It will take at least six months before a new FDA director is chosen.

4. Dr. Anthony Fauci would appear to have lost control of the ACTG system, where all government drug protocols are performed.

5. As Jim Eigo and Mark Harrington have discovered and told us, this ACTG system refuses PWA or activist input while it continues to perform multimillion-dollar protocols that have poor enrollment because they are not designed for human beings and which, in many cases, are inhumane because of the poisonous doses it needlessly insists on administering. The Principal Investigators (PIs) who run the ACTGs blame us for this poor enrollment and threaten to take away our Parallel Track—the first humane distribution of promising treatments during this entire plague.

6. Mark and Jim have also discovered that NO NEW PROTOCOLS WILL BE COMMENCED ANYWHERE FOR AT LEAST NINE MONTHS because the ACTGs have decided to move their data base from one center to another. When the new center (in Cambridge) is up and running, it will most likely take another year to organize and recruit for the new protocols. While they do this housecleaning, we're supposed to lie down and die FOR ALMOST TWO YEARS.

7. The horrid possibility exists that the main reason the ACTGs are changing data base centers is because the one they have been using (at Research Triangle in Raleigh-Durham) has been unable to adequately process or interpret all the data collected up to this time. This means that there is a good chance that everything NIAID and the ACTGs have told us about all the treatments they are shoving into our bodies may be based on USELESS OR FLAWED DATA. This means THERE IS A GOOD CHANCE THAT AFTER NINE YEARS OF AN EPIDEMIC THEY KNOW ABSOLUTELY ZILCH ABOUT ANYTHING. (After all the billions of dollars the ACTG system has cost, all we have is a little news about AZT.)

8. There are still huge areas of AIDS that remain unresearched to this day. This is BASIC RESEARCH that should

have been done years ago. Kaposi's sarcoma, for instance. Opportunistic infections. Cofactors. How the virus causes AIDS in the first place. *Whether* the virus causes AIDS in the first place. All our pressurings to please get to work on these still bring no results. Now they are telling us that we have to wait two more years before the ACTGs can get their act together.

9. ACT UP members were told by ACTG chief Dr. Dan Hoth in no uncertain terms that we are unwelcome at ACTG meetings, despite an invitation by Dr. Fauci. It is obvious they don't like us and are afraid of us and jealous of our success in obtaining access to the FDA, the pharmaceutical companies, and the Parallel Track—all of which threaten their Ivory-Tower work, where they play Frankenstein, or should I say where they play Fischl.*

10. I come back to Point One. This President, like the inhumane monster who preceded him, has given no evidence that he cares about AIDS. In a long discussion I had with a top congressional aide, I was told that the problems I have listed above pertain as well to every other aspect of the health-care delivery system. This system is a shambles, a mess, a tragedy, is out of control—any way you want to describe it. Thus there is little hope that AIDS will be singled out for preferential treatment over other health crises or emergencies. Indeed, as we all well know, there is less chance. IT IS DOWNHILL FROM HERE ON IN.

In other words:

Dr. Samuel Broder of the National Cancer Institute has said AIDS can be cured. Yet every impediment imaginable is being placed in the way of our receiving this cure.

WHAT CAN ACT UP DO IMMEDIATELY?

I propose that our new agenda is cut out for us.

1. We must immediately begin a dynamic, orchestrated effort to demand full participation in the decision making and operation of the ACTG system; if we do not get it, then let the ACTG system be dismantled and transfer its resources to our Com-

---

*Dr. Margaret Fischl of the University of Miami, together with Dr. Paul Volberding of the University of California at San Francisco, were the two principal investigators of the first AZT study, which recommended that extremely high doses of this drug, which many came to consider problematic, if not downright poison, be the standard treatment for everyone infected.

munity Research Initiatives. Pharmaceutical companies will then come to us when they see how much faster we can get results than the ACTGs.

We must threaten the very existence of ACTGs everywhere unless we are allowed to fully participate in the design of protocols, including the choice of drugs to be tested and the dosage amounts. If this is denied us, then we must begin a campaign to warn people everywhere that their lives are in danger if they enroll in ACTG protocols. We can no longer tolerate Dr. Hoth and his PIs playing God with our lives. It is apparent that to them we are completely expendable; they are only interested in obtaining data, by very foul, cruel means. Jim Eigo, Mark Harrington, Ken Fornataro, Rebecca Pringle-Smith, and the NIH's own biostatisticians have demonstrated not only that past trial designs have been unethical but that changes could be rapidly and effectively made which could drastically accelerate the process of providing the answers we all need. The resistance to this change comes from PIs and other AIDS bureaucrats growing rich on existing government contracts.

2. We must commence a series of zaps against local New York ACTUs, particularly those where inhumane high-dose AZT is still maintained, despite concrete evidence that much lower doses are more effective. Can you believe they haven't even changed to low-dose AZT in their own stupid trials?

Why should we sit quietly by and send people to their deaths? Indeed, there is now talk among PIs and government investigators of continuing their present methods on "less well-informed populations"—thus taking advantage of entire groups unable to receive adequate medical care otherwise.

Yes, WE MUST REFORM THE ACTGs—OR DESTROY THEM. They aren't working, we know how they can work, and if they won't listen to us we must take our bodies elsewhere. ACT UPs in other cities, particularly L.A., are already militantly radical on this issue.

■ ■ ■

On a personal note, I think ACT UP/New York is itself, at the present moment, encountering troublesome problems of its own. I think we have lost a certain amount of focus, and our ability to follow through on ideas and plans has weakened. We seem unable to mount as many major demos as we have in the past, certainly not with the frequency or enthusiasm that we once commanded.

At the same time, I think we are entering an era when demonstrations and zaps must be even more carefully created to arouse interest from a bored media. What we have accomplished recently, and a miraculous accomplishment it has been—Parallel Track, getting Jim Eigo and others on official committees, forcing the FDA into listening to us and acting on our advice—was accomplished because we were able, at the same time as we fielded our experts, to use our numbers and our actions as a *threat*. This good cop–bad cop, one-two punch, is developing into our most effective plan of action.

But I believe we've now arrived at the point where, if our success is to continue, we must field even more experts. Threats are most effective when backed up with concrete demands and suggestions on how to achieve them. Jim, Mark, Iris Long, Ken, and Rebecca are overwhelmed in creating these agendas. TOO FEW ARE DOING TOO MUCH OF THE WORK. We desperately need more people willing to devote the time and energy to becoming the experts that Jim, Mark, Ken, Peter Staley, Garance Franke-Ruta, Scott Slutsky, Stephen Gendin, David Kirschenbaum, Jon Engbretzen, and a few others have become. Remember—none of these knew a damn thing about treatment issues not so long ago. But they took it upon themselves to become experts.

Most of our members come only to weekly meetings. Many never speak at all, even if their minds are racing with suggestions. Some speak too often and only to criticize or complain. Many don't even stay around for very long. The room begins to empty around nine, and by the end, when important issues are often voted on, the room is almost empty.

Compared to our total numbers, few participate actively in committees. And yet it's in our committees that so much vital work is done (and where friendships are most often made). Our committees must be reinvigorated and reinfused with our famous energy that was fueling us just a year ago. Treatment + Data, Media, and Actions all need as many members as they can get. Without our committees functioning strongly, we are less strong.

I wonder if we might consider forming an emergency committee to immediately discuss ways to strengthen ACT UP and how to perhaps reapportion the division of labors. Or perhaps a more effective starting point would be devoting an entire meeting on another night to just this brainstorming. We have enormous reserves of personpower and brainpower, but a lot is slipping through the cracks. I know many people feel frustrated—they want to work, to commit time and energy, but they are befuddled about how to plug into committees or to raise issues on the floor. Monday-night meetings can be very daunting; I know they are for me. I'm often nervous about speaking up.

One thing I often hear is that the meetings used to be more fun. Why? Were people a little looser, and did we agree with each other more? There needs to be a discussion on how the meetings are run. And what we can do about the confusion that often reigns on the floor, on the Coordinating Committee, among the facilitators who, in an attempt to keep order, often overlook goals and resort to "process" instead.

Everyone needs to rethink her or his commitment to ACT UP. How much time can we possibly devote? How interested are we still in what we all came together for originally? My own committment has been to research and cure, because when these are successfully accomplished there will be no more AIDS. But I know that others are interested in issues equally pressing— how to deal with the here and now of AIDS, and all the attendant tragedies inherent in that homophobia. Perhaps we might talk about forcing ourselves to be ruthless in addressing only those issues that other organizations are not attending to (even though they might not be doing as good a job as we could). We only have so much energy. We must not dissipate it.

How can we outreach to our friends who were once with us and need to be encouraged to come back? Should we think about our Affinity Groups, particularly if they are a vehicle for instant actions or ongoing focus on particular issues? (I personally think ACT UP should party more together. We work so hard and play so little.)

Am I alone in thinking that we have become, as a group, more conservative? (Or are we just tired, a little bit burned out?) It has recently seemed to me that we've often chosen the path less energetic, less controversial. Often we have many new members voting, members not up to levels of political anger or militancy that older members remember. Many are the votes in which the number of abstentions speaks more of caution than of being not fully acquainted with all the necessary information. How can we educate ourselves—in both areas—so that we don't step back, but step forward?

We must never lose sight of our goals. Or of what we have accomplished. And, in the two and a half short years of our history, we have done more toward ending the AIDS epidemic than any other organization, group, individual, politician—you name it—around. Our accomplishments have been historic, unprecedented, monumental. We must build on them. In the past we have been very good at self-criticism and self-correcting and changing course to accommodate changing times.

■ ■ ■

Personally, ACT UP gives me my greatest energy and my greatest reason for being alive. We have already proved so much to the world and to our fellow gay men and lesbians. Mark Harrington is fond of saying the world's revolutions did not happen when there is no hope. They happen when there *is* hope, and when the system can't keep up with the rising expectations of the maligned and the downtrodden. We have discovered there is hope that this epidemic, as Dr. Broder says, can be cured. We must clutch this hope every day to our hearts and use it, as we have done so often, to fuel our anger and our fury. What we are entitled to—what is just out there, over there—is being denied to us and we demand that it be ours. It's there, still out of reach, but coming closer. We can't stop now. We've started the revolution. We can't quit until we finish it.

WE MUST MAKE TOMORROW HAPPEN TODAY. AND WE SHALL!

It's heartbreaking for me to read any of the many letters like this that I wrote to ACT UP. There was such *hope* then. To tell you now that ACT UP actually accomplished many of those revolutions in the bureaucratic system seems almost beside the point, remembrances of things past. Yes, we accomplished much that involved superhuman efforts. And *still* we have so little. What a condemnation not only of bureaucracy but of the effectiveness of grass roots organizations. And of democracy itself.

For the first few years of ACT UP's existence, it was my life. I cared for little else. As in the early days of GMHC, there was such an abundance of visible, tangible love and cooperation among so many that it was almost total joy. Each week hundreds of men and women with a shared goal and much energy and determination to achieve it came together. I've never seen the likes of it. It was more inspiring than GMHC's formation because there were many more of us, and many of us were women. And there was *anger*. As I'd got tired of saying, GMHC became—with such speed it was frightening—a very passive, very timid, bunch of pastoral workers. Could people *really* face death with such acceptance? Evidently.

There were ACT UP meetings, it seemed, almost every night, including weekends. Meetings for planning, meetings for painting posters, meetings for civil disobedience training, meetings to learn and teach ourselves about science and treatments and how the NIH worked and what all those acronyms I so blithely tossed into my letter meant and how they were operated, and chapter and verse on why they didn't work and how they must be changed so that they might. . . . Oh, it was all very heady stuff. We planned for that day when we'd be listened to, when it would be *our* decisions that would right the wrongs and eliminate the endless delays. We often met in our first office so late into the early hours that the landlord asked us to move.

There have been and no doubt will be many discussions on what happened to ACT UP, to this miraculous outpouring that was one of the most remarkable occurrences in gay history. ACT UP is still in existence, of course, and I don't mean to sound its death knell; I'm speaking specifically of those halcyon years of its youth and growth, when *change* seemed possible, when there was no "No" we'd acknowledge. Depending on whom you talk to, we got three or four or five good years, which is more than most grass roots organizations ever have. And it was during those years that we made history.

Infiltrating the system, demanding and receiving a seat at the table, many seats at many tables—we thought all this wise at the time. It was only in hindsight that I saw the danger. It's easier to be angry and pressure people when you don't know them personally. When you know them, it becomes more difficult. And once you sit down with them at that table, you're inevitably and irretrievably co-opted and corrupted by the very system you started out to challenge and hold accountable. (This is precisely what's destroyed GMHC's effectiveness.) But I learned this after the fact, as I learned too late so many of the lessons of activism.

I cite as my best example my own relationship with Tony Fauci. Before I knew him personally, it was in no way difficult for me to come after him like a maniacal tiger.* As I came to know him over the following years (now that I'm HIV positive, he's even one of my doctors), even though I'm just as furiously angry at him for what he does and doesn't do, it's become painful for me to call him names. When I do criticize him in print, I find myself hoping he doesn't see the piece. He's a nice man with a lovely wife and he works seven days a week and rarely sees his kids. I have to remind myself that my idol Hannah Arendt pointed out for us all how nice people can perform so many evil deeds.

---

*See "An Open Letter to Dr. Anthony Fauci," page 193.

In any event, as I've said, ACT UP nurtured a group of young treatment activists who went out and sat at those tables and became bureaucrats. When others of us saw it happening and realized it could only lead to crippling us, they disagreed. Better to be on the inside, they all said. Did we *all* have to go inside, I inquired. They felt the more, the better. I went in for a while myself, until I realized I could be more useful yelling from the outside. So I went out again. And have tried to stay out. By the time the Clinton administration came along, ACT UP's Treatment + Data Committee had angrily split itself apart, and many of its "smartest" members formed an independent group, TAG (Treatment Action Group), which now acts like a mini government satellite. TAG breaks my heart. It's as if they'd never been in ACT UP at all, as if all their experiences in grass roots activism taught them nothing.

So all those smart young men and women aren't in my life anymore. I'm angry at them for what I think has been a massive case of selling out. But I miss them. I'd looked upon them as my children. Now I knew how my parents must have felt when I left home and proceeded to do absolutely everything they didn't want me to. I guess I'll never learn that fighters don't necessarily continue to fight in the same way. It's difficult, short of mandatory conscription, to hold a fighting force together, focused on the same goals and using the same tactics.

But, boy, for a few minutes there we sure *believed:* ACT UP would change the world! Hope's what keeps you going, and I still have a bit of it left. But nothing like what we had in those early ACT UP days. Perhaps hope is the childhood of any movement, perhaps its adolescence, too. Maturity doesn't eliminate hope so much as it puts it in perspective. It's *there,* and it's essential and useful and all that. But it doesn't invigorate anymore. The rent's paid only by sheer hard, grueling, and grungy noninspirational *work.* It's when this dawns on many members that they start to disappear.

I'm often asked why I don't start *another* organization, that with each of these earlier ones I must have learned enough, finally, to put together *something* that works and stays working and where divisiveness won't, in the end, destroy. The trouble is I don't know what other kind of organization to start. I don't know what tactics to try that we haven't already tried, in ACT UP or GMHC. And I'm tired of working with people in groups. People in groups don't show off people as individuals in the best of lights. Democracy is a strange, peculiar animal. It's like a virus itself: Just when you think everyone's got their finger on its focus, it mutates; it builds up resistance to the very proteins that should give it health—energy, fresh blood, new ideas. It's as wickedly elusive as hope and as toxic as a lie. If I started anything new, I'd have to find a way to foster elitism, be a dictator, and rule with an iron fist. I don't want to do that (though some have thought I do). But I suspect that's the only thing that might work. Because I don't think democracy does. It certainly doesn't work for gays and lesbians.*

This particular letter to the floor shows an ACT UP already established and beginning to show the wear and tear. Meetings of over five hundred people were the norm, and it's very difficult to control, corral, and inspire so many people into regular cohesiveness.

The talk of reforming or destroying the ACTG (the identical controversy is still going on today, joined now by the very doctors who run this even more useless and expensive monster) and the establishment of more efficient community-based research groups (still the best idea and still an idea looking for a life healthier than AmFAR's feeble attempts have brought it) gives an idea how ambitious and knowledgeable we'd become.

The ACTG was the first place we managed to infiltrate. Today there must be dozens of "activists" on its various decision-making committees. To what use? To what end?

*See "Whose Constitution Is It, Anyway?," page 177.

Dear Paul

Dr. Paul Volberding
San Francisco General Hospital
995 Potrero Avenue, Building 80, Ward 84
San Francisco, CA 94110

Dear Paul,

Several months ago I wrote to you requesting that I be allowed to speak at the International AIDS Conference this coming summer in San Francisco, of which you are cochair. You were kind enough to call me immediately to say that you looked favorably upon my request.

I did not expect to be turned over to a committee of gay Uncle Toms, led by Dr. Wachter and Mr. van Gorder.

As the founder of ACT UP, of which there are now a great many active chapters around the country, and the cofounder of Gay Men's Health Crisis—the two most important AIDS organizations in this country—I believe I am entitled to a little more respect than I have experienced with these two, culminating in my request being denied.

I think you will find that it will prove a big mistake not to have honored my fervent solicitations. By snubbing me in such a fashion you have slapped in the face not only me and what I have stood for these past nine years, but every other AIDS activist. I trust that with the publication and circulation of this letter, ACT UPs everywhere will now commence their planning to join my call to action—at the conference—to let you, your committee, your conference, and the world that is watching know that, once again, an attempt has been made to silence us.

It is constantly amazing to me how often—when the offer is made, the hand extended, by those of us on another side of this battle, to cooperate—the chance to work in tandem is so casually and carelessly rejected.

Vito Russo, my good friend, who *was* chosen, was never consulted by your people, and, indeed, as your committee was informed, is not even interested in speaking, preferring that I do it. The fact that none of your people even bothered to talk to him is further proof that you are afraid of what I might say, which is greatly troubling.

Everyone had hoped that your conference, of all conferences, and in your city, of all cities, would allow the chance for divergent opinions to be aired publicly. Evidently such is not to be the case; and once again we face a conference homogenized, made bland, and blanched of open discussion of the many divisive issues that prevent AIDS from being cured.

I can assure you that you will now find it will be a conference otherwise. You have, in effect, thrown down the gauntlet, and I intend to see that it is taken up.

If you wish to view this letter as a threat, please do so.

Over years of fighting on a daily basis I've discovered you can't always be the good boy, calling every shot correctly and doing the right thing every minute of every day. You're bound to commit acts you're not particularly proud of. This is one of those acts—even though I believe what resulted proved useful.

While I can't apologize for the passion that led to this

letter's writing, and while I guess you can't be a fighter without being a little threatening now and then, I can see this threat sounds a bit more on the self-serving than on the warrior side.

I wanted to speak at the damn conference very badly. I wanted to scream at all those asshole doctors and researchers and scientists that they knew better than anybody how awful everything was—so why weren't they speaking up and out! I'd begun to notice I was a good speaker. I found I was becoming somewhat of a public figure. I was being sought out more and more by the media. At first I found this unsettling and uncomfortable. Then I wondered if this visibility was handing me a certain power I should learn to utilize as effectively as possible. What better forum than this international conference for my ideas, my thoughts, my opinions? For identifying our enemies? For calling a plague a plague?

I'm often asked how I have such a good relationship with the media, in that I appear so often. I think the reason is that I speak out forthrightly, and say, with no bullshit, exactly what I think and feel and want. Also, I enjoy reporters, because they're writers, too; so they sense our relationship is not an adversarial one, as their relationships with most of those they deal with are.

The San Francisco AIDS Conference was obviously an important forum. I still long intemperately to speak at one of these international affairs. It seems to me that such an address to such a body would be an affirmation and acceptance, at last, of AIDS activism.

But it was not to be. Volberding, never my favorite AIDS tyrant (I was to call him San Francisco's most successful undertaker), bullshitted me into believing I would be allowed to speak, then sent two of his henchmen (Dr. Wachter, by the way, turned out to be straight and wrote his own book about this conference, a tepid affair—both the conference and his book) to set in motion a mechanism that would take the slot away from me. ACT UP was to be allowed to choose its own speaker. As I was always looked upon by many members as someone who had to be held in check, for fear I would take over the organization in some sort of coup d'état, I knew that once it was put to the floor to vote, I would not be the winner. Had I lobbied, I might have won their vote. But I could never bring myself to do that. With ACT UP, I always demurred when it came to this. A strange pride always silenced me. My mind would go something like this: If they don't choose me, knowing how much I want to be their speaker, I am not going to beg them for it. Perhaps I should have.

Vito, much beloved, was chosen. He didn't go, and the spot went to Peter Staley, a handsome young man who made a very moving and gutsy speech that received the large amount of media attention it deserved.

Always a man of my word, I followed through on my threat, which caused some useful repercussions, as you'll see a few pages further on. . . .

What Are You Doing to Save My Fucking Life?

4 December 89

Mr. Richard D. Dadey, Jr.
Human Rights Campaign Fund
1012 14th Street, N.W., Suite 607
Washington, DC 20005

Dear Mr. Dadey,

I am in receipt of your long letter, your bulging packet of expensively-produced direct-mail propaganda, and your invitation to attend a fund-raising cocktail party at the home of my friends, Herb Cohen and Danny Cook, at which you hope to induce as many as possible to join a "Federal Club" of $1,200 donors.

I have read all of your material. It is not very zippy, but this kind of stuff, for some reason, rarely is. You will forgive me, but even after reading it, and even after being cognizant of HRCF's existence for many years, and even after attending several of your lavish dinner-dos at the Waldorf, I am never quite certain *what* HRCF *does.*

Your long letter informs me that, in 1988, "as a result of the money and clout we brought to the table . . . in our legislative battles, stronger and more sophisticated relationships were developed with our nation's lawmakers." My goodness. How can that be so? Our relationships with our nation's lawmakers could not be worse.

Then your letter tells me: "Indeed the Campaign Fund moved into a higher echelon of influence and power in 1988. . . ." Higher than what? We are already at the bottom, in the cellar, of influence with our nation's lawmakers, our nation's President, our nation's Secretary of Health and Human Services, our nation's Surgeon General, and we would be at the bottom with our nation's Director of the CDC and Director of the NIH if our nation's President had seen fit to fill either of these positions.

In fact, both your organization and the gay community are, as I write this, probably in the worst shape and in more trouble than we have been during the entire length of this unendurable plague.

I resent your organization. I resent just about every gay and AIDS organization in Washington. For you see, I don't know what you *do*. I don't know what *any* of you *do*, down there. I think you must all go out to lunch a great deal with "our nation's lawmakers" and then think that you have accomplished something and made entrance into "more sophisticated relationships" and "higher echelons of influence and power."

You and we have done no such thing. You and we have accomplished dipshit. And what we have accomplished, minuscule though that is, has not been accomplished by any of you Washington ladies who lunch.

What are you doing about getting someone put in charge of AIDS?

What are you doing about getting us a good FDA Director?

What are you doing about getting us NIH and CDC Directors?

What are you doing about getting research *started?*

What are you doing about getting promising treatments released immediately?

What are you doing about the hateful ACTG system that is going to be the death of us?

What are you doing about conveying to "our nation's law-makers" with whom you are so buddy-buddy, that your constituency is furiously angry and will, or can, take very little more?

What are you doing that in any way conveys a sense of URGENCY?

I am told you have a new executive director. Why is he such a secret to the world? Why is he not on television every chance he gets, quoted in the press at every opportunity, conveying this sense of URGENCY? Perhaps he is too busy being a lady who lunches too.

I am aware that it is counterproductive to blast our own organizations, which are, I am always told, "doing their best" or "doing all they can"—with and for a community that is, for the most part, still, yet, continuing, in a state of denial that AIDS even exists.

But you are asking for our money and I am telling you that you are not doing your best, or doing all you can. None of our gay organizations in Washington is doing its best or doing all it can.

I say this because I have seen what ACT UP has been able to accomplish in the past year alone. It accomplished more than all of our AIDS and gay organizations have been able to accomplish in the entire duration of this epidemic. And we have no officers and no board of directors and we don't go out to lunch with anybody. But everyone sure as hell knows we're here. And what we do. And what we want. And everyone knows our demands are URGENT.

But ACT UP can't do it alone. And it gets precious little support from any of you Washington lunchers. The main battle to never put out of sight is that of research and treatment—for when they are successfully achieved, there will be no more AIDS. It is not enough to get Congress to appropriate money. You have to see that it is spent and spent wisely. None of you dimwits down there can ever think of this Big Picture. And almost all of the research is being conducted by second-rate yo-yos. And a huge amount of the research—still, yet, continuing—is NOT BEING DONE AT ALL.

What are you and all those other gay and AIDS organizations in Washington doing about any of this?

Dr. Samuel Broder has said AIDS can be cured. But just about every impediment imaginable is being placed in the way of our receiving that cure. What are you doing about it? Now that you have developed such "sophisticated relationships" and have "moved into a higher echelon of influence"?

WHAT ARE YOU DOING TO SAVE MY FUCKING LIFE!

The destruction of hope by the Bush years brought increasing rancor of gay against gay: It was as if we had nowhere else to unload all our tremendous disappointment and upset on but each other. We were the only outlet we could locate. I'm as guilty of this as anyone. I saw nothing I approved of being done by anyone and I let everyone have it with both barrels. I still feel this way. It is utterly disheartening that my own brothers and sisters seem so unable to get their act together in any unified or sufficiently effective fashion.

I guess I've felt this way since the very beginning, and I shouldn't unload this one on George Bush. So many of us. So little power. When will we claim it? It's there, just waiting for us.

We're still being represented in Washington by incompetent boobs, and I still haven't stopped dumping on them. We'd be better off if we didn't have any Washington organizations at all.

It's always seemed falacious to me that just because we're all brothers and sisters in this harsh world all gays should automatically love each other. Well, there's no community of people anywhere in the world in which everyone gets along with everyone else. I cannot imagine a life without criticism.

So I don't apologize for this letter to HRCF either. And I *still* don't know what this organization does.

I guess it's less self-damning when one sees that no other movement—be it of feminists, pro-choice people,

people of color, you name it—is in any better shape. The Reagan-Bush years saw to it that *every* non-conservative movement was effectively silenced. Those fucking Washington doors were sealed with cement!

A Call to Riot[*]

With this article I am calling for a MASSIVE DISRUPTION of the Sixth International AIDS Conference that is being held in San Francisco June 20–24.

Every human being who wants to end the AIDS epidemic must be in San Francisco from June 20th to 24th, at the Sixth International Conference on AIDS, either inside or outside the Moscone Convention Center or the Marriott Hotel, screaming, yelling, furiously angry, protesting at this stupid conference.

These are the facts:

1. A cure for AIDS is available much more rapidly than we are getting it. Treatments are available that we cannot get. Vital research simply isn't being done.

2. We are not getting any of this because of bureaucracy, red tape, and a President who, to put it mildly, doesn't give a shit. George Bush has even refused to speak at the opening of this conference. It is customary for a head of state to open these international conferences.

---

*_OutWeek_ magazine, No. 42, March 14, 1990.

George Bush has been a fucking shithead about AIDS, ignoring it just as much as his doddering, imbecilic predecessor with his Machiavellian wife.

3. The government's ACTG system for delivering promising treatments to those who desperately need them (which is administered by the National Institute of Allergy and Infectious Diseases, part of the National Institutes of Health) is a sham— a shocking, sinful sewer of ineptitude, run by idiots, nincompoops, quack doctors who should have their licenses revoked.

New research is on hold while they take a year off to sort out their fucked-up computer data base. Their research has not been adequately available to minorities, women, or children. Thousands of ACTG treatment slots are *empty.* Can you believe that there are thousands of vacancies for people to receive free drugs, and this asshole government and this asshole ACTG system doesn't fill them up? How fucking inefficient, and SAVAGELY INHUMANE, can a system be?

What *new* treatments has the ACTG system come up with in the four years of its dreary existence? NONE. NOTHING. NIENTE. NADA. Every drug that is presently available for AIDS has come from some source other than the ACTG system—a foreign country, a pharmaceutical company, independent research. You'd think such failure would make the ACTG less powerful. No way. To make certain we are exterminated a little faster, the ACTG has control over what new drugs are studied (or rather, not studied) and what research is funded (or rather, not funded). Thus, our lives are totally in its hands and its hands are killing us as sure as if they stuck daggers into our hearts.

4. The Doctor Strangeloves who control the ACTG system are the same Doctor Strangeloves who are controlling the agenda of, and shutting out any dissident voices from, the Sixth International Conference on AIDS.

5. These are also the very same doctors who are trying to screw us out of Parallel Track. (They don't like Parallel Track because they don't have control of it.) This historic and revolutionary method for getting more drugs into more bodies with more speed was conceived, fought for, orchestrated, and obtained by ACT UP. All you PWAs and HIV-Positives: All those

promising experimental drugs you can't afford to buy overseas or on the underground and you thought were waiting for us on Parallel Track? They just got snatched away. Just when we were about to get ddC and GM-CSF to follow ddI. Do you want them back? Then you fucking well better show up in San Francisco June 20 to 24!

6. TONS OF BASIC SCIENCE HASN'T EVEN BEEN DONE YET! Can you believe that?! I repeat: MASSIVE AMOUNTS OF RESEARCH STILL HAS NOT EVEN COMMENCED. NIH doctors know this! They know what should be researched and still it is not being researched! THEY KNOW IT! Can you believe such tactics, such an attitude?

And they have the money!

And people think we are being paranoid when we scream GENOCIDE!

7. The excuse they use is that GOVERNMENT RESEARCH IS INVESTIGATOR-INITIATED, NOT GOAL-ORIENTED. In other words, any stupid asshole can submit a grant proposal for funding, even if every lab in the world is already studying the same stupid thing; but God forbid something important needs to be studied and no one has submitted a grant to study it. God forbid Drs. Tony Fauci or Sam Broder or Paul Volberding or Margaret Fischl or Thomas Merrigan or Dan Hoth or Larry Corey or Martin Hirsch (some of these people are not your friends, no matter how nice you think they are) should then go out and LOCATE an investigator and hire her/him to research the question the way you hire an actor to play a part. *This stupid attitude could very well be the death of us. The research might never be done!* HOW MANY YEARS DO YOU HAVE TO PISS AWAY WAITING?!

8. This conference is going to be about as "International" as the Ku Klux Klan. Uncle George's Government now forbids anyone who has AIDS or is HIV-positive to enter his wonderful country. Uncle George is punishing us for having the naughty HIV virus in our system. Any foreigner who has AIDS or is HIV-positive and wants to come to the "International" AIDS Conference is forbidden entry past our Statue of "Liberty."

Thus, every foreigner with an ounce of humanity is staying home to protest this inhumanity.

Yes, huge numbers of foreign scientists, plus international AIDS and gay organizations, as well as many American ones, too, are all boycotting the Sixth "International" AIDS Conference.

In other words, THE SIXTH "INTERNATIONAL" AIDS CONFERENCE WILL BE A SICK JOKE.

Most of those there will be—like scabby strikebusters—the slick, heartless Washington bureaucrat representatives of Uncle George, and the expense-account rich hucksters from the greedy profiteering drug companies that suck our blood, and the thousands of representatives of an international media that still can't report AIDS with any accuracy or genuine understanding.

9. We are being royally fucked over, screwed to death, whatever you want to call being INTENTIONALLY ALLOWED TO DIE. This is no longer hyperbole, exaggeration, opinion—it is fact. The systems this government has in operation simply could not move any more slowly.

HOW MANY TIMES DO YOU HAVE TO HEAR THIS BEFORE YOU BELIEVE IT! AND RISE UP AGAINST IT!

THIS GOVERNMENT OF SHITHEADS WANTS US DEAD. WHY CAN'T EVERY GAY MAN AND LESBIAN GET THAT THROUGH HIS/HER HEAD? INDEED, UNCLE GEORGE WANTS ALL FAGGOTS, NIGGERS, JUNKIES, SPICS, WHORES, UNMARRIEDS, AND THEIR BABIES DEAD.

THE STRAIGHT WHITE MAN IS THE GAY PERSON'S ENEMY! HAVEN'T WE HAD ENOUGH PROOF? HOW MUCH MORE EVIDENCE DO YOU NEED? DO YOU HAVE TO BE LINED UP IN FRONT OF A FIRING SQUAD BEFORE YOU FIGHT BACK?

WE HAVE BEEN LINED UP IN FRONT OF A FIRING SQUAD, AND IT IS CALLED AIDS.

WE MUST RIOT! I AM CALLING FOR A FUCKING RIOT!

It is imperative that ACT UP chapters from everywhere and activists from everywhere and all their friends and families and all marchers and all screamers, FROM EVERYWHERE, be in San Francisco June 20 to 24 in front of all the TV cameras and photographers and reporters that will be there to see us. WE

MUST BE THERE TO LET THE WORLD THAT IS WATCH-
ING SEE THAT WE ARE FUCKING FURIOUS!

Would you believe that more people have already registered
for this conference than showed up in Montreal? That means
over fifteen thousand people have already registered.

Thus, a lot of sleazy, scabby, strikebusting people who are
not boycotting the conference will be there. Whether your organization is *officially* boycotting or not, IT IS VITAL FOR
YOU TO BE THERE INDIVIDUALLY.

*Because we are being given a rare and perfect opportunity to
act out our anger and fury where so much of the world's media
will see us.*

We accomplished miracles last year in Montreal. We got the
release of ddI, fluconazole, DHPG, low-dose AZT, AZT for kids,
and expanded access for EPO, and laid the groundwork for ddC,
GM-CSF and Parallel Track. We got all this not because they
were given to us generously; we got them because we fought for
each and every one of them like furies!

Now we must make history again. WE MUST SCREAM
AND FIGHT LIKE FURIOUS FUCKING GODDAMN TI-
GERS FOR OUR DRUGS AND OUR RESEARCH AND OUR
CURE!

WE MUST RIOT IN SAN FRANCISCO!

FROM ALL CORNERS OF AMERICA, AIDS ACTIV-
ISTS AND THEIR FRIENDS AND FAMILIES MUST
COME TO SAN FRANCISCO AND MAKE THEIR VOICES
HEARD!

BE THERE!

TELL YOUR FRIENDS TO BE THERE!

TELL YOUR FAMILIES TO BE THERE!

PASS THIS ARTICLE AROUND. (Make as many copies as
you can.)

REPRINT IT ANYWHERE AND EVERYWHERE YOU
LIKE. (Gay publications everywhere: Please reprint this article.)

LEAVE YOUR FARTS IN SAN FRANCISCO.

JUNE 20–24.

A MASSIVE DISRUPTION (outside *and* inside) of the
Sixth International AIDS Conference in San Francisco June 20th
to 24th.

MASSIVE! DISRUPTION! RIOT! LIFE!

Well, here it is: my Volberding threat in action. By now
I'd pretty much forgotten the threat part. I considered
this a genuine call to arms.

I hadn't given much thought to just what I meant by
"riot." Or rather I knew what I meant but what I meant
and what others thought I meant and what the word
means were construed very differently by many people.
I just wanted a gigantic ACT UP disturbance that, if it
worked, would not allow conference meetings to be held
in silence. I didn't mean violence, though I can see where
it's possible to read into my text that, if you are prone to
it, by all means . . .

All hell broke loose. This is one time when my hyperbole was taken for fact. San Francisco went nuts. The
local news programs were filled with stories about what
awful things might happen. Police were given special
training. The conference center was cordoned off and additional security was added. Everyone was expecting
bombs and fires and guns. They should have known that
gay people just don't do that sort of thing.

Many in San Francisco's gay community were very
angry at me. I was interviewed so much the frenzy was
whipped up even more. It almost was sort of funny turning on the evening news in New York and seeing yet
another preparatory precaution being made in San Francisco to make ready for what Kramer called for.

In the end, the only thing that happened was that
ACT UP's Peter Staley made a ringing speech, and a
projection of George Bush on the giant screen was ridi-
culed, and the Secretary of Health and Human Services,
the most inhuman Dr. Louis Sullivan, was booed so loudly
during his entire speech that though he continued un-
daunted to the end, his words were completely drowned
out. (The result of this was that Dr. Sullivan showed
scant attention to AIDS throughout his entire tenure,
and made no bones about the fact that he hated AIDS
activists and he was punishing us. A great attitude for a

doctor to take, particularly one whose own population—
Dr. Sullivan is a person of color—is particularly hard hit
by AIDS.)

I didn't go to San Francisco myself. I was told I'd be
arrested at the airport and detained until the conference
was over. It didn't occur to me to sneak in like a guerrilla
and direct my troops from some secret hideout. Or that
I could have given some nifty press conferences from a
jail cell. Some warrior me. It appears that Larry also just
doesn't do that sort of thing. More fool I.

I've often wondered why I haven't resorted to more
violent means. Or *somebody* among us hasn't done the
same. I remember at one ACT UP demo, one of our larger
ones, at City Hall in New York, a Brazilian journalist
asked me: "You call this a demonstration? In my country
when they raise the bus fare the people burn the buses."
I've never forgotten that. I've always wondered why,
even when we are most assuredly being murdered, someone among us doesn't start murdering back.

There were about five thousand people at that City
Hall demo. In a New York metropolitan area with some
one million gay men and lesbians, this is all we could get
to protest a hateful closeted Mayor who had done next
to nothing for us. No disruptions occurred in San Francisco either. There were plenty of activists milling about,
but by conference's end they all marched in solidarity
with the doctors attending the conference, led by Dr.
Paul Volberding!

Yes, I was beginning to see that activism in the gay
community had its limits—of participation and of effectiveness.

I tried to repeat this tactic in my next *OutWeek* column, "A Call to Riot—Part Two," urging one and all to
join ACT UP at quite possibly the most impressively
planned and executed demo we ever had—at the National Institutes of Health on May 21, 1990. Months of
excruciatingly detailed planning had gone into this one:
firecrakers and fireworks and smoke bombs in different
colors and armies of demonstrators, costumed in every
conceivable medical guise, who came from all over the

country. Everybody on our side did a grand job. No show at Radio City was ever better. The trouble was nobody from any other side showed up. There was hardly a reporter or TV camera to be seen or found. And because the NIH is far away, in suburban Maryland, with no passing pedestrians, there wasn't anyone watching us either, except for some employees looking out their windows. It was the Big Show that no one came to.

This lack of press attention was becoming a big problem. Our demonstrations were only useful if the world saw them. For a while, particularly after St. Patrick's, we'd been the media's darlings. Suddenly they were bored with us. When, to protest their ignoble ignoring of AIDS (many hospitals did, and still do), we picketed Memorial Sloan-Kettering in New York for an unprecedented round-the-clock four days (and I mean around the clock) and not even one local station ran anything (there seemed to be an unusually large number of fires that week), it was hard to deny our tactics were becoming less effective.

ACT UP began to hold special meetings to discuss what we should do to combat this and other internal problems beginning to become endemic. There were those who felt it didn't make any difference if the media didn't show up, that the demos were good for *us*, for self-empowerment. I thought that so much hard work, and expense, to put on a show just for ourselves, was navel contemplation of too high an order.

Internally, ACT UP was now beginning to show even greater signs of strain.

Something Rotten*

16 April 90

Something rotten is going on.

For a while I tried not to look at it directly. It would go away, I thought. Even though I was personally hurt and pissed off about some of the distasteful stuff that was directed at me, I figured I could live with it. I'm a big boy.

But it isn't only happening to me.

Now I realize that, as in some zit that isn't being squeezed, the amount of pus that is forming under the skin of ACT UP is getting bigger and bigger.

---

*Another of my "Letters to the Floor" of ACT UP. I labeled this one ". . . a personal communication between ACT UP members. It is private, confidential, and not for publication." Needless to say, the *Native* published it in its next issue. There was now a lot of love lost between ACT UP and the *Native* between just about everybody and the *Native*. Something went rotten with that paper, too, and it still is. AIDS was replaced in its columns and its editor's consciousness by Chronic Fatigue Syndrome as *the* thing that was threatening the world. After originally supporting us, the *Native* took to endless attacks, and eventually ACT UP declared a boycott, which I don't think has yet been lifted, on buying it. The *Native* has ceased in any way to be taken seriously anywhere and we are all the poorer for it. New York has no gay newspaper in which we can all talk to each other.

I was recently witness to a monstrous scene in a public restaurant, in which Marcia Levin* stood up and started screaming and hurling accusations and insults and condemnations at Yvonne Furst. I am very fond of Marcia and I am very fond of Yvonne, and both have worked like tigers for ACT UP. Was Marcia breaking down from the strain of tending to so many sick friends? Was it some isolated incident? Or was it indicative of something more pervasive, in all of ACT UP, something spreading around like the virus itself? Marcia was erupting like some volcano with years of boiling lava inside of her, desperate to explode. But why was she erupting hate at Yvonne—Yvonne who fights AIDS, as does Marcia, seven twenty-four-hour days a week?

What was this all about, indeed? Two of our most valuable members erupted, one of them spewing out hate like a viper and the other heaving wretched defensive sobs and tears as she is accused of being too obsessed with and elitist in her work, told that all the women of ACT UP hate her and nobody can work with her—in a Chinese restaurant, where we'd gone to have some r & r.

And since I have respected Marcia, I wondered if her actions were trying to unconsciously tell all of us who were witness to this unfortunate scene (some eight or nine of us) something about what was happening to all of ACT UP.

On another front, I was aware of the controversy surrounding Ron Worthington's work as Administrator. Those who dared to criticize the current state of office affairs out loud had been punished by being bad-mouthed themselves. Many members of the floor had been witness to some of this, but instead of helping Ron out with any of the less than glamorous tasks involved in running such a big and clumsy organization, they reacted by ignoring the issue altogether, with the result that we are more disorganized administratively than ever. And poor Ron, because this job means a great deal to him, has not known how to fight back except by stirring up the pot of drama queens himself.

On yet another front, the Majority Action Committee** seems to waste few opportunities to guilt-trip the floor over just about any issue they can.

---

*I've changed a number of the names in this letter.
**The Majority Action Committee was reserved exclusively for people of color.

Then there is the continuing saga of the castration of Peter Staley. Peter seems to be in great disfavor and to become more so with each week. Last week, the very mention of his name brought boos from several members. (Since when do we allow that?)

I think Peter Staley has done more for ACT UP than almost any other single person. But then it has become increasingly apparent over the past years that ACT UP finds it very difficult indeed to reward passion, competence, devotion, and service. ACT UP prefers to find a way to shit on anybody who works *too* hard for ACT UP. It seems to make no difference that we have been able to live so high off the hog because Peter's tenure as head of Fund Raising has brought us, in the past year alone, over $750,000, and that he has almost single-handedly developed our merchandising business. (Think of that the next time the treasury is bare—which, at the rate we are pissing it away, should be very soon indeed—and there's no money to pay for bail or transportation to an important action.)

Then there was the spectacle of Ron and others beside themselves in their haste to pour out their dissatisfactions about Peter Staley and others, including, I would guess, myself, to *Voice* reporter (and ACT UP member) Donna Minkowitz, who is preparing an article on the future of ACT UP. (Since when do we bad-mouth each other for public attribution?)

Now I am hearing utterly bizarre reports about what is happening at AIDS Treatment Registry. Jean O'Brien, who gave so much to us, and to whom we have given so much (most recently a grant of $25,000), cruelly insults and attacks a number of ACT UPpers, most particularly David Rothstein (once her particular favorite), who are working their asses off for her. She is also insisting that people who work for ATR distance themselves from any connection to ACT UP. Is this how she acts out her worries and fears for ATR's health and survival?

At AmFAR, an ACT UP member, Fred Pester, cruelly hires, terrorizes, and fires ACT UP members, chewing them up and spitting them out, destroying their health insurance benefits, wrecking their confidence.

A week or so ago I was bad-mouthed in the *Washington Blade* by a fellow member, Jim Rinaldi. (Since when do we bad-mouth each other *in public?*)

Then I discovered that the chairman of our Media Committee, Alan Duff, was informing anyone who interviewed me that I must not be identified as the founder of ACT UP.

This followed a number of months of my being screamed at hysterically by Marvin Furrigan—outbursts that I tried to ignore—as he tried to discredit my founding of ACT UP, inserting his personal vendetta in the minutes of a recent Coordinating Committee meeting.

Then I was shown "A Capsule History of ACT UP," put out by the Media Committee, in which my founding of this organization is never mentioned, nor is my name.

So now, I, too, am being thrown down the toilet, along with Peter.

When I was called by both *New York* magazine and ABC News on the same day telling me that Alan Duff had informed them that I was not the founder of ACT UP, and when I heard that Peter Staley's name had brought forth boos and hisses from the floor, I decided that I must write this letter to you.

Something very rotten indeed is going on.

I am appalled by the behavior that all of these incidents represent. They represent gay people, any people, at their shittiest. If we cannot respect each other's contributions, and give credit where it it due, and support each other, both publicly and within our own group, then we are going to lose this war against AIDS even faster than we are already losing it.

Is it because we are losing the war against AIDS that we are so punishing and hateful to each other? If that's so, then we are sick people indeed. And I fear for the survival of ACT UP. These are true signs of burnout and the end. These are signs of self-destruct.

On a personal note, I would like to say that I am going to proudly claim as long as I live that I founded ACT UP. I don't care what any of my enemies claim, or those who weren't even around at the time. Hundreds of people witnessed this creation, and I have consulted with enough of them to know that I am not in any way inaccurate in declaring that the organization would not be here today if I had not made the speech calling for its specific creation on March 10, 1987.

I have witnessed barbaric and dishonest attempts at "revisionist" history before. Indeed, I have seen my own contributions to the foundation of Gay Men's Health Crisis disparaged, ignored, and denied by those who came after me. I have poured the major part of my life these past ten years into trying to make history. I am proud enough of my contributions to want, nay demand, credit for them. I was screwed out of GMHC. I shall not be screwed out of ACT UP.

To those who wish to deny me this credit: Only death will shut this mouth of mine.

As far as the other matters I raise are concerned, on November 27, 1989, I wrote a long communication to the floor entitled "We Must Make Tomorrow Happen Today." I wrote at great length about my belief that ACT UP was in great trouble. A large committee was then formed to discuss and formulate ideas on how to grow and move forward. This large committee met for endless hours and months. Every single one of their suggestions was voted down by the floor with a speed and a distrust and a refusal to discuss them that were awe-inspiring.

I have no more suggestions to make.

I think we are turning rotten at our core. I think we are hitting out at each other more and more blindly and turning each other into the enemy. We have had absolutely no reason to distrust each other, but that is what we have learned to do.

I weep for us.

Here, in a nutshell, is gay politics personified—for all I know, perhaps all politics personified.

When I think of reasons for my lessening involvement in the day-to-day activities of ACT UP, this letter comes closest to explaining why I weaned myself away. Somewhere a few years into its history ACT UP's membership became less inclined to work together. It just happened. Beyond the usual ongoing discussions we had about everything, there appeared no apparent evidence of schism or disagreement about policy or direction. It was almost as if one day a new page was turned and a new chapter started being written. Maybe, to the clairvoyant, it was all there from the beginning. Pollyanna me, for the longest time, thought anything wrong could be put right. I was wrong. Or rather I saw that it would take more energy to make ACT UP into the fighting machine I wanted it to be than it would take to find the very cure for AIDS itself. While I loved being a part of that wonderful organization when it was wonderful, I had to face up pragmatically to the fact that when it started being less wonderful, my energies could be put to better use elsewhere. For instance, writing a regular column for a gay publication (as I did for *OutWeek* and would do for *The Advocate*) seemed more beneficial than writing letters like this one, where I sound like an old-maid schoolteacher.

The scenario I describe sounds like a soap opera parody. My naive expectation that ACT UP would behave any differently from the way the world behaved strikes me now as a dose of double standards. To this day there's been no way to fix its problems—problems that in one way or another festered at and destroyed other chapters around the world as well. I wonder if perhaps we might just have been very very lucky that those early days of GMHC and ACT UP went as well as they did, before things turned sour. Maybe, people being people, we got more than we had a right to expect.

This time round, when the paternity of an organization I felt was there because of me was questioned, I determined to fight back. There was, and remains, great ill will between me and GMHC, not only because it's never done what I founded it to do, but because they have managed over the years to eradicate just about all traces of my having ever had anything to do with the place. A year or so before this present letter to ACT UP, I'd been forced to write a stinging rebuke to James Pepper and the rest of the then GMHC board for an attempt at just this same sort of revisionist history:

"Increasingly I have noticed in the press that several present and past board members—particularly Judge [Richard] Failla—have taken to referring to themselves as a 'founding board member of GMHC.' And now Mr. Pepper's letter refers to a classroom 'dedicated to the co-founding Board.'

"For the sake of all future historians, and to protest against the sleazy posturings of Judge Failla and Mr. Pepper, I would like to state the following facts. Gay Men's Health Crisis was my idea. I called together five friends to hear about it. I gave it its name. There was no co-founding *board* of GMHC. GMHC was officially founded by six men: Nathan Fain, Larry Kramer, Dr. Lawrence Mass, Paul Popham, Paul Rapoport, and Edmund White. This happened in my apartment, on January 4, 1982, although various groups had been meeting together since the first get-together, also in my apartment, on August 11, 1981.

"The first board of directors, which was eventually formed in May 1982 (and did not include Judge Failla), was composed of Paul Popham, Larry McDevitt, Brad Frandsen, Joe Paschek, Nathan Fain, Larry Kramer, Dr. Lawrence Mass, Harry Diaz, and Joe Hernandez. On August 23, 1982, Harry Diaz and Joe Hernandez resigned and Robert Wachter, Enno Poersch, and Richard Failla were elected."

The business about ACT UP hurt me. A few people believed that ACT UP was founded by nobody and that it had sprung full-grown from the head of Zeus. There's no question a movement starts because the timing is right and energy is out there waiting to release itself and coalesce around some entity. There's also no question, though, that someone has to unleash all this energy, and I'd never doubted that it was my speech* that led to ACT UP's formation, which I carefully monitored and supervised, as I had the early days of GMHC.

Perhaps this sounds egocentric. I don't know. I'm not so saintly as to believe people should do things without rewards and recognition. I'm much too insecure for that. Like any creative person, I want to see the results of my ideas take form and grow and prosper. And to be allowed to be proud of them. I don't think I could do much anonymously. People do much better work when they're rewarded. I'm no exception.

---

*See "The Beginning of ACTing UP," page 127.

After this letter's appearance, no one at ACT UP said anything in opposition.

I've been a reader and a writer for too long not to know how history can be, and most often is, written—filled with lies—and that you better get your version on the record before you die. Gay history is particularly bad at recording anything with any accuracy or consistency. Already in the history of AIDS I've read too much that proclaims some person's deeds, or certain events, that are pure fiction. I can imagine some future historian winning a Pulitzer or Bancroft for a ten-volume tome on the plague, filled with nothing but errors. For instance, I find it sadly amusing how many doctors and scientists, when queried today, maintain they saw their first cases—and sounded their first alarms—in 1980 or 1981. Utter bullshit. If as many of them had seen as much and spoken as bravely, we wouldn't have a plague today.

Time Out for Depression[*]

With this award, I am leaving AIDS activism and gay activism.

In 1983, after working very hard to start GMHC, I was pushed out of the organization that meant so much to me.

Several weeks ago, I was denied the paternity of ACT UP.

This morning I received a letter signed by all the people of color at GMHC, calling me a racist; I had tried to right what I considered to be extremely bad treatment by GMHC of one of my old friends, Susan Richardson, who is a woman of color who worked for them.

I think we are all going crazy.

In *The Sound and the Fury*, William Faulkner wrote: ". . . no battle is ever won. . . . They are not even fought. The field only reveals to man his own folly and despair, and victory is an illusion of philosophers and fools."

For ten years we have had only agony and rejection, as the virus got completely out of control. I have come reluctantly to the heavyhearted conclusion that the system will not move for us, that the system cannot be made to respond and save us, that

---

*Remarks delivered upon being presented with, and not accepting, the Michael Hirsch "Person of the Year" award from Body Positive, May 17, 1990.

330

the world will not perform the humanitarian acts that are essential to our survival.

We have lost the war against AIDS. Millions of people who need not die so young will die so young. I see no way that these millions of deaths can be prevented. Even if a cure were found tomorrow, the system would not test and make it available fast enough to save us.

There is only strife and bickering and distrust and death: That is all we have and all we have to look forward to. Our Presidents and our governments have turned us against one another and, in our utter despair, we make each other the enemy.

Michael, from one fighter to another—we have lost. We could not fight hard enough. We were too poor and our forces were too few.

I *was* depressed. Burn-out is something I never allow myself, so even now I won't concede that's what was happening. I remember jotting down the few words of this speech only hours before the ceremony. The room was very quiet as I spoke, and Colleen Dewhurst, God love her, ready to present me my award, was left holding it and left also to move the ceremony along in a more festive spirit as I bolted from the room. I heard resounding applause as she said something like, "We must never give up the fight."

Michael Hirsch had been someone who never gave up. I remember how he used to call me in the very early days, from his job—I think he ran a phone-sex service of some sort—and tell me his plans for fighting so that attention would be paid. We joined together once to plaster flyers on the St. Mark's Baths demanding they be closed. When he couldn't get any organization to be as strong as he urged them to be, he started his own organization. Even when he got sick, he never stopped. He was arrested at an AIDS convention in Washington for overturning a table belonging to the wretched Burroughs-Wellcome Company, which, true to form, pressed charges—against a sick man!—and Michael wound up in jail, to be sprung by his courageous doctor, the wonderful Dr. Barbara Starrett. I remember her, from a pay phone at the Washington Hilton, screaming at the police: "But you are incarcerating a man who is dying!" Even now, I wonder how many doctors fight as hard for their patients as Barbara did and does.

Once again I seemed to have fallen victim myself to the very standard I put forth: It's okay to criticize. Funny how I never seem to think about how criticism can hurt. As the contents of this book amply demonstrate, I've lobbed enough tomatoes and eggs at enough people and organizations to get my due share lobbed right back at me. Over the years I've maintained, not without honesty, that when this happened it didn't bother me. Usually it didn't. At this moment in time, I guess it did. Something entirely unrelated also did. Why was I one of so few people doing what I was doing? *That* was beginning to bug the shit out of me. Why are there so few gay men, HIV-positive or not, who are out there screaming and clamoring for a meaningful system for finding a cure? I don't think what I'm doing or saying is in any way remarkable. So why am I relatively alone on this front line?

I remember some guy coming up to me on the street outside my neighborhood Gristede's and effusively thanking me for "what you're doing." I found myself, literally, screaming at him, something along the lines of "Fuck you! Why aren't you doing it, too!" Oh, I'd said much the same in my writings, but now I found myself screaming it on street corners and as I slammed down phones. Yeah, I was depressed. And I didn't have ACT UP to go to every week to calm me down.

Many think I was kicked out of ACT UP, as I was separated from GMHC. This isn't true. ACT UP actually (and sometimes unfortunately) doesn't have a mechanism for removing members. I just stopped going to meetings. I'd drop in on T+D now and then, but even that became a tremendous chore. "Process"—that awful contrivance which is Satan's version of Robert's Rules of Order—has taken over, as I guess after a while it takes over any group of more than three. The endless interminable arguments, over how to spend twenty-five dollars or, to quote Paul Rudnick, "that funds be raised to purchase rubber dental dams (a safe-sex device) for the indigent citizens of El Salvador" were too much. Yes, my main, and previously most successful, support system was gone. I was on my own now.

AIDS: The War Is Lost*

I am fifty-five years old. When I started fighting AIDS, I was forty-four years old. I don't feel fifty-five years old. I feel not much older than most of you. That happens to some people, if they're lucky, as they grow older—they somehow stay young inside. But I know I must look ancient to you, and yes, I have seen so much you haven't seen that I am old in many ways that you can't be yet.

I have discovered—and this only over the past ten years—that the world is not a very nice place and that people, all people, are often not very nice people. And this has not been a nice lesson to learn, and perhaps not one that should be presented to you—you who are full of hope and just starting out in the world and on the journey that I started when I left Yale in 1957, before most of you were even born. Yes, that makes me feel very old, knowing that I can never be so young again, and so full of hope as you are now.

---

*I called this my Student Speech: Since June 1990, it's been delivered, in one form or another, at Oberlin, Amherst, Bowdoin, the University of New Hampshire (which was kind enough to print it up in a handsome volume they distributed widely), New York University, Yale, and a few others I can't remember at this moment.

I hope you are full of hope, and will remain so, even after what I tell you, because hope is the only thing that keeps us alive. And yes, believe it or not, despite everything I know and everything I have been through and learned these past ten years, I still have hope. Even though, as I want to talk to you about tonight, the world has lost the war against AIDS. AIDS has won.

I'm going to put all my statistics up front, give them to you now, and try not to give you any more. I've learned that statistics can be made to lie any which way you want them to, and I, like the government, have certainly learned how to use them to my advantage; but what I am going to give you are a few statistics that can't lie, for anybody.

There is one new HIV infection in the United States every fifty-four seconds.

There are 267 new cases of AIDS every day. That amounts to some eight thousand cases every month.

There is one AIDS death every nine minutes.

At least four in every thousand college kids are now infected.

That means at least two or three or four of you here tonight are now infected.

Don't feel safe. Please, the rest of you, don't feel safe. The incubation period of the AIDS virus is very, very long. When I first started hearing about and fighting against what was to be called AIDS, there were only forty-one cases. When I first started getting really scared and vocal, there were one thousand. We are rapidly approaching 200,000 cases of full-blown AIDS, with up to six million people already infected with the HIV virus—nobody knows how many and nobody really knows how to count them.

And the fastest-rising risk group in the major cities is now heterosexual women. In New York City, the percentage of straight women coming down with AIDS has risen from 3 percent to 7 percent.

The World Health Organization now estimates that three million women are already infected with HIV.

The first 100,000 cases took nine years. The next 100,000 cases will only finish accruing in two years. If the health-care system of this country almost collapsed under the intolerably burdensome weight of 100,000, it is terrible to imagine what another 100,000 will do.

And the terrible thing about these numbers is that they're low. The Centers for Disease Control, which keeps the talleys, relies on doctors reporting all their cases to them. As we're finding out, many doctors, for various reasons, aren't reporting their cases. They haven't time, or they're protecting their practices or their patients. So all of these figures, which are known to be low, are also known to be imprecise. They're mostly based on extrapolations from small samplings from isolated areas or from the cases that doctors do report to authorities. We also know that large numbers of those infected never see a doctor.

Now I'm not going to give you any more statistics. No—I'm going to give you one more: By the year 2000, the World Health Organization estimates that, the world over, there will be 20 million people infected with the AIDS virus.

No—I'm going to give you another statistic. An important one. This is going to be the last one, I promise. One out of four households in America has now been somehow touched by AIDS.*

That is an awful lot of grieving families, grieving very silently.

AIDS is an epidemic—now a plague—that need not have happened. It was obvious to enough people from the very beginning what would occur unless measures of warning and education were taken immediately. But because AIDS was then striking down mostly gay men, the forces of bigotry were powerful enough to prevent such measures from being taken—indeed, are still fighting powerfully to prevent such measures from being taken.

AIDS has taught 25 million gay sons and daughters a scary lesson. Many of the parents of 25 million gay sons and daughters don't want to take care of their children when they are ill. In

---

*My editor, as editors the world over are sure to do, has asked me if I would please attribute these statistics to something official-sounding. I would if I could remember where I'd found them. Over the years I'd made it my habit to jot down the highest number to date, of whatever it might be—deaths, infections, heterosexuals, students—whenever I heard or read it, and then insert it in the next article or speech. I usually neglected to jot down the source, or, if I did, it invariably got misplaced somewhere along the journey from composition to delivery to typesetting. But the numbers were definitely taken from some acceptable source. As I mentioned in my introduction to Part Three, I no longer bother much with statistics.

fact, this country will do almost anything rather than pay attention to AIDS: It will not educate people or support adequate funding for research and treatment; it will not do anything about lessening the cost of what meager treatments there are, which are so expensive that most of those with AIDS simply can't afford them; and it will not exert pressure on the second President in a row who pretends that AIDS—ten years into a plague—isn't even here, and refuses to put someone with brains in charge of it.

Can you imagine: A plague is raging and there is no one in charge of it?

Can you imagine: We're in a war without a general?

Can you imagine: Parents are letting their own kids die and not doing anything about it?

Can you imagine: In a time of plague there is only minimum, sporadic, uncoordinated research conducted, for the most part, by second-rate yo-yos, if it is conducted at all?

Can you imagine: Lifesaving drugs (some even owned by the government) are priced so high that most of those who desperately need them can't afford them?

Can you imagine: There is no endorsement of full-scale education, safe-sex guidelines, condoms?

Can you imagine: The second compassionless President in a row refuses to put anyone in charge (as he did immediately for scandals involving illegal drugs, HUD, savings and loans)? He has appointed another in a long line of useless Secretaries of Health and Human Services, has installed a compliant Surgeon General (getting rid of Dr. Koop, an exceptionally useful one), and has removed the head of the Food and Drug Administration just when, miracle of miracles, he was beginning to do something effective. Until last month the President hadn't even appointed a director for the National Institutes of Health.

Can you imagine $1 billion, so far, thrown away on a system of government-supervised networks of local hospital treatment centers that has, for five years now, simply not worked, functioned, got off the ground? God forbid they should test anything but their beloved AZT, which has seen a 50 percent rise in lymphomas in those who manage to survive it. God forbid they should run studies on any of the fifty to one hundred drugs backed up in the NIH pipeline. God forbid they should run tests on combinations of therapies. God forbid they should test treatments for the Opportunistic Infections most AIDS patients die from. God forbid they should acknowledge any treatment from abroad. God forbid they should test drugs *not* manufactured by one of the companies that have just about every principal investigator at every hospital and university and medical center and government agency *on their payrolls* as "consultants." (Talk about "conflict of interest"! Just about very AIDS investigator receives fees from one or more pharmaceutical manufacturers.)

Thus we are hardly further along on the road to a cure than we were five years ago when this system was set up to research and locate this very cure.

As matters now stand, 20 million people are going to die.

And yet one of the top NIH AIDS experts, Dr. Samuel Broder, has said publicly that he believes AIDS can be cured.

Yet every impediment imaginable is being placed in the way of our receiving this cure.

Why? Because AIDS is still thought of as a gay disease. While it remains predominantly heterosexual in Africa, while straight cases in this country continue to rise slowly, it has served the conservative, right-wing agendas in America to maintain that AIDS is a gay disease. And faggots are this era's niggers and kikes. An officially sanctioned scapegoat to sow hatred seems, historically, always to be necessary in this country and this world. Since it's now illegal to discriminate against Jews and blacks, let's go after the queers.

(Gays keep congressional bigots inordinately busy. Senator Gordon Humphrey offered amendments two years in a row denying federal health-care funds to any organization that used the terms "normal, natural, or healthy" to describe homosexuality. Senator Armstrong offered a broad amendment to the Americans with Disabilities Act, which protects people with AIDS, to remove protection for gays whether they had AIDS or not. The inhuman monster Jesse Helms got an amendment passed that requires all government-funded safe-sex materials to in no way mention, illustrate, or discuss homosexuality or the way gays have sex. Way to stop a plague, America. Thanks, Mom and Dad.)

I have a friend in ACT UP who is twenty-two years old. He is very sick. He's from a small town in Massachusetts. I asked him, How did you get infected so young? Didn't you know what was going on? Surely word must have reached your town to be careful. And he said, No, he hadn't known anything when he made love for the first times in his life. When I meet kids like this, on their way to death before they even know life, I want to put a gun to the heads of people like Reagan and Bush and Cardinal O'Connor and Ed Koch and Jesse Helms and Abe Rosenthal, who was editor of *The New York Times* during those first years when that newpaper—"all the news that's fit to print"— refused to write anything about AIDS, and force them to come face to face with these kids who are going to die because their leaders refused to allow a country to be educated and warned.

On Wednesday, November 15, 1989, at 7 P.M., in Springfield, while leading a candlelight vigil at Southwest Missouri State University in support of my play *The Normal Heart*, a young student organizer—someone your own age—had the house where he lived burned down by local bigots. Springfield is the home of the Assemblies of God, a fundamentalist religious group. *The Normal Heart* is about how and why AIDS was ignored from Day One. It shows two men kissing. It shows two men getting married. It shows one person losing the person he loved most in the world. In six years and over six hundred productions, including those in Russia, Poland, Israel, and Catholic Ireland, there has never been an incident. (Indeed, in Ireland, the government even paid for the production because they thought it such a valuable educational tool.) It's used in many colleges and schools as a textbook. It's been chosen one of three plays to inaugurate the new Roumanian National Theater. But in our own wonderful country, a Missouri state representative named Jean Dixon used the same argument Helms used to remove the exhibition of work by the gay photographer Robert Mapplethorpe at the Corcoran Gallery in Washington—that taxpayers' money must not be used to "promote" homosexuality. Talking about something is evidently equal to promoting it. As if people didn't have their own minds.

(When told about the fire, Jean Dixon professed sadness but claimed the student leader, Brad Evans, was a "satan worshipper." She then insisted on studying the bodies of his two cats killed in the fire, and proclaimed that she thought he was into animal sacrifice as well.)

There are 25 million gay people in the United States. That is no small number of taxpayers. Twenty-five million gay men and

lesbians have every right to see our lives dramatized, photographed, painted, filmed, exhibited, read about, promoted—and
protected. We have a right to be taken care of when we are ill
just like straight white heterosexual middle-class males, the ruling class in this country. Indeed, the American Revolution was
fought by citizens over just this issue: taxation without representation.

So let's not talk about "the rights of taxpayers to determine
how their money is spent," as Representative Pat Williams of
Montana did, referring to heterosexual taxpayers. And let's not
take any more polls about whether "taxpayers" or editors of
Newsweek or viewers of "Entertainment Tonight" approve of
gays. It's illegal to take polls about whether people approve
of Jews or blacks. (And if these polls were taken, I think Jews
and blacks would lose.)

And let's not trot out that old chestnut: Gays are abnormal.
Twenty-five million is too large a number of folks to be caused
by anything but normal statistical differences. And don't claim,
as Representative William Dannemeyer has in his recent book,
that homosexuals can change (we can't and don't want to if we
could), so aren't entitled to rights. Jews can convert to Christianity, too, but still they're protected against discrimination.

A black kid is murdered in Bensonhurst, a Jewish kid gets
mauled in Brooklyn, fourteen school kids are killed in upstate
New York in a tornado, and the law and the media are there in
droves in a minute. Gays are murdered regularly and no one is
there at all. The FBI in Missouri refused to investigate who
burned down Brad Evans's house. No reporter has *ever* asked
Reagan or Bush a question about AIDS at a Presidential press
conference.

I seem to have spent a lot of time talking about hate and
discrimination, rather than about AIDS. But then it has taken
me ten years to realize that AIDS, in every possible way, is a
metaphor for hate, the hatred of the ruling class for the minority.
And this minority now includes not only gays but also Hispanics
and Africans and Afro-Americans and women and *children* and
people who take drugs and men and women who prefer not to
get married and women who find themselves selling their bodies
for money. Somehow this mixed salad of people is tossed to-

gether and instead of being heralded—as this country and its leaders are always so proud of proclaiming—as part of the big, wonderful "melting pot," "the rainbow coalition," "the thousand points of light," "the gorgeous mosaic" that makes America brave and great and strong and true, they are relegated to that now hateful category of *minority:* the expendable ones. The ones who can be left to die. The ones who can be, intentionally, left to die.

For make no mistake, I now know that intentional genocide is going on.

Otherwise so many people would not be left to die.

Otherwise the leader of a country would put somebody in charge of a plague.

Quite simply, some bookkeeper has discovered that it is cheaper to let us die then to try to save us, to keep us alive.

You think research is going on full-speed, no-holds-barred, all-stops-out at the National Institutes of Health, once thought of as the most famous, the premier science and health facility in the world? There are *twenty-nine* vacancies for scientifically trained personnel at the Division of AIDS at NIH. Nine of these are for department chiefs. But no one is being hired, because there is a hiring freeze. And no one was applying for these jobs anyway, because people can make so much more money working in the private sector, why would anybody who is any good want to work at the now second-rate NIH? Way to stop a plague, George Bush.

(And, by the way, George, twenty-five thousand Americans have died from AIDS since you took office. Oops—another statistic. Well, it just slipped in.)

I am only telling you what six federal studies and more than fifty congressional oversight hearings have all told the President: The research on AIDS is uncoordinated. No one is in charge.

And you thought there was major research going on in Washington toward finding a cure? No, sir. No, ma'am. There is one billion dollars being pissed down the toilet at the National Institutes of Health, where there is no one in charge of AIDS and where there are so many committees and committees within committees and peer reviews that it is truly impossible, and unnecessary, for anyone to ever have to make a decision.

Can you imagine that a system is set up so that it is not necessary for anyone to make a decision? That is what has happened to government in our country.

And that is how the Holocaust—the big one, of Jews and gays and gypsies in Europe during World War II—that is how the Holocaust was allowed to happen: good men and women just doing their jobs, good family men who had families to protect and who were part of huge bureaucracies and who were only following orders from someone higher up. The great philosopher Hannah Arendt, whom I hope you are studying and revering, has written about this, most specifically in her book *Eichmann in Jerusalem: A Report on the Banality of Evil*.

In America, yet another holocaust is going on. Good men and women with families to feed and who are part of huge bureaucracies are keeping their jobs by doing—or not doing—what their superiors are instructing. And the superior at the top, the President, is telling them nothing, so it is nothing that is really being done—even though these good family men and women know that more and more people are coming down with AIDS and dying from AIDS. When I ask Dr. Anthony Fauci (who is in charge of the choosing and testing of new AIDS treatments for our government and whom Bush has called "a hero") if he has told Bush how awful everything is, Fauci says that you do not talk to the President that way.

This is how Hitler's henchmen followed his orders.

By now you are thinking this is sounding farfetched and I am going crazy comparing our Presidents to Hitler. I beg you to locate another book, in addition to books by Hannah Arendt. This one is called *Modernity and the Holocaust* and it is by Zygmunt Bauman, who is Professor of Sociology at the University of Leeds, and is published here by Cornell University Press. This is the first full academic explication of a theory I have held for a long time and wrote about in my own book *Reports from the holocaust*. Bauman takes my theory a step further. He maintains—God help us all—that, in the modern world, holocausts are inevitable; that modernity—the progressive triumph of modern civilization, the determination by some to create more perfect worlds—has brought with it systems of bureaucracy that result in calculated exercises of bureaucratic moral indifference that can be generated on a massive scale. Bureaucracy of course does not reward competence and originality—only compliance. Bauman's conclusion is that *society now functions to render moral norms inoperative, rather than to enforce them.*

And that is what has happened. A society which hates gays has allowed them to become this decade's Jews. And just as Jews were joined in the extermination camps by others who were not Jewish, so gays are now joined by many, many others who are not gay. And yet there is no condemnation of all this. Morality and moral norms are not operating. Just as the world sat by while millions of Jews and others were murdered, so this same world is sitting by as millions of gays and others are murdered.

Let me illustrate.

Three years ago, almost four, when ACT UP found out that government research was not going on—despite the appropriation by Congress of sufficient funds—I decided I had to go to Washington and try to unravel the trail that led from the White House to the various agencies. I had naively believed that just because the money we'd fought for so desperately for so many years had been appropriated, something was being done with it. ACT UP had discovered that it wasn't—that the system of official AIDS treatment centers the NIH had set up was receiving millions and millions of dollars ($47 million at that time; it's now up to a billion) and had nothing but vacancies. Hospitals that were supposed to be treating two thousand people were treating ten. I am not exaggerating. Hospitals like Sloan-Kettering in New York were receiving a million dollars a year and treating ten people in a program funded by NIH for several thousand.

I believed that the NIH would be spending this money. For three precious years I and others sat by and waited for their results, thinking they were doing their work. How many dear friends died while I and others sat by not paying attention, not having the energy or courage to get on the phone and inquire politely: "Please, sirs, can you tell me what you're doing with all that nice money Congress gave you?" How could we have been so lazy and irresponsible and *trusting?* Gay people, of all people, should know better and know how not to trust. Where were we all? Where were all our gay and AIDS organizations? Where were our people in Washington? Where was I? For I blame myself more than I blame anyone else. I had trusted too!

My first meeting was at the White House, with the President's Domestic Policy Advisor, a man named Gary Bauer, who advised Reagan on AIDS.

It's an awe-inspiring experience to actually walk up to and into the White House. Past the gates, past the guards, into that very place itself. I grew up in Washington, and my father worked for the government, so perhaps the symbolic act meant even more to me.

Gary Bauer was, and still is, a small man, with hooded, beady, untrustworthy eyes. He is so slight and dainty that I thought for a moment, succumbing to a stereotype, he might be gay. Then I thought, No, he is the kid who was always called a sissy growing up and now has undying hatred for gays because he was always thought to be one. For I had read and heard the many awful things he'd said about gays, about AIDS being God's revenge on us. Yes, someone who worked for the President had actually said things like this publicly.

It was a most peculiar interview. I was coming for help, but I knew he was a man who hated me and my people. He knew that I had access to the media (indeed my interview had been set up by *Newsday*) and that he could no longer say the hateful things publicly he'd said before he worked at the White House. I asked him if Reagan's ignoring AIDS was intentional, and he answered that he had not seen enough evidence that the Black Plague was going on, and therefore it was receiving sufficient attention. He was particularly interested to hear from me that current evidence indicated the gay male population of the major cities was on its way to becoming totally exposed to the virus. I asked him why the President had refused to put anyone in charge—to appoint an AIDS czar. He told me the President *was* the AIDS czar. I asked him why the President had not read Surgeon General Koop's Report on AIDS or the National Academy of Sciences AIDS report—both of which were then almost a year old and both of which begged for immediate, all-out action—and Bauer responded that the chain of command dictates that, in matters of health, the President talk only to his Secretary of Health and Human Services, then Dr. Otis R. Bowen. Bauer referred to AZT as ACT. It was perfectly obvious that he loathed homosexuals. (Indeed, he now works for something called the Family Research Council, and he appears quite regularly on TV

shows as a hate monger.) And this was Reagan's AIDS adviser—
a President we now know was ruled by his advisers.

Continuing my journey through the bureaucratic labyrinth:
Dr. Bowen, the Secretary of Health and Human Services,
wouldn't see me. He was Reagan's *third* Secretary of HHS, and
he was supposed to be in charge of all AIDS matters. During his
entire term of office, he was never heard to say publicly one thing
about this disease. The Secretary of the main department of your
government in charge of AIDS—the one single man who can report to the President on the state of this nation's health—had
never been heard to say anything about AIDS—and this was the
beginning of the seventh year of this plague.

There is now no question in my mind that Gary Bauer (who
ruled Dr. Bowen as John Poindexter ruled his Ollie North and
others, both probably never bothering to tell the President anything, feeling in their heart of hearts that they were performing
acts the President would approve of) made it clear to Bowen that
AIDS was not a top priority to be discussed with the President,
or anyone else.

You think it is different now? The new Secretary of Health
and Human Services, Dr. Louis Sullivan, actually has *opposed*
the AIDS Research Bill. The Bush Cabinet is much better on
rhetoric than the Reagan Cabinet, but just as do-nothing behind
the scenes. Dr. Sullivan has been surrounded by a staff of pro-
tective right-wingers. Of all places in the cabinet, HHS is one of
the most tricky, for this is where abortion is dealt with. And very
early on Dr. Sullivan put his foot in his mouth, if you remember,
by favoring abortion and then backtracking. This so terrified the
White House that they surrounded him with a staff so conservative that AIDS is rarely spoken of either.

I *was* allowed to meet with the Assistant Secretary of HHS
under Reagan, Dr. Robert Windom. He'd never worked in government. He was a private physician from Sarasota who came
to Washington because he contributed $55,000 to his idol's cam-
paign fund. He was described to me this way by a top legislative
congressional aide: "If his IQ were any lower, you'd have to water him."

You laugh, and Dr. Windom was in charge of our lives! An
uncaring, dumb stooge who knew next to nothing about AIDS
was in charge of my life and in charge of your lives, particularly

the two or three or four or five or six of you in this audience who
are already infected.

Dr. Windom reported to Dr. Bowen, who reported to Gary
Bauer, who reported to the President.

Dr. Windom had an assistant named Dr. Harmison, who also
wouldn't see me. Dr. Harmison, it was well-known, did not like
gays. My gay congressional contacts—and we have many gay
people working on the Hill—described Dr. Harmison to me as
"evil." "You cannot say enough bad things about Lowell Harmison," I was told by more than one. His biggest paranoid fear
was that gays would donate blood in order to pollute, intentionally, the nation's blood supply.

Dr. Harmison reported to Dr. Windom, who reported to Dr.
Bowen, who reported to Gary Bauer, who reported to the President.

Bauer, Bowen, Windom, Harmison. These were the four top
men in charge of AIDS in the U.S. government, the government
of all the American people. Two bigots, one not-very-smart man,
and one coward. And I knew more about AIDS than any of them.
Indeed, any one of you here who reads the newspapers and
watches TV knows more about AIDS than any of these four
monsters.

Next I went to the National Institutes of Health. The NIH
receives some $7 billion *each and every year* to look after the
health of the American people. "To improve the health of the
American people" is the wording of its charter. The then head
of the NIH, whose name was Dr. James Wyngaarden, was never,
during his entire tenure, heard to speak out publicly about AIDS.
The biggest plague of modern times, a transmissable virus in-
fecting a new person every single minute, and the man in charge
of the nation's health never said a word about it.

Dr. Wyngaarden reported to Dr. Windom, who reported to
Dr. Bowen, who reported to Gary Bauer, who reported to Reagan.

The NIH looks like a college campus. Very picturesque. It's
really made up of twelve institutes, which are sort of like dorms,
or frat or sorority houses. Very manicured and lovely.

Ten years ago, when AIDS was first noticed, and you would
have thought NIH would jump on it fast, here is what happened:
You would have thought that because there was a cancer in-

volved, called Kaposi's sarcoma, AIDS should have gone to the institute in charge of cancer, the National Cancer Institute of the National Institutes of Health. The NCI is the richest fraternity at NIH. In 1981, when AIDS first showed up and should have gone into this rich fraternity, the head of this rich fraternity didn't want it. So he blackballed it. He had $1 billion of research money "to improve the health of the American people" and this man, whose name was Dr. Vincent T. Devita (who resigned in 1987 to take a job running Memorial Sloan-Kettering in New York at a reported $400,000 a year—that's the kind of money you can jump to from a government job paying $80,000 a year if you are a good bureaucrat who is compliant and obeys, who never makes any waves), knew AIDS was a smelly political hot potato and so he passed the buck to a poor relation, a much smaller institute named the National Institute of Allergy and Infectious Diseases, which had a budget of only one-fourth that of NCI and which was not nearly such a popular fraternity to rush and was then run by a man named Dr. Richard Krause, who was a closeted gay man and so terrified of being discovered to be gay that he didn't want AIDS in his fraternity either. But since his frat had no choice but to rush this new member, he quit instead.

He was replaced by the man who is in charge now, the man who probably has more to say about AIDS and my life and the lives of all of you who are in danger than any single person in the entire world. His name is Dr. Anthony Fauci.

At that time, Dr. Fauci reported to Dr. Wyngaarden, who reported to Dr. Windom, who reported to Dr. Bowen, who reported to Gary Bauer, who reported to Reagan.

Now Dr. Fauci reports to Dr. Mason, who reports to Dr. Sullivan, who reports to John Sununu, who reports to Bush. The names may be different, but the effect is the same. Dr. Mason is a Mormon (Mormonism is a religion that particularly hates gays), and Dr. Sullivan is surrounded by his conservative right-wing staff, and John Sununu I shall talk about in a moment, and the President is still not being informed. Are you beginning to see what Hannah Arendt and Professor Zygmunt Bauman mean when they talk about the banality of evil, about how holocausts can happen and are bound to happen in this modern bureaucratic world?

All it takes is one person somewhere high up in the chain of command who hates, and everything and everyone else just falls into line all the way down to the bottom of the heap.

Professor Bauman puts it very bluntly:

> When the modernist dream [of creating the perfect society] is embraced by an absolute power able to monopolize modern vehicles of rational action [the press; public opinion] and when that power attains freedom from effective social control [a weak media, or one controlled by conservative forces, as ours is] and non-interference, the passive acceptance of those things by the population at large—genocide follows.
>
> All these factors and forces are fully "normal." They are constantly present in every modern society and their presence has been made both possible and inescapable by those processes which are properly associated with the rise and entrenchment of modern civilization.

Nobody here is *really* saying, "Go out and kill the faggots and the niggers and the spics and the junkies and the whores and the illegitimate kids and the unmarried mothers," but, in fact, that's just what they are all saying and just what is really happening.

It is now a recognized fact that Franklin Roosevelt did less to save millions of European Jews from their deaths during World War II than was recognized at the time or for many years afterward. Two distinguished books go into great detail. *While Six Million Died* by Arthur D. Morse came out in 1967 and *The Abandonment of the Jews* by David S. Wyman, a professor at the University of Massachusetts, in 1984. Both books are devastating to read. I grew up worshiping Roosevelt; he was the man, the President, the humanitarian, who could do no wrong. American Jews, particularly, worshiped him. What blind fools we were. Morse puts it quite succinctly: "Since [Roosevelt] was afraid that the Jewish issue was a political liability, he helped to doom European Jewry by inaction even as he proclaimed America as the asylum for the oppressed." The man in Roosevelt's government responsible for the Jewish "rescue" issue was named Breckinridge Long. According to Wyman, Long does not appear to have been "overtly negative to Jews simply because they were Jews." He does not appear to have been anti-Semitic.

What is clear is that his was the desk at which all help, all suggestions, all possibilities to save the Jews stopped. Nothing proceeded any further, to any superior or to Roosevelt. He performed the same services for Roosevelt—sweeping a particularly uncomfortable issue under the rug—that Gary Bauer performed for Reagan. And that John Sununu performs for George Bush.

John Sununu. The state of New Hampshire has little to be proud of in sending this son to Washington. His will be a name that will lead to as much infamy as that of Breckinridge Long and Gary Bauer in the history books. He will join the list of murderers. There is no question in the minds of anyone in Washington that Sununu's mission is pandering to the conservative right. The AIDS issue is as much a political liability to Bush as the Jewish issue was to Roosevelt. Every glimmer of progress on AIDS—in funding, in leadership, in responsibility—has been dashed in the office of John Sununu. This is not opinion; this is fact. The former governor of the state of New Hampshire is a murderer.

This is how a *New York Times* reporter described George Bush, on Monday, October 29: ". . . a prisoner of his Presidential staff and the information and strategy they funnel to him."

Don't tell me it can't happen here.

So what do we do? One American in five personally knows someone who has AIDS or is HIV-positive. (Oops, another statistic. Forgive me.) That means one out of every five of you with me here knows someone who has AIDS or is HIV-positive. That is an awful lot of silent Americans. An awful lot of Americans who are silently grieving.

So, what do we do? Lie down and die? Many people do. Most people do. It's very hard for minorities to organize. They have enough trouble existing in this world as it is. Many of them are very poor. A lot of them don't speak English. Most of them are, in one way or another, afraid. Life is very terrifying for many, many people. That's why it's so easy to kill so many of us off. That's why it's so easy to evict us or cut benefits or eliminate social programs—and cut, cut, cut, and trim, trim, trim. Most people are afraid to fight back. Most people don't like to make waves. Most people don't understand they have power. The Constitution gave us power.

It always amazes me when I tell people they have power and they answer: "Power? Me? What power?"

Your voice is your power. Your collective voices. Your group power. Names all strung together on membership lists are power. Bodies all strung together in a line are power.

I know that it's not easy, that it's harder than ever. The fight against the entrenched by the dispossessed is never-ending and exhausting. Shortly after I came back from that fateful, awful trip to Washington, I formed ACT UP—the AIDS Coalition to Unleash Power—and we have bodies all strung together in a line and we have loud, angry, obnoxious voices and in almost four years we have achieved considerable power. I also know that many of us are extremely tired. I also know that more and more of us are getting sick and dying faster than we can replenish our ranks. I also know that AIDS is getting worse and worse. I also know that, in New York City, now, you cannot get into hospitals and emergency rooms, and that dead bodies are now found in doorways. I used to think that ACT UP could save the world, that if there were an ACT UP in every city and on every college campus, the system would have no choice but to respond. It was in a similar fashion that this country was extricated from the war in Vietnam—by a growing grass-roots movement that grew and grew. I see ACT UP growing, but I see AIDS growing faster. There are already more Americans dead from AIDS than Americans who died in Vietnam.

You are all so young still, and though I feel young, feel not much older than you, I know I am, and I know my body is now infected with HIV and my dreams are nightmares that I didn't have when I was your age. I know I'm very tired, and I know that my fellow fighters in ACT UP chapters around this world are tired, and I fear for the future of 20 million people unless by some miracle in some laboratory somewhere a cure is discovered soon.

I don't know what it takes anymore to rouse you to join this fight, to realize that it is the most important fight in the world today—that you must put aside or combine this with other fights which perhaps appeal to you more, fights for civil rights and equal opportunity and pro-choice and anti-smoking. Whatever is important to you, I ask you to fight for that *and* against AIDS.

For a *transmissable* virus is going around, and nothing is stopping it. And as I have talked to you some sixty new people have become infected and some five people have died, and two or three or four or five or six of these new infections are in college students, young men and women just like you, perhaps you. . . .

I wonder if you can put yourself in the place of my young friend Mike, who is just one or two years older than you are, who graduated a year or so ago from Ohio State. He is smart, very bright, and very handsome too. Everything in the world to live for. He graduated and went out into the world, filled with hope and enthusiasm and energy. He came to New York, to Columbia University, and he fell in love with another smart and enterprising and handsome young man. And, knowing about AIDS, they decided to live with each other and be faithful to each other. They set up house together, like people in love want to do and often do. And then Mike's lover came down with AIDS. Because no one is safe now, no one who has had sex in the past ten or fifteen years. This is a very slow virus, which often hides for a very long time. Mike took care of his lover devotedly, hoping against hope that someone might know more today than ten years ago, and that his lover might survive and their relationship survive. But his lover got very, very sick. He could not seem to get any better. He got worse and worse, and when they thought it could not get any worse, it got worse. This is a horrible illness, wasting, wretched, painful, ghastly to watch and to witness and to endure. And expensive, so expensive—with the medicines one must have costing thousands of dollars and insurance companies only paying part or not paying at all because the drugs are experimental and not approved yet by that slow process in Washington that must approve everything before an insurance company is *forced* to pay. Two young people just starting out in life cannot afford to be sick from AIDS. One night Mike came home and found his lover had taken an overdose and had left him a note saying good-bye. Mike ran to his body and realized that he was still breathing, that he was still alive. And then began the most torturous moments of Mike's life. Should he let him die? Should he call emergency and try to save him? Save him for what? For more of this awful, hateful, wasting, wretched illness? Let him die, one voice said. But what if he got better? What if a new drug comes along in the next few months? Save him, another voice said. Oh, yes, save him, because . . . because this is the man I love and the man I want to spend the rest of my life with. Can you imagine having to deal with a decision like this? Mike is only a year or two older than you are. What would you have done?

He saved him. His lover was saved and lived six more tortured months in excruciating and wretched discomfort and pain before he died. And to this day, Mike has not forgiven himself for not letting his lover die the first time round.

I guess it's when I hear experiences like this that I get more energy to keep on fighting. More than any statistic, these are the things that hit home. How can life be so cruel? How can we not fight against this? How can we not keep hoping that a government and a President and a John Sununu and a country—finally—will pay attention?

Only an all-out effort by the President and federal government in concert with governments around the globe can now defeat AIDS. These alone have the resources and authority to win. President Bush must put one person in charge of AIDS and grant that person emergency powers to cut through the red tape. And AIDS must be made top priority.

Anything less will condemn 20 million people to death.

As matters now stand, I believe there is nothing at present or in the near future that is going to save the lives of those presently infected. Despite what you read or hear or see or are told, AIDS is not a manageable disease, and I don't see anything that makes me think it is going to be a manageable disease in my lifetime or the lifetime of the other 20 million infected. John Sununu knows this. George Bush knows this. Every doctor in every hospital knows this. And now you know it too. Twenty million people are going to die. Will you be as silent as your President? Will you be his accomplice in this holocaust?

The fact that the war against AIDS has been lost doesn't mean we stop fighting. In fact, it's just the reverse. We have to fight even harder because the odds are so much worse.

There are no new tactics for this fight. The oldest tactics on the books are still the ones that work the best. They require that everyone get involved in participating in the struggle. Groups that are powerful—Jews, Protestant Episcopalians, Catholics, the NRA—are powerful for this reason: because they have strong memberships that contribute time and money and their professional skills. It's those professional skills we are particularly lacking. Most of the people fighting on the front line are, quite frankly, the young. We don't have the Wall Street lawyers and the accountants and the doctors and the people who have not only the money but the contacts and the power. We don't have as strong a base of powerful gays as the Jews do of powerful Jews. And Washington knows it.

ACT UPs everywhere are going through a tough time. Everyone is angry—and for good reason—and the anger is hard to channel productively, particularly when people are tired and when we perceive, correctly, that not much is happening that's going to save our lives.

I hope that what I have said somehow reaches a part of you and that you will join our fight.

A new statistic has just come in: One out of every 250 people in the United States is now infected with HIV.

One day, out of the blue, an invitation came from a student at Oberlin College. Would I come there and make a speech? I usually turned down requests to do this sort of thing. It's a lot of work, writing a speech, and I don't particularly enjoy traveling anymore, and it really knocks the hell out of a writer's writing schedule. I can't remember why I accepted. I thought if I could write a speech that I could use in different places, it would give me a chance to get to the kids. Periodically I feel guilty that I don't put myself out there more. I think it's important for older gays to be role models for younger ones and to be seen publicly by those who aren't gay. And judging from the amount of mail I get, it's very much appreciated by those just coming out or those simply being a young gay man or lesbian in this world. (I certainly could have used a few visible role models when I was at Yale and tried to kill myself because I thought I was the only homosexual in the world.)

Oberlin was a very exciting experience. Peter Staley came with me; he'd graduated from Oberlin, and after his own speech, he was received like a hero. (Such a good role model was he that Oberlin sent four full buses to ACT UP's NIH demo in Bethesda.) Their largest auditorium was standing room only, and I got a standing ovation. That was certainly encouragement enough for me, and I soon found myself speaking at a pretty impressive roster of America's institutions of higher education. My, how things had changed!

This speech has always been important to me. I'm criticized so often (particularly by Jews) for calling AIDS a holocaust, or intentional genocide, as if these things simply could not happen in this day and age. When the British AIDS activist Simon Watney told me about Professor Bauman's book and I read it, I realized I had the dynamite I needed to blast away this opposition convincingly. And that became the basis of this speech.

So I thank that young man from Oberlin for the invitation, and for rousing me out of my funk.

It wasn't long before I found myself getting bored giving the same speech over and over. It was too much like being an actor, giving a performance again and again, trying to find a way to repeat what went well. It didn't seem right—giving a performance. Soon I found myself trying to write something new for each occasion. And it wasn't long before I was back to turning down invitations because of the amount of work it took to write something new.

I must also say I began to feel that my climactic message—all that "your voices are your power" stuff; "join ACT UP and save the world"—were hollow words I knew I was having more and more difficulty believing myself. Although I may not have been going to meetings, I very much wanted ACT UP to keep on going (I still do and it's still trying), but I had to face up to the fact that

ACT UP was not saving the world. It was even having great difficulty saving itself.

Could it have saved the world? Absolutely. Could there have been a cure by this time? I have absolutely no doubt in my mind there could have been.

A "Manhattan Project" for AIDS*

I am so frightened that the war against AIDS has already been lost.

It is beyond comprehension why, in a presumably civilized country, in the modern era, such a continuing, extraordinary destruction of life is being attended to so tentatively, so meekly, and in such a cowardly fashion.

The armies of the infected, their families, loved ones, and friends no longer know how to deliver their pleas for help. Every conceivable method has been attempted, from quietly working from within to noisily demonstrating without.

Millions of people who need not die so young will die so young. As things stand now, everyone who is presently infected can reasonably expect to die. So desperate is the situation that Dr. David Baltimore, president of Rockefeller University, has called for a "Manhattan Project" for AIDS, an equivalent of the scientific effort that produced the atomic bomb. He's right. Only the federal government can manage the project to find, as

---

*The op-ed page of *The New York Times*, July 16, 1990.

quickly as possible, the cure that top scientists believe is there and that could stem the ocean of death.

The number of those infected with AIDS is now so terrifyingly large that, even if a satisfactory treatment or cure were found tomorrow, there is no system in existence anywhere in the world that could deliver it in time to save so many people. The numbers of those facing death from AIDS are so large that eyes should glaze—with tears.

In America, 212 new cases of full-blown AIDS are diagnosed every day; there is one AIDS death every twelve minutes, and a new case of infection every fifty-four seconds. At a minimum, one to one and a half million Americans are infected.

A report by the American Council on Science and Health predicted that one in every twenty-five New York City residents will have AIDS in the next ten years. Last week, another story revealed that AIDS is already the leading cause of death among black women between the ages of fifteen and forty-four.

Worldwide, 386,588 cases have been reported in 151 countries. The World Health Organization estimates that this number is now at least 700,000, and that 6 to 8 million people have the virus that causes full-blown AIDS. By the year 2000, the infected population will approach 20 million.

All of these figures, which are known to be imprecise, are also known to be low. They are mostly based on extrapolations from small samplings from isolated areas or from cases that doctors report to authorities. We know that many doctors and patients do not report their cases, and that large numbers of those infected never see a doctor.

A transmissable virus is loose in the world. It may be one or several. It is completely out of control. Short of a cure, there is no way it can be stopped—not by mandatory or volunteer contact tracing, partner notification, quarantining, incarceration, or legislation. It is out there, everywhere, and it is rampant.

We are living in a time of plague, and two Presidents in a row have refused to stem it. Their refusal to act will cost taxpayers a fortune—easily more than the entire cost of the savings and loan bailout.

Six federal studies and more than fifty congressional oversight hearings have all concluded the same thing: The research on AIDS is uncoordinated and the funding cycles are inefficient. No one is in charge.

President Bush has done as little about AIDS as President Reagan. Twenty-four thousand Americans have died from AIDS since he took office. After stumbling on abortion, the Secretary of Health and Human Services, Dr. Louis Sullivan, has meekly followed the lead of the White House on AIDS, even though many sense he would like to perform adequately.

It is suspected that the real villain of the piece is John Sununu, the White House chief of staff, whose mission seems to be appeasing the conservative right. The result is the perpetuation of a federal policy on AIDS that was crafted by Ronald Reagan's AIDS adviser, Gary Bauer, who is now more visibly displaying his rhetoric of hate as head of the Family Research Council.

Ten years into this plague, the federal agencies dealing with AIDS are mired in such bureaucracy that it is next to impossible for them to respond to the crisis. There are so many committees and committees within committees, peer reviews and interagency task forces that few can sort them all out.

Paths of least resistance are the chosen norm. Imagination is not encouraged and exchange of vital information is often nonexistent. The two most important agencies, the National Institutes of Health and the Food and Drug Administration, are both still lacking a permanent director. Rivalries and distrust between them are embarrassingly, visibly rife. International fistfights over who should get the Nobel Prize for AIDS research has destroyed trust universally. Pharmaceutical companies now test their drugs abroad rather than confront the American maze.

The bureaucracy is so byzantine, nobody can or has to make a decision.

Research is delayed not only by a lack of any coherent plan and mature guidance, but also by a lack of first-rate personnel. The chief NIH laboratories have twenty-seven vacancies for AIDS scientists. Vital studies that many assume are being done are not.

Conflict of interest is rampant. Just about every major AIDS researcher with a government grant is also on the payroll of a major pharmaceutical manufacturer as a "consultant." Thus, the only drugs that are being tested are ones controlled by these same manufacturers. Hundreds of promising treatments developed by the less well-connected are simply ignored—and people continue to suffer and die.

President Bush and Dr. Anthony Fauci of the NIH have constantly assured us that more has been learned in record time about AIDS than any disease in history, that everything that can be done is being done. Dr. Fauci, a dedicated and overburdened scientist, is no doubt trying to calm the waters for his boss, the President, who once called him a "hero." But a real hero must tell the truth, even when it is unpopular.

Huge areas of AIDS still aren't understood. Yet government grants that would locate and assign a researcher to a specific AIDS problem are prohibited by some funding regulations.

Dr. Fauci's $500 million program for conducting experimental drug trials at local hospital sites around the country, the AIDS Clinical Trials Group, has fallen tragically short of its goals. Slots for tens of thousands attract only hundreds, mainly because most people with AIDS are excluded from the trials by a battery of illogical and murderous restrictions.

And recent editorials in *The Lancet* and the *Journal of the American Medical Association* seriously question the usefulness of AZT, a twenty-five-year-old, exceedingly toxic antiviral treatment on which the NIH spends billions of dollars. AIDS doctors and patients desperately need something more effective, but they won't get it until the AIDS drug pipeline is rerouted and streamlined.

Stopping the tragic delays in research and treatment—delays which are mostly bureaucratic, not scientific—seems impossible. The President is not interested, and while Congress votes money for the war, it abdicates responsibility to see that these precious funds are spent wisely.

To top it all off, the media have yet to expose most, if not all, of the wrongs enumerated above. They reserve their energies for criticizing the tactics activists have used to compensate for the media's shameful silence.

Only an all-out effort by the federal government can defeat AIDS. It alone has the resources and authority to win. President Bush must put one person in charge of all aspects of AIDS and grant this person emergency powers to cut through the red tape. And the President must take up Dr. Baltimore's call for a "Manhattan Project" to find that cure.

Anything less will condemn millions to death, and the war against AIDS will indeed be irrevocably lost. And history will record that it was lost because two U.S. Presidents and the entire federal government surrendered.

The Deadly Reality of Research into AIDS*

I know that many of you believe that hundreds of millions of dollars are being spent wisely and well on conquering AIDS, that the battle against this scourge is in good hands and that we are close to finding a cure. Well, I must disillusion you.

I recently attended a meeting of America's leading AIDS doctors and researchers, convened by the National Institutes of Health. It was a very depressing meeting.

There is no good news about any treatment to conquer HIV, the human immunodeficiency virus that causes acquired immune deficiency syndrome.** There is not even anything on the horizon that anyone is really excited or hopeful about. And, worst of all, there is the growing sense of unease, so palpable you can almost touch it, as it begins to dawn on everyone what a few had

---

*The op-ed page of *The Philadelphia Inquirer*, December 30, 1990.

**Editors now routinely insist upon definitive causative terminology like this. HIV probably does cause AIDS (and probably with a cofactor). Most of the time I'm pretty convinced. But I trust so few people, and what they say and how they perform—after seeing them, working with them, and/or knowing them over these years—that it wouldn't surprise me if AIDS was caused by something still completely unknown and out of left field. The practice of scientific research in this country simply does not inspire confidence, in any way. Nothing surprises me anymore.

only whispered about in private: Nobody knows what to do next, what to study, what to research, what to do for the millions of people already infected.

AZT (the only antiviral approved by the Food and Drug Administration) is not the wonder drug that many had hoped it would be. It's becoming more and more apparent that AZT's effectiveness is confined to a fraction of those taking it, and only then at a very specific moment in the patient's illness, and only then for a very short period. AZT intolerance, AZT lymphomas, and AZT myopathy (deterioration of the muscles) are occurring in far too many of those taking it. Early returns on two other antivirals in the research pipeline (ddI and ddC) have been challenged. It is clear that none of these drugs is going to be the answer that will cure the 20 million people who the World Health Organization has told us will be infected globally by the year 2000.

So just where do we stand in the battle against AIDS? Here are a few frightening facts:

• After eleven years—during which an epidemic went from a pandemic to a plague—there is no one leading the fight against AIDS. The second President in a row has refused to put anyone in charge of it, as he has done for scandals involving illegal drugs, HUD, and the savings and loans. Can you imagine winning a war without a general? Without even any majors or captains? Thus what is being done is completely uncoordinated. Indeed, because of this leaderless state, much of the most basic research on what makes the HIV virus tick has not even been begun.

• Because there are still too many unanswered questions, it is impossible to develop proper treatments or create the cure that many top scientists say is possible. And most of the research that is being done is not being conducted by our very best scientists. The real brains and biggest guns in scientific research, in virology, immunology, infectious diseases, biochemistry, are not researching AIDS. Thus many people with AIDS are undergoing medical treatment based on sloppy experiments conducted by second-rate scientists.

• The research that is being supervised and the treatment recommendations that are being passed out originate at an agency whose reputation has been tarnished in recent years—the National Institutes of Health. Once considered the premier scientific research facility in the world, NIH is now a place where, among other tragedies, one of its most brilliant lights, Dr. Robert Gallo, is under congressional and institutional investigation for possible scientific fraud. Like AIDS itself, the NIH is also leaderless. Two years into his term, George Bush has yet to name a permanent director.

In addition, there are twenty-nine scientific vacancies in the Division of AIDS at NIH. Seven are high, important, vital, supervisory positions. There is also a hiring freeze. Even before the freeze, no one was applying for these jobs because they can make more working in the private sector and NIH is no longer considered a great place to work.

• Congress has voted billions of dollars for various AIDS programs, but Bush and before him Reagan and their powerful Office of Management and Budget have seen to it that much of this money is never released for spending.

• People are conducting their sexual activities based on the deductions of epidemiologists at the Centers for Disease Control in Atlanta. These people (who are often very wrong—remember the swine flu epidemic that never was?) have told the world that oral sex is low-risk behavior. Now comes word from a San Francisco study that oral sex might be dangerous.

Because of all this, I believe that there is absolutely nothing at present or in the near future that is going to save the lives of those millions of people who are now infected with HIV. By "save" I mean just that, not just the extension of life by the added months that AZT or other drugs might offer.

AIDS is *not* a manageable disease (despite what is repeatedly told to us by government officials and their apologists), and I see nothing on the horizon that makes me, a person who is HIV-positive, think it is going to be a manageable disease in my lifetime.

The government's AIDS bureaucracy goes around calming the waters, telling congressional committees, newspaper reporters, and television audiences around the world that all is well, that things are looking up, that progress is being made, that the cure is just around the corner.

Every person we've put our trust in has misled us about the extent of this plague and about the outlook for a cure. Do not believe anyone who is saying that matters are under control, that we have learned more about this virus in record time than any other disease in history, that we are spending more on AIDS than any other illness. These are all lies.

What we know is this—a transmissable virus is going around. Nothing is stopping it and there is, as of yet, nothing to stop it.

There is one new HIV infection in the United States every fifty-four seconds and there is one AIDS-related death every ten minutes.

We also know that at least two or three of every thousand college students is now infected and one out of every four households in America now knows someone who has been touched by AIDS.

And we know that 63 percent of all people with AIDS are people of color and 14 percent of those with AIDS are women.

In the next ten years, 80 percent of all HIV infection will be heterosexually transmitted. Ten million children will be infected and two-thirds of all AIDS cases will be among women and children.

Twenty million people will be infected by 2000. As matters now stand, they are going to die.

Reading these two op-ed pieces, for two of the most respected newspapers in the world, is a sobering experience. Here were all my charges—many of them most strong and compelling—and these editorials might just as well not have been written, for all the attention paid to them. It's when you see this so blatantly that you wonder, How much longer can I go on, could anyone go on, in the face of such overwhelming and continuing apathy? Throw in the sponge or towel or whatever it is you throw in—perhaps it is both; well, throw them both in. Enjoy what time is left, as free from the aggravation of this apathy as you can make it.

I am writing these words on a lovely April day in 1994, a Sunday morning. I have just retyped the preceding two editorials so I can submit a clean manuscript to my editor. I have not slept all night, because while taking a shower at 2 A.M., I discovered a blotch on my left leg that I am convinced is a lesion. I am afraid to call and wake up any of the people I know who could tell me whether my self-diagnosis is correct or incorrect. Everyone who is HIV-positive or has AIDS has been through episodes like this. Every bump and splotch is redolent with deathly possibilities. Only this time I'm convinced I'm right. After all these years I think I know an incipient lesion when I see one. I get out of bed as the sun is coming up and walk my puppy over half of downtown New York, accustoming myself to my new condition. Now I have AIDS. I have Kaposi's sarcoma and I have AIDS. What will this mean to my life? I have a lover now, for the first time in years. We're remodeling an old barn in Connecticut. Will I live to see it? Since KS can move swiftly, should we immediately sell the house before any more money is poured into it? Should I tell him that I think we must part now? Oh, the scenarios become torture.

I interject the above because it is 1994 and these editorials were written in 1990, four years ago. There is still no adequate treatment for KS. There is no decent antiviral to attack HIV. There is no government program that would make sense to anyone but a nitwit. The third President in a row is full of shit on this issue. Anything, everything, I've written and said since 1981 might as well have been flushed down the toilet. I might as well have spent all those years and all that energy doing something pleasurable. If I'm going to die, I certainly could have had more fun.

I could have written every word of both these pieces in 1981, or yesterday.

What is wrong with this country of ours? Oh, what is wrong?

I'm impressed not only by the urgency of these pieces, but by their tone. No hyperbole here. Calm, reasoned, edited. Not the crazy Larry so many of my critics so quickly summon up.

What difference does it make—the tone, the voice, the vocabulary, the reason? What difference that these calm and measured sentences appeared in *The New York Times* and *The Philadelphia Inquirer* instead of the *Native* or *OutWeek* or *QW* or *The Advocate?*

We are going to be allowed to die and that is that.

■ ■ ■

A few words about Dr. Robert Gallo, since he's mentioned in the *Inquirer* piece, and about Dr. David Baltimore, since he's mentioned in the *Times* piece.

Dr. Gallo was reported by various journalists— among them John Crewdson of the Chicago *Tribune*, Nicholas Wade and Philip Hilts of *The New York Times*, and Charles Ortleb of the *New York Native*—to have stolen the HIV virus from the French team, in order to claim its discovery for himself. It was a good story for all of us for a time—scientific chicanery in a time of unattended plague, in a race for the Nobel Prize. What richer paranoid scenario in a plague providing many? This possibility was compounded by Dr. Gallo's own personality: He is a proud man, considered by many to be a genius, with a certain difficulty in relating to and talking to others, and particularly maladroit in dealing with the media, especially one attacking him with much hostility. He was, in effect, his own worst enemy.

Initially I went along with those against him. Then— thanks to an exceedingly detailed screed by Crewdson of what he considered irrefutable evidence—I got to read the record and to see that both evidence and charges were exceedingly complicated and guilt far from clear. Then discoveries were made in both French and NIH lab records that appeared to indicate that whatever had been done, it was not premeditated. I don't pretend to understand the science of it, but viruses were evidently contaminated, as quite often happens.

For me and for all people facing death, all this was and is almost irrelevant. For the many years these charges were hanging over his head, Dr. Gallo—this smartest of scientists who, no matter what he did or did not do, had been responsible for some of the most important AIDS breakthroughs—was interested only in clearing his name. He could not concentrate on his research or on running his laboratory of many dozens of scientists at the National Cancer Institute. This was a terrible loss. Who knows what he might have discovered during those years when so many journalists and a wretched congressman named John Dingel were hounding him?

Dr. Gallo has recently been exonerated by government investigators. Nicholas Wade, in a *Times* piece, then called him the first hero of AIDS. (Without in any way mentioning that Gallo was called something quite the reverse only weeks before and in these same pages. So much for all the news that's fit to print.)

Representative Dingel has also been front and center in putting Dr. Baltimore, also considered by many a genius who might have helped to save us, out of commission. Dr. Baltimore, already a Nobel Prize winner (for helping to discover the very reverse transcriptase that has turned out to play so important a part in understanding the HIV virus) and, until Dingel got through with him, the president of Rockefeller University, is probably the most distinguished scientist in the world who's said publicly he thinks AIDS can be cured and has some ideas on how to do it. You'd think this alone, in a man of this caliber, would make someone of importance, like a President of the United States, certainly a congressperson in the House of Representatives, jump at the chance to put Dr. Baltimore in charge of *something*. Well, think again. Dingel, who has great power in Congress, would not allow this over his own dead body.

Baltimore's crime is, in the face of a plague that is heading for a billion people, so puny and unimportant as to almost not bear elaborating upon. He defended a colleague who may or may not have fudged some data on her thesis. When confronted with this, Baltimore became stubborn and, like Gallo, too filled with hubris. Hubris makes congresspersons (and the media) go for the jugular. Dr. Baltimore's been pretty much out of circulation.

The world has been deprived of two of quite possibly the finest scientific minds available to save us.

It is often most difficult not to believe that everything connected with AIDS is a giant plot against those of us who are sick and against our, or its, *ever* being cured.

No wonder one looks for the mastermind. No wonder one believes quite easily in paranoid scenarios. No wonder one believes in intentional genocide.

A close friend far more cynical than I advises me to temper my praise for Baltimore and Gallo, saying that they are creatures of sheer ambition who do not care whether we live or die except as an intellectual challenge or feather in their self-promoting caps, that, yes, a good case can be made for our being deprived of good scientific minds, but that these men are in no way heroes or martyrs, and if they really cared about saving humanity, they would have found a way no matter what their additional burdens. I state his case. I also remember that this was a country that, when it *wanted* to win a different war, invited a known Nazi, Dr. Wernher von Braun, to work on our space program.

And no wonder one continues to imagine incurable lesions in the dead of night.

We Killed Vito[*]

My name is Larry Kramer. This is very difficult for me.

The Vito who was my friend was different from the one I've heard about today. Since I hate old movies, I wasn't in his home screening crowd. And I didn't play card games on his nights out with the boys. My Vito was the friend who called late at night and read me the long angry letters of protest he constantly wrote, or mailed me the printouts of his furious speeches. We talked constantly about gay politics, about our organizations and our leaders. He was the only person who agreed with me unequivocally on everything I did and said. We even talked about the content of this speech.

We killed Vito. As sure as any virus killed him, we killed him. Everyone in this room killed him. Twenty-five million people outside this room killed him.

Vito was killed by 25 million gay men and lesbians who for ten long years of this plague have refused to get our act together. Can't you see that?

---

*Delivered at the memorial service for the much beloved film historian and activist, Vito Russo, Cooper Union, December 20, 1990. Reprinted in *The Village Voice*, February 20, 1991.

Vito was the most beloved gay man I've ever known. And gay men killed him. And lesbians.

When will we get our act together? When will we take responsibility for our lives? And our community? And our future? What does it take? When will the Dick Jenrettes and the Barry Dillers and the David Geffens and the Lily Tomlins—and where is Vito's great buddy Lily today?—and the Calvin Kleins and the Bill Blasses and the Bob Grays and the Whitney Houstons and the Carol Bellamys and the Liz Holtzmans and the Jodie Fosters and the Ed Koches stop pillaging and robbing us blind and stabbing us in the back?

There are no more than five thousand gay men and lesbians fighting to keep us alive in this entire country. Really fighting. Not being dilettantes. Fighting on an everyday, week-after-week basis.

By the refusal of those who should be leaders to come forward to lead, and fighters to come forward to fight, Vito was murdered. By his very own.

Can't you see that?

Because so few of us are fighting for treatment and a cure and research, there was no treatment or cure for Vito.

Can't you see that?

There could have been a cure by now. There should have been. It shouldn't still be in the same mess it's in today. In ten years, we're nowhere. Nowhere. Anyone who tells you otherwise is a liar.

Vito devoted his life to fighting for us. And we let him die. Time and again he sacrificed his own career when he felt it was more important to protest or write an article or make a personal appeal that might help further the cause of gay rights or help for AIDS victims. That's right. I said victims. We are victims. Of our very own. We're killing each other.

Can't you see that?

Ten years into a plague and our organizations still don't talk to each other. And our boards of directors are still incompetent. And our leaders are cowards, or weak tokens, or idiots. We are still the most leaderless 25 million history has ever produced. If Moses or Jesus or Joan of Arc came along to lead us, we'd shit all over them and throw them out.

For ten years of a plague we have refused to organize and find ways to designate leaders to negotiate for us in the corridors of power. So we don't have any power. Surprise, surprise.

When Vito was offered the morphine drip for the first time in the hospital, his great friend, Arnie Kantrowitz, asked him, "You know what this is for?" Vito shook his head Yes. Then Arnie asked him, "Do you want it now or do you want to stay a little longer?" Vito somehow found strength to whisper back, "I want to stay a little longer."

Don't you ever forget those words. "I want to stay a little longer." Because, at some point, we're all going to face that question and we're all going to want to answer it with the same words. "I want to stay a little longer."

There ain't no cures yet, boys and girls. There should have been by now. There would have been by now if we were all straight and white and male and middle-class. There would have been by now if 25 million gay men and lesbians had their act together. But we didn't. And they shit all over us. Day after day they shit huge turds all over us. And Vito's dead. And everyone in here knows plenty who are dead. We killed them. And I'm going to be dead. And 20 million HIV-infected by the year 2000 are going to be dead.

Can't you see that?

They haven't even done the basic science yet. That's what they think of us. How can they discover a cure when they haven't even done the basic science yet? They don't do basic science for faggots and queers and niggers and spics and junkies and whores and bastards. And we let them shit all over us. We let them kill us, too. We're very generous.

If we don't let them kill us with HIV, they kill us with gay bashing. Or taking away our insurance. (Vito didn't have any insurance. He had to declare bankruptcy so he could qualify for Medicaid and Medicare. He had to scrounge around for decent care, and he was not allowed to earn any money.) Or not writing about us in the newspapers. Or portraying us as freaks on movies and TV. They throw a million turds at us. There's going to be a benefit screening of a movie called *Silence of the Lambs*. The villain is a gay man who mass murders people. AmFAR is holding the benefit. Thanks a lot, Mathilde Krim. Thanks a lot, Arthur

Krim, for financing the movie. Thanks a lot, Jodie Foster, for starring in it. Vito really would have screamed about that one. Who says we're not killing each other?

Can't you see that!

You want to stay a little longer? Then you better plug into the activist community somewhere. And work your butts off. You've got brains and abilities. You've got something to contribute.

Make it better!

Because the few of us still fighting are tired as all hell and dying faster than we're being replaced. Vito is dead. You can't replace Vito. And we killed him. We all killed him. We didn't fight hard enough to save him. Even those of us who are fighting are not fighting hard enough.

And everyone here knows it. You all know it!

Did you love him? You're here because you said you loved him. How much did you love him?

I think most of us are full of pious shit. We come to services like these and most of us didn't do one goddamned thing to help save the loved one we came here to mourn.

If Vito meant anything to you, go out and emulate him. Do what he did. Get your hands dirty. Fight in his memory. If you don't know what I'm talking about, learn.

Then you can say to Vito: So long, Vito: this one's for you.

I find it hard to take memorial services—the whole experience is too macabre. Everyone sits there, no one making the connection between why the person died and how little the "mourner" did to save the life of the person they've come to mourn. The two times when I agreed to speak I decided to deal with just this issue.*

There's not a person in the world who knew Vito Russo who didn't love him. And who doesn't still miss him terribly. His early death was a monstrous loss; he was *the* great role model, inspiration, activist, loving

---

*See also "Who Killed Jeff?" page 426.

friend, film historian. The Great Hall at Cooper Union was packed for his memorial. When I got to the meat of my remarks, I sensed the utter silence that I was learning occurred when I said things in an unexpected way. I could sense people almost holding their breath. What was I saying that was so shocking or unbelievable? I always mean everything I say. I don't say it to shock. I say it because that's what I'm thinking. Most people don't say what they think.

There was a blasphemous amount of applause at the end, which totally surprised me. I'd expected people to throw spoiled tomatoes or rotten eggs.

I'm also told that many were appalled, and still hold it against me, again and still using their disapproval of my tactics as an excuse not to fight as hard as *they* can.

More about some of this when I discuss my unpleasant experiences with Jeff Schmalz's memorial.

Thanks a Lot[*]

1 April 91

Ms. Joan Tisch
The Regency Hotel
540 Park Avenue
New York, NY 10021

Dear Joan,

It has been an awfully long time since we had our lunch, which I considered such an exciting and hopeful one. Since then you have not responded to my numerous calls and letters.

This is a last-ditch-stand letter, an imploring, begging, on-my-knees plea. I am pleading with you. I beseech you to ask your husband to meet with me.

George Bush must hear voices such as Bob's. Bush must put someone in charge of this plague. Unless he hears the pressure from people such as you and yours, everything is going to stay

---

*A letter to Mrs. Preston Robert Tisch, a GMHC board member and the wife of one of the richest men in the United States.

as dreadful as it is. And all your work at GMHC, no matter how
fine, no matter how generous, will be for naught.

I have not much left in me, either activist-wise or (probably)
health-wise, and it is going to be one of my last all-out endeavors
to get Bush to pay attention to AIDS. I think it can safely be
said that he is really worse than Reagan. Of Reagan it can be
said he was out to lunch; George Bush is not and is obviously
very aware of how awful everything pertaining to AIDS is and
still chooses to do next to nothing. He talks a better game, but
the words are not deeds.

This weekend I had a secret meeting with several officials
from the U.S. Department of Health and Human Services. All of
them are involved with AIDS. They asked for this confidential
meeting. They came to me as the founder of ACT UP. They came
to me because they don't know what else to do. In effect, it was
a last-ditch attempt for them, too. They told me horror story
after horror story. How nothing can get done. How Dr. Sullivan
is prevented from doing anything. How all the offices set up to
deal with AIDS are not functioning. How inept many of those
placed in charge are. It was terrifying to hear. Everything one
suspected, of course, only worse. And they came up to New York
on their own time and their own money to try to get us, the
activist community, to somehow do something. But the activist
community is powerless in or anywhere near the White House.

Last week I heard all the latest figures and predictions for
the near and far future, both for the city and the country, in a
speech by Dr. Ernie Drucker, one of the most prominent of epidemiologists. They are all worse, more horrible than anyone expected. It can be said that nothing is working: education,
condoms, safe sex. If we think New York is plague city now, we
have seen nothing. Tisch Hospital, already overburdened, will
not know what hit it.

I am not overdramatizing. You know that. Why is it so difficult for you and Bob to see me? More important, why is it so
difficult for men such as Bob and Larry to talk to Bush about
this? Is not Bob the Mayor's representative in Washington?

At our luncheon, I proposed that Bob should take with him
to a meeting with Bush a group of those best equipped to impress
Bush. I don't have to be there. I just want it to happen and

succeed. We can all sit down and put our heads together about
who the best people would be. Big deals like your husband.

Why are you giving me such a hard time about this? In the
many months that have passed since we met, do you know how
many tens of thousands got infected, got sick, died?

Joan, you, Bob, and Larry have the power to do something,
really do something, about all of this. I beg you to use this power.
I beg you and Bob to talk to me personally. I am not a horrible
person. I am just someone who is very afraid of death, someone
who sees nothing but death, someone who wants his community
to live, and someone who thinks he sees how certain actions can
achieve results. I had the original idea for GMHC. I had the
original idea for ACT UP. Obviously I am no fool. Please, please!
Ask Bob if he would hear me. If you really want to be heroes, if
you really want to go down in history as having been inspirational and contributed something to AIDS, and this city, and this
country, let us meet and discuss this and plan a plan of action.

F or many years it was next to impossible to get any
people of power or wealth to join the boards of any AIDS
(or gay) organizations. With the arrival of Joan Tisch and
Judy Peabody on GMHC's board, this situation changed.
Joan was a volunteer, and the story is she'd come in and
stuff envelopes one morning a week and nobody knew
who she was until one day someone happened to notice
she was always picked up by a chauffeur and asked,
"What's Joan's last name?" And somebody else looked it
up. Nathan Kolodner, the board chair, was informed, and
before you knew it Joan stopped stuffing envelopes.

Joan's husband, Bob, was a member of Reagan's cabinet as well as brother to the even richer Larry Tisch,
and I urged Nathan and his successors, Joy Tomchin and
Jeff Soref, to put Joan to better use than just coming to
board meetings—and the same for Judy Peabody, a well-
known, well-born, and extremely well-connected New
York socialite, married to someone even more so. These
two women, who between them and their husbands know

just about everyone there is to know, could easily help get a message into the White House. I managed to have lunch with Joan to put forth my request for a meeting with her husband, and a meeting with Judy to somehow summon in her chips in this area, too. Neither to any advantage. Neither woman desired to help in any way remotely approaching this fashion. Repeated requests, with as much charm as I could muster, also failed.

I have come to resent these rich people who, in their limousines and fancy clothes and big hair, come slumming to take care of the dying faggots and other poor people. I find it more and more condescending. One call from Bob Tisch, or his brother Larry, or both of them, to George Bush, or now Bill Clinton, telling the President to take, once and for all, a leadership position to end this plague would do more than all their checks put together. Joan and Bob's son, Steve, whom I believe is straight, has been board chair of AIDS Project Los Angeles, which has been as cowardly as GMHC in lobbying in Washington. He doesn't ask his father or his uncle to make any phone calls either.

It is incomprehensible to me to have such power and not to use it. Or should I say it is revolting that they have such power and choose not to use it in behalf of AIDS.

And because people like the Tisches and the Peabodys are affiliated with the likes of GMHC and APLA, other rich benefactors, like David Geffen and Barry Diller, follow suit and blindly climb on board, never knowing exactly what these organizations do and don't do, and what their money is buying besides a tax exemption. When I criticized Barbra Streisand for giving millions to these two groups, she had no idea they were "so unpolitical."

A recent *Advocate* column I wrote (which is not included in this book), entitled "After Seeing *Schindler's List*," compares GMHC to Dachau and APLA to Auschwitz. "They're our exterminators . . . the places we send all our 'Jews' to so that they can be put to death quietly, so that no one can hear our agonizing screams in the dead of night. These AIDS organizations are our censors, our thought police, our SS. They stomp out disruptive explosions. They tranqualize the infected lest the rest of the world hear or see anything too uncomfortable or embarrassing. . . . By their total inability to confront the very system they were founded to hold accountable, the [boards, the executive directors, the management of the] GMHCs and the APLAs of this world usher us into the gay gas chambers, which they've built with our very own money. God forbid they should put up a fight . . . God forbid they should be Schindlers."

It does not go down well with many people when I criticize these benefactors. Well, with the lack of any response whatsoever from Joan Tisch, I found I was getting warmed up.*

*See "No Sense of Urgency," page 383.

Genuine Thanks

7 August 91

Mr. Richard L. Gelb
Chairman, CEO
Bristol-Myers Squibb
345 Park Avenue
New York, NY 10154

Dear Mr. Gelb,

It is almost two years to the day since I first wrote you suggesting that ACT UP join with Bristol in a joint cooperative effort to hasten your drug, ddI, to market.

Thus I thought another letter was in order, to congratulate us both—Bristol and ACT UP—upon reaching our desired objective: imminent FDA approval and your license for wide distribution of this useful treatment.

I think it is most important—and that is why I'm circulating so many copies of this letter—for as many as possible to know that cooperation with ACT UP can be so productive, and that we are not the enemy so many choose to view us as. We are most grateful to you and all your associates for instinctively trusting us from the beginning, and listening to us, and learning from us about so many

379

of the matters that no pharmaceutical manufacturer can ever know, but needs to know, before and while conducting trials aimed at obtaining the best results in the targeted communities.

I can honestly say that the Bristol–ACT UP relationship was almost totally ideal. The goal was never lost sight of, and the process of working together never broke down. We respected each other and carefully considered the other's point of view.

Truly, this coalition, this result, and this experience have been historic. Would that other drug companies would be as trusting, or as attentive to our advice! And would that our President—a Yale man like us both—could fully comprehend the horror of this plague amongst his people and work as compassionately to end it as have ACT UP and Bristol.

We have created the model for testing all future AIDS drugs; now we must hope and pray and fight that others follow it.

Thank you.

P.S. The biggest thank you for our assistance that Bristol could arrange would be to price ddI so as to relieve the afflicted communities from the grotesque price of AZT.

I include this letter to show how it could go when it went well. This was ACT UP at its best. And shows what we could do. And did. (And still do.) I don't know if even any cancer advocates have achieved this kind of direct cooperation with the drug companies. It was, is, remains truly innovative.

When I get low I can throw shit on things. What great contribution has ddI made to the conquest of this plague? And all the drugs that ACT UP has fought so hard for— only a few have proved more than marginally useful. And what about all the treatment activists playing doctor? A lot of us know more than a lot of the doctors, who for too long a time haven't really bothered to learn or teach themselves as much about our illnesses as they should.

But isn't it a tricky business, playing God? It's one thing to read up on something and self-medicate. It's quite another to dispense "wisdom" to everyone. Do AIDS activists, including myself, go too far, recommending treatments questionable at best, bad-mouthing treatments that might be helpful? The results of studies are endlessly questioned, which is fine; but—again—questioning is one thing and making statements of fact based on them is another.

It's hard not to pass on our strong opinions to anyone who asks for them. And many people ask for them. I still get a lot of calls and queries. It's difficult to constantly remind myself I'm not knowledgable enough to speak out definitively. Over these years there have been treatments the activists trashed, which, for that reason, were buried for good. Years later it's been realized perhaps they shouldn't have been dismissed so quickly; they should have been tested further, in other combinations or dosage amounts, for instance. In my own case, I certainly spent a lot of wind denouncing AZT. What an irony, then, when I found myself having to take it, not primarily as an antiviral, but to raise my dangerously low platelets—which, for the moment, it has done.

When I mentioned to Simon Watney how I felt guilty that we might, along the way, unwittingly have passed along, or advocated, some bad advice, he dismissed my feeling this way: "An argument that seemed right at one stage may be wrong at a later stage. We must constantly be able to change with the volatility caused by government inaction. No! Absolutely not! No guilt if what we recommended turned out to be incorrect."

There is certainly far more blood on government hands than ours. Perhaps activists are often a better source of information. It's a complicated issue. People have to realize they're going to have to make their own decisions and to inform themselves as best they can— things they don't usually want to do. Patients are all too often much too ready to let doctors dictate their treatment. In the past, doctors have resented outside information such as activists are providing. With AIDS they seem all too happy to delegate this onerous responsibility to someone else, almost washing their hands of it. Then, if anything goes wrong, they can blame the activists. And many of the activists, particularly of late, are certainly as blameworthy as many of the doctors. It's the hardest thing in the world for patients to accept the fact that, in the end, there's no one to listen to who can guarantee anything. And we all want guarantees so much.

Better-designed trials, for ddI and other potential treatments, was also a major ACT UP victory. But it's also turned out to be a hollow one. It's all well and good to have wider participation, by gender and geography, for instance, and to eliminate when possible (and it is possible more times than not) placebo and various other forms of "blinding" and "double-blinding"; but the bottom line is that there still aren't many drugs worth testing, in a well-designed study or any other kind.

This letter was written at a time when it still hadn't hit home that the most basic of scientific research was lagging so far behind, indeed simply wasn't being done at all, and that we activists were really fighting the wrong battles. We were ahead of ourselves. We'd barged inside expecting research to be much more advanced than it was; we had yet to discover that it was farther behind than even we imagined possible. And at this advanced date in the history of a plague!

It was when we could ignore this reality no longer that AIDS activism took yet another nosedive. There wasn't, and hasn't been, enough energy to go back to square one again. And square one is where we have to return to.

An enormous and very expensive infrastructure has been set up to maintain a status quo that doesn't work, but in which too many now have vested interests they can't afford to abandon. So the labs are there, but without experiments to conduct in them. And the protocols for testing drugs have been designed, but without any new candidates to test in them. That's why AZT keeps getting tested and retested, in yet new combinations. There's nothing new to look at.

And that's pretty much where things still stand—exhausted and diminished ranks of activists, minimum pressure, little innovative research, snail-paced progress. And idiots, as always, minding the store.

No Sense of Urgency[*]

I've been in Washington for almost two months. I saw—once again—how little is being done for us. I have no doubt the 40 million of us the World Health Organization now tells us will be infected by 2000 (I personally believe 40 million are *already* infected) are going to die.

I look at the two organizations I helped to start, GMHC and ACT UP—my children—and I ask myself: What have we accomplished?

And I am forced to answer: Very little.

People are still dying like flies. The White House is still as inaccessible as the moon. We have been unable to make the world pay attention, much less care. We are still pariahs. We have not stopped this plague.

Not only my organizations, but AmFAR, AIDS Action, NGLTF, HRCF, minority task forces, AIDS Institutes, Presidential AIDS Commissions, and on and on and on—none has done much good.

---

*Tenth Anniversary of GMHC Speech, Cathedral of St. John the Divine, November 22, 1991. The service was officially called "The Gathering of Remembering and Renewal," and its catchy motto was "Remember, Respond, Resolve."

I don't believe that education works very well, and we're putting so much trust in it. Education did not stop Magic Johnson from getting AIDS. Nor Kimberly Bergalis. The World Health Organization says Africans know how AIDS is spread, yet the spread stops not in Africa. The figures are marching inexorably faster than we can ever stop them by education.

I'm not certain I know what safe sex means. I wonder if it's easier to get this disease than we try to convince ourselves is the case. I believe we do not understand how this disease, in all ways, is spread. I don't believe the blood supply is safe. Four hundred thousand people in France were, only a short time ago, given infected blood because of stupid bureaucrats. I don't believe any statistic put out by our government. There is no way to explain or extrapolate anything remotely resembling an accurate estimate of how many of us are sick.

I don't believe much of what any government agency tells me about *anything:* AIDS, statistics, safety, sex, *anything.* If you'd spent as much time as I have, these past ten years, dealing with these bureaucrats, you'd know how second-rate so many of them are; how mentally, intellectually, morally, and spiritually bankrupt so many of them are; how immature, inexperienced, naive, and badly educated in their fields so many of them are. How could anyone possibly trust a government that puts out a definition of AIDS which denies that women get it?

I do wish everyone would cease calling AIDS an epidemic. It is not an epidemic. An epidemic is a few cases of something rare that weren't around yesterday. A plague is something sweeping through the world—uncontrolled and uncontrollable. To deny that AIDS is a plague is denial of the highest order.

So ten years into a plague, here I am—and I have to tell you that it is exceedingly weird to picture, ten years ago, the start of GMHC in my living room, and to be here in this cathedral tonight—here I am telling you that everything we have done and we are doing is useless and that we have no choice but to start all over again in our fight.

The only thing that is going to make this plague go away is a cure at the most, and successful treatments at the least. And research is the one area, in all these ten years, we have ignored.

Because of this, research into AIDS is still in the Stone Age.

Because of this, there is not one drug that is any good.

Everything we've been waiting for is turning into a dud.

I believe the American Foundation for AIDS Research should have been in the forefront, being the watchdog on AIDS research. It is painful for me personally, but I must finally face up to the fact that someone as clever and well-connected and appealing as Dr. Mathilde Krim, and her partner, Elizabeth Taylor, have proved little more than dilettantes. It never even occurred to Elizabeth Taylor, who has a daughter-in-law positive for six years and now with AIDS, even to request a meeting in the White House with her fellow actor Ronald Reagan, who got us into this mess. I look at the long list of famous names on AmFAR's national council. I ask myself: What have any of these people done for AIDS: Woody Allen, Warren Beatty, Burt Bacharach, Roslyn Carter, Mrs. Michael Eisner, Douglas Fairbanks, David Geffen, Katharine Graham (who could call the President and eat him for lunch), Marilyn Horne, Angela Lansbury, George Hamilton, Lady Bird Johnson, Michael Sovern, Barbra Streisand, Jack Valenti, Raquel Welch?

As always, I ask myself: Why must the activists be the only ones who go after the Presidents who murder us?

I believe the board of directors of Gay Men's Health Crisis, like AmFAR's, is composed of well-meaning but utterly misguided healthy people who have no sense of urgency, no sense that tomorrow will not be here. This board, like AmFAR's, has no important player with AIDS on it. No wonder these organizations have no sense of urgency. And yet they make nothing but important decisions for people with AIDS.

Well-meaning. Boards of GMHC, boards of AmFAR, boards of this and that—filled with the well-meaning. Every one of these people knows people in positions of great power. And not one of them will get on the phone and call these people up and say, "Let's all work together to get to George Bush and demand help!"

Brooke Astor was quoted in the paper talking about the New York City fiscal crisis in the seventies and how New Yorkers from all walks of life banded together to fight for this city. "Labor unions, financiers, artists, writers," Mrs. Astor said, "one just doesn't see that kind of rallying together today. I don't really know why."

Two years of my begging GMHC board member Joan Tisch for a meeting with her husband, Bob, one of the richest and most powerful men in the world, have resulted in nothing. Joan Tisch, I don't think you or your husband want to end this plague.

Why haven't you, Bob Tisch, and Dr. Saul Farber,* the head of your hospital, and Dr. David Rogers and Dr. David Ho and Dr. June Osborn and Dr. Mathilde Krim and David Geffen and Dick Jenrette and Barry Diller and Elizabeth Taylor and Pat Buckley and Judy Peabody and Michael Sovern and Barney Frank and Gerry Studds all talked to each other and gone as a group to tell George Bush that because no one in his dumb administration talks to anyone else and because no one is in charge of a plague, 40 million people are going to die?

Shame on you, Bob Tisch. Shame on you, Joan Tisch. Shame on you, Mathilde Krim. Shame on you, Judy Peabody. Shame on you, David and Barry and Dick and Douglas and Elizabeth and Raquel and all the rest of you. Good fortune has presented you with wealth and prominence and power and a platform and a voice, and you refuse to use them to end this plague.

It's ten years since that first meeting in my living room, and everyone still doesn't get it!

Everyone will call me nuts—boy, this time Larry's really gone too far and flipped his lid; now he's even biting all the hands that are giving us our only handouts. Everyone still spends their time and money and energy taking care of sick people instead of fighting for a cure. Instead of fighting against a President who doesn't want us cured. The fact is that changing diapers, eroticizing safer sex, passing out condoms, placing endless ads in the *Village Voice* are not stopping people from dying. They just make you, the healthy ones, feel better.

There's got to be a higher vision for your reason for being! You've got to want to end this! Instead I see layer upon layer of bureaucracy, hordes of employees, and thousands of volunteers spending hours and days at endless meetings—just like all the bureaucrats in Washington—meetings that have nothing to do with ending this plague. Plus all those useless, well-meaning

---

*Dr. Saul Farber is the head of the New York University Medical Center. Its Tisch Hospital is named after Bob and Larry Tisch, the latter of whom is also on the New York University board.

board members who have absolutely no sense of urgency, no sense of urgency, no sense of urgency, no sense of urgency, that 40 million people will die in a few short years' time.

I tell you, it would make not one single bit of difference to the progress of this plague if GMHC wasn't here, and, yes, if my beloved ACT UP wasn't here.

We suffer one defeat after another, one death after another, one monster in the White House after another, and we take it, we lie down and take it, and our boards of directors and our national councils go home to apartments on Park Avenue in their limousines instead of driving directly to the White House.

Dr. Fauci, little Napoleon, the government's great apologist, now admits publicly that AZT and ddC and ddI don't work. Merck just canceled their L drug. There is not one drug that is any good! Everything we've been waiting for is turning out to be a dud. Did you think a cure was going to appear by itself, miraculously springing full-blown out of the head of Zeus Gallo? I am telling you research on this disease is still in the Stone Age! Why? You think it's because science has to take its own time? Wrong! It's because nobody's in charge of anything! Nobody is watching the pot not boil. Nobody is sending the blokes into the lab with the requisitions—study this! We know what has to be studied. It isn't being studied. The full pathogenesis of this virus still hasn't been studied. Pathogenesis means what's really happening inside us that leads to disease. It's usually the first thing that's studied. Ten years—it still hasn't been studied.

Where were you, Mathilde? Where were you, everybody else? We are in the midst of a huge war and there is no general.

I go to the NIH, and one office doesn't know what the next office is doing. Or has learned. Or has accomplished. It is as disorganized as that. I have dinner with Dr. Gallo and he tells me something exciting, and when I ask Fauci, "Did you hear what Bob Gallo told me?" Tony says, No, it's all news to him. And this complete and utter lack of communication exists from the highest to the lowest.

For years I have been calling, begging, pleading for a Manhattan Project for AIDS. Why does every board and every organization ignore such an obvious suggestion? Why does no one join me in this call? Bob Tisch, if the value of your real estate is going down because of AIDS, and this city, of which you are unofficial Mayor, is going down the toilet, and your hospital is so filled we can't get into it, why don't you and Dr. Farber join me in this call for a Manhattan Project? Bob Tisch, I implore you from this pulpit in this house of God to call this meeting!

Let me try and put it one last way. If we spent half as much time, energy, and money fighting for a cure as we do fighting conservatives on testing and condoms and education and where should the international conference be held and who can legally attend, we would have that cure by now, and the science at NIH would be better than the food at Bob's Big Boy. We are fighting for everything but that cure, and we no longer have time to fight all these lesser battles.

And you don't want to fight for that science and that research and those treatments and that vaccine and that cure. Because it requires a real shakeup of the political and medical establishments and you don't want to get your hands dirty. You only want to feel good and virtuous, which comes from attending events like this and writing a few small checks.

I don't want your dollars to help me die! I want your dollars to help me live. I don't want your dollars to build GMHC another building! I don't want your dollars to ensure job security for a bureaucracy growing so huge I am sorry I started this damn organization. I want your dollars to save my life and save the lives of 40 million other people, which you can do without buildings and a staff of thousands. You can do it with ten, twenty, a hundred important powerful board members who are willing, finally and at last, to open their mouths!

And it is up to all the rest of us everywhere to pressure them until they do!

Well, now you can go home and say, "I heard Larry really going crazy, out of his mind again." And you'll ignore me again until, ten years from now, when you gather here for another one of these tender meetings of "Remember, Respond, Resolve" and you'll say, "Oh, Larry Kramer, thank God we don't have to listen to him anymore."

J eff Soref, GMHC's board chair, and Tim Sweeney, its executive director, invited me to speak at a service to mark the tenth anniversary of both AIDS and the organization. I must admit I was surprised by the invitation and more surprised when, after I told them that if I did accept they probably wouldn't like what I said, they both said I could say anything I wanted to. Indeed, they both preferred I make an angry speech.

A generous offer, a dangerous request. It resulted in a remarkable experience.

I expected many in the audience to walk out while I spoke. I thought at the time this was the angriest speech I'd ever made. (How often, I note, I felt this about a particular speech.) A recurring cough, which was beginning to accompany me everywhere, was hyperactive, and I was doped up on cough suppressant medicines and sprays, giving my voice some kind of weird breathless quality. When I ascended to the high pulpit of the Cathedral of St. John the Divine, which looks down the long nave from such a great height, I was terrified. The place was packed with some four thousand GMHC supporters. I didn't know if I could get my voice up and out there, into that huge void. Plunging in, I heard my words rolling down and out and into the darkness, amplified as they boomed on and out. It *sounded* phenomenal. All this gave me courage and strength. I couldn't see anyone's face because the place was so dark, but every once in a while I could hear loud applause, the first occurring when I went after Elizabeth Taylor. Expecting boos and hisses and getting applause momentarily floored me. The more names I named and the more I tacked accusations to them, the louder the applause. At the end I'd made arrangements to sneak out quickly via a side door. But there was such an overwhelming ovation I could not escape the realization that once again the anger I was voicing was not just my own. Walking out past what was now a crowd standing and *cheering* me, I felt like a movie star myself. I couldn't believe it. These were GMHC's *supporters?*

When I recently played the tape of that evening (which GMHC so generously provided all participants) to check that the above text was accurate, I smiled as I

discovered how most of the following speakers, including
Peter Jennings and various GMHC board members, had
rejiggled their remarks, on the spot, to rebut me. I certainly had thrown this memorial off course!

I mentioned in the speech that I'd just returned from
Washington. Indeed, I'd spent the previous months trying to live in the city where I'd grown up. I'd packed up
my computer and a lot of my gear and sublet a nice fur-
nished apartment, fully intending to stay indefinitely. I
spent all my time meeting with anyone and everyone I
could get near who was involved with AIDS. I felt, and
still feel, that it makes more sense for anyone fighting for
any issue to be headquartered in Washington. That's
where whatever action there is takes place. But the
longer I stayed there, the more nuts I became. It was
agonizing to see so many gay men and women in that city,
living in the closet, in no way fighting for our issues,
indeed quite often opposing them; and equally depressing to see those gay people who maintained they *were*
fighting for our issues: bureaucrats as compliant and
manipulated as every other straight-suited government
employee. Yes, indeed, I saw how little was being done
for us. And a lot of this lethargy and denial could be put
at the feet of our very own. Just being in this town, my
health, both mental and physical, began to suffer. I was
battling nigh unto irresistible impulses to slug almost
everyone I met. That stupid cough appeared. An old boy-
friend invited me to what sounded like a romantic weekend in Virginia, only to bring his trick. Even my sublet
turned against me—a gas leak was discovered, and I'd
evidently been inhaling gas since I arrived. Finally I
packed my stuff and came back to New York. At least I
can yell my head off in New York.

Name an AIDS High Command*

There is no way that, as presently constituted, our government's research establishment can accomplish President-elect Clinton's goal to find a cure and vaccine for AIDS.

How is it possible, then, to find a cure in such a swamp? Here are some suggestions:

The President must grant emergency powers to those working on the cure for AIDS. No cure, no useful vaccine, will come without such freedom. The unbearable weight of laws, prohibitions, and rules accrued over decades—many no longer even applicable or sensible—are an intolerable impediment to progress. Emergency powers are also essential to whip a moribund bureaucracy into shape in a time of plague.

A list of unanswered questions must be agreed on. It is clear how little we know about AIDS—about how it is caused and develops in the body and about the HIV virus that seems most implicated in its cause. The available drugs and treatments have been developed from hypotheses that are unproved or have turned out to be wrong. It is now tragically obvious we must go back to square one.

---

*The op-ed page, *The New York Times*, November 15, 1992.

Identify the leading scientists in the world best able to investigate and research these unanswered questions. This is the easy part. Put them to work forthwith to answer them. This is the hard (and expensive) part.

Establish a joint chiefs of staff for AIDS. As a war must have generals, so must a plague. An AIDS czar is no longer enough. These joint chiefs would comprise the AIDS czar and the chiefs of AIDS research, drug development, drug approvals, and clinical trials.

The czar (the name of the fine former Surgeon General, Dr. C. Everett Koop, is being mentioned by the Clinton people) would deal with the mountain of nonresearch problems: insurance, Medicare, education, immigration, discrimination, and needle exchange, to name but a few. He would also be the country's AIDS spokesperson.

It is unlikely that a czar adept at these problems would also be expert at riding herd on scientific research. Dr. David Baltimore should be made chief of AIDS research. Dr. Baltimore, one of the most brilliant minds anywhere, and who won a Nobel Prize for a discovery that has greatly advanced AIDS research, believes AIDS is curable. He is also under a cloud because of allegations of scientific fraud on the part of a colleague. He should be given the chance to rehabilitate his reputation. This would be a heroic opportunity for him to do so.

Dr. Robert Gallo of the National Cancer Institute is in a similar position. Dr. Gallo, who probably knows more about HIV than any other person in the world, has been hauled through the mud by critics who have accused him of everything from scientific fraud to cooking the books. We would do well to remember that the U.S. invited a Nazi, Wernher von Braun, to come here and build our space program. The transgressions of Dr. Gallo and Dr. Baltimore, if indeed there were any, are tiny compared to von Braun's. It is a sorry state of affairs when we must render useless our finest brains just when they are needed most.

Dr. P. Roy Vagelos would be an ideal choice to be chief of drug and vaccine development. As head of Merck, the drug company, Dr. Vagelos is greatly respected by his peers. He is a great believer in cooperation and has the personality to inspire it.

Dr. David Kessler should be made chief of drug approvals. Dr. Kessler has been a better director of the Food and Drug Administration than anyone in recent memory, but the antediluvian agency is beyond streamlining.

Admiral James Watkins, who was superb on Ronald Reagan's Presidential Commission on AIDS, should be made chief whip. Research depends on pressure. A drug's effectiveness can be learned in six months, not six years. Similarly, it should not take decades for scientists to conduct their experiments; there comes a point where caution and cogitation become criminal. The chief whip should join the other chiefs in overseeing the network of clinical trials, which are currently a multibillion-dollar fiasco under the supervision of the National Institutes of Health.

All AIDS research activities must be consolidated. There is no sensible reason why the Centers for Disease Control and the Defense Department and the numerous institutes that comprise NIH all should be researching AIDS. Such duplication is shamefully wasteful.

There already exists an Office of AIDS Research, at the Institute of Allergy and Infectious Diseases at NIH, under the supervision of Anthony Fauci, a brilliant scientist but a less than brilliant administrator. The NIH, despite its reputation, is the high church of a research system that by law demands compromise, rewards mediocrity, and actually punishes initiative and originality.

While one would like to yank the entire research setup out of this monstrous bureaucracy, one can only pray that such joint chiefs, answering only to Mr. Clinton, would find a way to use the best and scuttle the worst. No less than the lives of the expected 150 million* HIV-infected people worldwide are at stake.

I'm often asked: What would I do if I were in charge? Specifically.

*Each week, it seems, brings a new figure, from some organization or individual, the lowest ones always coming from the CDC or WHO, and the highest—still—that of one billion—from Dr. Haseltine.

This op-ed piece is an edited-down version (one never appears in the *Times* unedited) of what I'd do, more or less. It always seems so simple to me. Why does everyone make it into something so very complicated? Somebody smart has to be put in charge. And this somebody has to be given emergency powers (as those in charge of the original Manhattan Project were given emergency powers) to get on with it in the fastest and most expeditious way he or she sees fit. Identify the unanswered questions. Locate the smartest experts in those fields. And get the whole thing away from the strangulating cesspool that's the NIH and all those meddling hands in Congress. Yeah, it's real easy. If America hadn't turned into the most labyrinthine bureaucracy since nineteenth-century Russia.

The piece ran as part of a series the *Times* put together on issues for the President-elect to consider, called "Bill's List." I was actually invited to write it. I now had friends on the op-ed page (who unfortunately are no longer there).

This op-ed piece, as all the others that preceded it, anywhere, made not a damn whit of difference. For all I know no one even read it. (God knows the *Times* op-ed page is, on a daily basis, so infernally boring you can't blame the public for skipping it.) You'd think that being published in such a presumably prestigious place would bring at least some word of mouth. You would be wrong.

It's interesting to note that, in one way or another, many of these ideas have been put into operation, but not in any effective fashion—because the most important point is lacking: the granting of emergency powers. There is an AIDS boss, Kristine Gebbie, attempting to ride herd on all the agencies, but she hasn't been given any power by President Clinton to achieve anything; so she can draw upon only her voice and powers of persuasion to make the many competing players in the drama of this plague get along with each other, or even meet with each other on a regular basis (which they do not).*

---

*Gebbie "resigned" in July 1994, after so much protesting against her by AIDS activists that—reportedly—the White House finally asked for the resignation.

There is a new Office of AIDS Research, but no David Baltimore to run it. Instead, it is run by Dr. William Paul, a NIAID scientist who brings to this new position no prior experience in overseeing anything so important or wide-ranging—a nice man, I'm told, a lamb where a tiger's needed.* Gallo's been semirehabilitated, but he does seem much the worse for wear. Vagelos has established some sort of consortium of drug companies meant to cooperate with each other and share their AIDS research, but once together they don't seem to be able to think of anything very constructive to do except study all their already over-tested products *yet again*. Kessler's started his own drug committee to find out ways to speed new stuff into testing. This would be a great idea if there were anything to test and if Secretary of Health and Human Services Shalala hadn't put so many duds on the committee. Watkins doesn't want a part of any more AIDS committees—which is too bad, though who can blame him. Dr. Harold Varmus, the new NIH director, and David Baltimore's "friend," has done nothing to rehabilitate him. The longer Dr. Varmus runs NIH, the more I wonder if he cares about AIDS at all.

Why is the granting of emergency powers imperative? Because there are so many laws on the books now that a committee has to meet, discuss, and approve before any scientist can even go to the toilet. Hyperbole? If you were a smart doctor, would you go to work for a research facility (the NIH) with outdated equipment and a system of requisition that takes a year to get you a microscope or two years to get you a couple of monkeys? Where they pay you $60,000 a year when you can make $200,000 a year in private practice, at a pharmaceutical house, or at a major medical center? Where you have to beg your lab chief every time you need a new piece of software or a lab assistant or want to take a trip to a scientific conference? Where every expense has to be reviewed by four

*Eight months into his job, Paul—with a multimillion-dollar budget at his disposal—had yet to hire a single scientist or offer any notion or plan of what the fuck he might start to do . . . someday.

committees and then voted on by another committee and then submitted to an outside budget office, which, after studying it, has to pass it on to yet another office for final approval, after which it's finally sent back to your home base? Where after all this you still might not get the actual money, depending on the whim of your lab chief or how much remains unspent in the kitty?

And this is *before* you have to deal with getting permission to test anything on or in a human being or an animal. Seventy-five people will then have to travel to Bethesda, four times a year, three days each time, at taxpayers' expense, to vote at "Institute meetings" before you can lay a finger on a fly.

A cure? Not in our lifetimes. For anything.

There has never been a cure for any major illness to come out of the NIH.

Say this last sentence three times, out loud, real loud.

■ ■ ■

If 1992 seems slim on entries, it's because that was the year of *The Destiny of Me*, my companion play to *The Normal Heart*. *Destiny* was particularly painful to write, complete, and get on stage. While it received many awards and the best reviews I've ever had in my life, it represents so much of my life that was difficult to live through that I don't think I was ever able to watch a performance comfortably. I tried to look at my life and my family in as honest a fashion as I could—what my life as I've lived it has been like. It was an attempt to write my *Long Day's Journey into Night*. My brother liked it, my sister-in-law didn't, my mother thought it was a work of fiction, and Dr. Fauci, who's in it too, was more generous than he had to be. Perhaps because it's an unrelenting play, it's had relatively few productions around the world, compared to *The Normal Heart*. (But then my favorite child, *Just Say No: A Play About a Farce*, which is *nothing but* laughs, has had the fewest productions of all!) Barbra Streisand and Columbia Pictures have bought the film rights to both *The Normal Heart* and *The Destiny of Me*. (I love the notion of Barbra playing my mother.) Yes, Barbra and I somehow managed to get back together. Working with her on the screenplay of *The Normal Heart* was an exciting experience, a description of which doesn't quite belong in this particular book. I know she worries that I talk too much. So far I've only said the nicest things. (And meant them.) But if she's reading this, let me say: Barbra, if you don't film *The Normal Heart*, and film it well—watch out!

Thanks a Lot II

4 January 93

Mr. Philip J. Hilts
The New York Times
Washington Bureau

Dear Phil,

Your one-sided hatchet job on Dr. Robert Gallo was appalling.

This man knows more about the HIV viruses than any other single individual in the entire world. I don't care if he robbed Fort Knox. We can have the Nuremberg trials later. After the cure is discovered. (I remind you that this is a country which *invited* Wernher von Braun, a Nazi, to get our men on the moon.)

It is almost as if a conspiracy is afoot, to see to it that absolutely everything that could help end the AIDS plague is placed out of whack or commission. (Are you on Dingel's payroll? Pat Buchanan's?)

You are the AIDS reporter in Washington for the most powerful newspaper in the world. A new AIDS story breaks there at least once a week. But it never appears in the *Times*. What kind of reporter are you? Obviously a very lazy one. You cover

none of the conferences, none of the hearings, none of the legislation, none of the lobbying, none of the personalities. (The Fauci
story you should have written five years ago had to be assigned
to Jeff Schmalz.) There is a plague going on, but not in the Washington pages of the *Times*.

The Gallo story is a modern tragedy. I don't know if he did
anything wrong (no panel, commission, or Crewdson article has
convinced me) but he has, to all intents and purposes, been ren-
dered useless. Why aren't you writing about *this* tragedy, about
the moral implications involved, about the sad plight in which it
puts all of us, including Gallo, when an instrument of possible
salvation is cruelly cut down? Isn't that what a REPORTER is
supposed to do? Where I grew up (which was Washington), it
was.

I hear you are marrying Carissa Cunningham. She is a wonderful woman. You don't deserve her and she must be very desperate. I hope she will teach you how to to do your job with
intelligence, constancy, and compassion.

You are a pinhead.

cc:
Arthur Sulzberger, Jr.
Max Frankel
Joe Lelyveld
Phil Boffey
Jeff Schmalz
Nick Wade
Tim Westmoreland
Rep. John Dingel
Carissa Cunningham

It speaks poorly of me when I say this letter is among
my favorites. And that I delighted in circulating it in
AIDS corridors and those of the *Times*. This wretched
human being, Hilts, their AIDS reporter who never
writes about AIDS, has probably done as much harm
against us as Jesse Helms. So to get my rocks off in even

such a puny, pathetic way as this gave me pleasure. And still does so: I giggle when I read it. Hell hath no fury like a faggot scorned.

But he's still there, old Phil, still not filing any AIDS stories, still driving another nail in our coffin. He married Carissa, who had worked for GMHC and AIDS Action Council. I guess whatever fire and brimstone, anger and compassion I recall her as having had, she left at the office.

If *Times* history is any guide, Phil should be getting a promotion to some sort of editorship any day now.

Colorado*

5 January 93

Dear Alice, Arthur, and Andrew,

What has upset me—as much as your going to Aspen in the first place—is your determination to *justify* your actions. Suddenly, you have a philosophy that is against boycotts. Your sympathy for the people of Aspen, who voted against the bill (then how did the damn thing get on the ballot in the first place, if everyone in Aspen was so friendly?), to me is equally amazing. Your feet have dug themselves in because you know you have upset me and your never-ending overweening pride forbids you ever to say you're sorry.

You just don't get it, you just don't get it, you just don't get it. How many essays and plays and books and articles and TV appearances do I have to make? It's as if you've never heard one single word I've said. You carry my message? You don't know what my message is. Can't you see how you slap me in the face,

---

*A letter to my brother, sister-in-law, and nephew—written upon the occasion of their departure to ski in Aspen, Colorado, after that state had overwhemingly voted in favor of antigay legislation.

kick me in the balls, knock all the wind out of my gut? Obviously not. It doesn't have anything to do with boycotts or the people of Aspen, it has to do with showing me some respect. I am the most outspoken activist on these matters in this world, and for my own family to flaunt their opposition to me is like spitting in my eye.

I didn't make a big deal about asking you not to go. I just made the request and then watched to see what would happen, hoping you had learned something, knowing that you hadn't, that the overarching superiority that must be the foundation of your relationship to *everyone* would find its automatic way to ignoring everything I've stood for.

At first, after you left, I decided to let it go. Then it began to bother me too much. I can't let the people I love so much continue to diminish themselves so totally in my eyes, become so *small*. Because that's what you do to yourselves. I lose respect for you.

If I compare this whole fight for gay rights and the neglect of AIDS with Nazi Germany, you scorn my parallels. I can't make you see that gays are today's Jews. I and everyone I know and care about is dying or dead or sick, or will be. If Colorado isn't brought back into line, similar measures to declare open season on us will be on the ballots in a dozen states within the year.

On his death bed in St. Luke's last week, my friend Stephen Harvey, the curator of film at MOMA, begged his friends to see to it that the Aspen Film Conference and the Telluride Film Festival would be canceled this year. *On his death bed.* How can you go to a place like that when people feel this way? It shouldn't make any difference what you think; it should make a difference to you what *we* think. What you care personally about boycotts and the people of Aspen is irrelevant.

I spent New Year's Eve with Tom Holtz. Do you remember him? He is my oldest gay friend, through whom I met David Kessler and Lou Miano and Leon Lambert and Barry Fifield. We'd lost touch, and now he lives three blocks from me and weighs 120 pounds. We gathered around him, a group of old friends who, thirty years ago, were young and full of fun and energy and hope. Now we are all old and despondent. It was like a grotesque, awful movie as we reminisced about the old days. Tom, a Harvard man, can't afford the new Blue Cross rates and has no health insurance. He can't afford to go to his doctor.

When I came home, I found myself reading the latest copy of *The Advocate*. The year-in-review issue. A few letters had been published in response to my interview—a few more who hate me even more now for what I do and say and how I act. Then I read the death list of people well known in our community. There were six columns. I found myself underlining how many I knew. Charlie Barber. Bob Caviano. Ken Dawson. Melvin Dixon. Denholm Elliott. Paul Jabara. Randy Klose. Mark Kostopoulos. Scott McPherson. Tommy Nutter. Carmelo Pomodoro. Tom Rubnitz. Clovis Ruffin. Danny Sotomayor. David Wojnarowicz. (Year after year, how many dead friends' names do I have to list for you?) I started to cry. It was 4 A.M. The first day of the New Year. I was going into a second day without enough sleep. You know what that does to you. I put out the lights and tried to sleep. And I found myself thinking of you, of our problem, of our unresolved problem. Not speaking to you for so long. Not returning your phone calls. Not knowing how to talk to you or say all this shit again, yet once again. Not having much energy or appetite for doing it one more time anyway. Thinking: I don't want to have to go through this again. I don't want to. It's just easier not to talk to you anymore, ever. You know that's what I do when I can't fight back anymore. I take my marbles and go home. But where is home? You are home. What's the use, I found myself saying. What is the fucking use? They don't get it and I can't make them get it and they will justify their actions until the day I die. And then came those most awful of thoughts, that come in the dead of night, when one is tired: I wish I were dead. I'm going to kill myself. I'm going to go into the kitchen and take a knife and slice my wrists. This time I'll succeed. And I start to shake. And I have to start that litany that some shrink somewhere once taught me, that litany that I make myself go through when I get too low, when I lose faith in myself and in my mission and believe that my presence here on earth has accounted for naught: I make myself promise me that I will be allowed to kill myself only after I finish the next work, the novel that will tell the world everything I know and feel and will be my life's summation, then it will be okay to die, but not until then. I've performed this trick on myself a couple of times now. Just finish *The Normal Heart*. Just finish *The Destiny of Me*. Now it's just finish *The American People*.

But then you wouldn't understand what any of this has to do with fighting the Colorado law, would you?

This letter could no doubt be better written. I have agonized over it too long and can't find the tone I seek. I just want it over with. I want to get back to my work without my stomach hurting and my sleep disturbed. I simply will not be treated in this way, in any of these ways. I am not begging anybody to love me, Arthur. I know you love me. I would not be writing this letter otherwise. And I am not punishing anyone, Alice, except myself. For expecting more from those I love, whom I believe should know better. More fool I.

Andrew, your jokes about sending my boys to picket you are beyond tacky.

Why can't any of you understand that what I am talking about is death. The text, subtext, metaphor, totality, end result of all of this is death. Colorado right now is death. Your brother, your brother-in-law, your uncle is dying. And he is trying not to. Why is that so hard for all of you to understand?

Why?

In case you're wondering what the status of my relationship with my family is, right now it's fine and we're together and loving once again. But it hasn't been so long since we were back on our old stamping grounds. Over Colorado. I stopped talking to the lot of them. For about three or four months. My brother was going to go skiing there no matter what, as he's done every year in recent memory. With his wife and two of his three children.

After receiving this, my niece, Rebecca, dropped out, followed by my nephew, Andrew, then finally Alice. Arthur went alone. He's as stubborn as I am, and no brother was going to dictate to him what to do. Not only did he go once, he went back several times. Oh, I was livid. I believe it even made the press somewhere: gay activist's brother skis in Colorado. He felt that Aspen was on our side and sent me lots of clippings from the local papers supporting those of us who felt so strongly.

But that wasn't good enough for me. It was a long time before my own stubbornness allowed for a rapprochement. Once again, somewhere along the line he called me or I called him and we made our peace and we're back to our loving relationship once again.

I include this letter because I've always gone on so about gay people standing up to their families, harsh and painful as it might be. I've always maintained we shouldn't keep anything away from them that's going to gnaw at our own innards and make us miserable. I hate to hear of gays who won't tell their parents and relatives of their homosexuality, for fear it will hurt them somehow. Well, it hurts us more not to tell them—not only that we're gay but what our fight is all about.

My family has certainly had a hard time of it from this writer amongst them. I've used them relentlessly in much of my work. I owe them all a debt of gratitude for allowing me to criticize them so publicly. I know it hasn't been easy for them, particularly for my sister-in-law, who felt particularly wounded by references to the early years of her marriage in *The Destiny of Me*. I'm sorry she doesn't hear the loving comments about her in the final scene.

As I get closer to a death I fear is coming, I find I have less interest in the part of me that needed, for whatever reasons (many of them certainly valid), to push so much into their faces. By now, we've worked out whatever it is we've had time to work out. Now we're on the end of our journeys with each other. I find myself urging that we get over whatever it was that bugged us about each other in earlier days. And to enjoy what time we've left together.

Thanks a Lot III

12 January 93

Mr. Robert MacNeil
MacNeil-Lehrer News Hour
356 West 58th Street
New York, NY 10019

Mr. Jim Lehrer
Ms. Judy Woodruff
3620 S. 27th Street
Arlington, VA 22206

I have been wanting to write this letter for quite some time.
Your January 6th segment on "special interest" groups now compels me at last to do so.

Why were gays not included? Everyone else was. What kind
of oversight or slap in the face was this?

Why were AIDS activists not included? Surely this is a "special interest" group that Clinton has made huge promises to?
What kind of oversight or slap in the face was this?

406

I state—without any hesitation or equivocation or caveats—that the MacNeil-Lehrer News Hour has the worst record on gay and AIDS coverage of any news program, on or off the networks. Even local stations and the tabloids do better than you do.

It is truly shocking and I wonder why.

Robert MacNeil, you have an openly gay son, Ian. (An enormously talented young man he is, too.) Are you so ashamed of him that you cannot bear for your program to deal with issues that remind you of him? Do you not ever worry that he might come down with AIDS? Or be fag-bashed? Or denied his rights as a human being? Surely such a father, so concerned, would insist on reporting on these issues on his very own program.

I find this huge hole in your coverage so grotesquely hypocritical that sometimes I want to throw something at my TV set when, week after week, month after month, you—who pretend to be so all-inclusive—continue to ignore this plague of AIDS, and refuse to acknowledge gays as the important political force we at last have become. (Six percent of Clinton's vote came from gays, a bit more than the Jewish vote.) How dare you continue to ignore us?

And when you do deign to do an AIDS story, you always manage to get the wrong people on to speak, the bureaucrats. And you never confront them with any but the most banal of questions, and you accept all their answers without question. You act so bored, as indeed anyone would be listening to the likes of Matilde Krim or Tony Fauci, experts in the art of saying nothing on the record (or off it either).

I am ashamed of all of you, who claim to be liberals and human beings. I am even more ashamed of Robert MacNeil, the father of a gay son.

And as we enter the thirteenth year of the AIDS plague, and as another President proceeds to slyly sweep AIDS under the carpet (talking a very good game to the contrary), I wonder when and where our help, and the truth, will come from.

PS: I am making a speech to the Gay and Lesbian Journalists Association at the Gay and Lesbian Community Center at 7 P.M. on Sunday, January 17, and I shall read them this letter.

As you can see, I write a lot of letters. Let me tell you there is no better way to get rid of your anger when something annoys you than by writing a letter to its perpetrator and then sending carbon copies to everyone who's his or her boss or peer or competitor. I highly recommend it as a good way to start your day. It really makes you feel like you're accomplishing something.

The "MacNeil-Lehrer News Hour" has long bugged the shit out of me. Here is this pompous bunch of windy self-styled liberals who night after night completely ignore gay and AIDS issues as if we didn't exist. When I learned that MacNeil had an openly gay son, that did it for me. My dam burst.

The whole issue of how the media reports gay and AIDS issues has rarely been dealt with adequately. I spend a lot of time going after the *Times* because it's supposed to be the paper all other opinion makers really follow and notice and quote and emulate and all that stuff. If the *Times* runs a big story on something, then all the other news suppliers feel it's all right for them to do the same. Since no TV news program has this kind of clout, we sort of let them *all* get away with their crappy, lousy job.

Peter Jennings and "ABC Nightly News" have generally done the best job of the three prime-time newscasts. But George Straight, their science reporter, who's been covering AIDS since the beginning, is visibly tired of the story and stays away from it more often than not. Beth Nissen on "ABC Nightly News" does good stories. "Nightline," on the other hand, sucks. If Ted Koppel isn't homophobic, as I'm told he isn't, then why does it always sound like he's in such pain whenever he utters the word "gay" or "homosexual"? "Nightline" has done more programs on Bosnia in six months than they've done on AIDS in twelve years. Tom Brokaw is so-so, but "NBC Nightly News" has a great science reporter in Bob

Bazell, though he's allowed very little time for AIDS. CBS is the worst. Dan Rather and Connie Chung are so relentlessly heterosexual. And don't you just want to wipe that shit-eating grin off Dan Rather's face! And since Susan Spencer was moved off science, they really don't have anyone who's any good.

CNN is a special case. Their stuff always smacks to me of being vaguely, almost imperceptibly, conservative and right-wing. But it's easier to get a story on CNN than anywhere else; they do have that gaping, hungry twenty-four-hour maw to feed. Frank Sesno is a jerk and Judy Woodruff is ex-MacNeil-Lehrer. "Crossfire" is a no-win situation, I don't care what anyone says. Larry King's heart is in the right place, but not very often. Of all the networks, CNN—on all their programs—manages to find the biggest bigots to tell the "other side" of the story.

A special place in the pantheon is reserved for Phil Donahue, who, from the very beginning, has done more for AIDS on television than any other single person. Year in, year out, he's been front and center on this issue, with compassion, understanding, and the willingness to be on "the right side" when it means a lot of grief for him, per-haps even losing him the ratings race to Oprah Winfrey, who, on AIDS, is inhumanely negligent. She's lost members of the inner circle of her staff to AIDS; not even that prompts decent coverage from this woman.

Magazines are worse than newspapers and television. *Time* and *Newsweek* ignore gays and AIDS on a consistent basis, as do the lesser newsweeklies, the wretched *U.S. News & World Report, The Nation,* and *The New Republic;* and of course at *Harper's* and the *Atlantic* we simply don't exist. *The New Yorker,* under Tina Brown, has improved greatly over the Shawn-Gottlieb days, but strangely enough they've not honored AIDS with one of those in-depth pieces they're so famous for. I can't think of one single magazine, even something as "love you all" as the *Utne Reader,* that acknowledges us in any decent and regular way. And somebody ought to go up to Pleas-antville with a posse and string up all those closeted queens who put out the *Reader's Digest.*

It's amazing how many of the reporters we so admire have never or rarely reported on AIDS or gay issues: Diane Sawyer, Barbara Walters, David Brinkley, William Safire, Anthony Lewis, Russell Baker, Tom Wicker, Calvin Trillin, Frances FitzGerald, Maureen Dowd, Meg Greenfield, Murray Kempton, Gary Wills, David Halberstam—oh, it's a very long list that could go on and on. . . .

I believe all of this appalling behavior by the journalistic community can be traced to the even more appalling behavior of *The New York Times*. As I said, the *Times* is the yardstick by which all others measure their coverage. It's as simple as that. This is a country which glories in playing Follow the Leader. If the *Times* isn't writing about it, no one else feels they have to, either. What's more, the *Times* and its editors and its publishers know this, which makes matters even more disgusting. God, how I hate how this newspaper, decade after decade, has treated us.

It's interesting to note, as a finale to this tirade, that the best AIDS reporting anywhere continues to be done, as it has been since the beginning, by the same three women: Laurie Garrett and Catherine Woodard at *Newsday*, and Marilyn Chase at *The Wall Street Journal*. (Marlene Cimons of the *Los Angeles Times* used to be on this list, but she doesn't seem to write about AIDS very much anymore.)

To get back to the MacNeil letter: MacNeil answered, in the highest of dudgeon, with a very angry letter indeed, in which he included a list of what must have been all the dates that the words "AIDS" and/or "gay" were so much as mentioned on their program. Fortunately (agonized inveterate viewer that I am) I remembered enough to write back, in as blistering a fashion, saying that he was full of shit, that most of his instancings hadn't been stories at all, just mentions, and that the ones that were stories or segments were flabby, flawed, and soft in the ways I then enumerated for him. Then I outlined a dozen story suggestions. I sent copies of my letter to some fifty journalists and editors and every likely candidate I could think of. *New York* magazine's Intelligencer column ran an item, but that, I thought, was it. And the program certainly didn't get any better.

And then in May 1994, Ian MacNeil, the son, came to New York with the London production of *An Inspector Calls*, for which he had so magnificently created one of the finest sets ever seen on a theater's stage. *The New York Times* decided to do a story on father and son. David Dunlop, an openly gay *Times* reporter, remembered my early correspondence with the father and told the reporter writing the father-son story, Georgia Dullea, about it. And there in the pages of *The New York Times*, a year and a half after writing it, was a discussion of my letter, with Ian MacNeil refusing to criticize me, or my tactics. "He created Gay Men's Health Crisis and ACT UP, for God's sake. . . . Part of all that is to use any weapon anywhere to publicize the AIDS issue. And if that includes saying Robert MacNeil doesn't love his son because he's gay, then he'll say it. . . . Heaven knows whether he believes it or not. That's almost irrelevant within the politics of what he's talking about."

I cite all this to make a point: This letter was finally paying off, not only in this important mention in the *Times*, but in the public comment that its appearance at last provoked. So write those letters! And don't forget to send copies to everyone important you can think of!

Ian MacNeil also complimented me outlandishly. This had other repercussions, sadder and more touching. It went like this.

For some time now I've been stymied as to what to do next in the way of activism. Something new, something fresh, something more invigorating is required, and I can't seem to come up with whatever it should be. Oh, I know what it should be. I just can't bring myself to do it. Here is Ian MacNeil, in the pages of the *Times*, calling me a brilliant political lifesaving strategist, and I say to myself, Okay, Larry, now's the time to go out there and, finally, lead the underground guerrilla movement that you know is needed, that you know is the only thing that will work now to pierce the endless lethargy and provoke a cure.

I called one of the gutsiest activists I know and we had a secret lunch to discuss all this, and what happened is what always happens: We were too skittish about doing what really has to be done—intimidating public displays that could scare the shit out of people to such an extent that they'd see that pressure was put on the White House to finally make a cure for AIDS a top priority (instead of not on their list at all). Bombs, fires, guns, explosions, tainted blood—all of these are needed, and it is indicative of how incapable of utilizing any of these tactics I am that I can write about them so openly.

And the funny thing is I just know that if I, a Jew, had been fighting for the birth of Israel, I would have been a member of the Irgun,* their guerrilla underground that did all those things.

■ ■ ■

There were many festivities connected with our historic march on Washington in April 1993. One of them was a dinner at the Library of Congress honoring HHS Secretary Donna Shalala. It was to be her first public appearance speaking on AIDS. I'd tried to get in touch with her since her appointment, to no avail. She didn't return calls or faxes or letters. Her rudeness by this time was annoying me. Her staff was no better. No one would talk to the activists and no one would talk to me. By this time it was beginning to be obvious to me that Bill Clinton, as far as AIDS and gays were concerned, was a big dose of hot air. Oh, he said all the right things, but there was no action where it mattered. But because he was saying what we wanted to hear, the usual tactics of confrontation and embarrassment wouldn't work. Very clever of him.

I decided to put on my own demo at this dinner, which was blithely billed as "Our Place at the Table." I'd never done anything like this before, I mean by myself. I was actually kind of nervous. Since it was a dinner sponsored

---

*See also the ending to "Oh, My People," page 191.

𝕯onna 𝕯o-𝕹othing WORKS FOR
Bill the Welsher

It has been six months since **Bill the Welsher** got elected. It has been five months since we heard **Donna Do-Nothing** would be Health Secretary. WHAT HAS SIX MONTHS BOUGHT US? **Bill the Welsher** has announced **no AIDS programs**, nor put in place **ANYTHING** that would change, end, alter the horrors of the last 12 years. **Bill the Welsher** has announced **no AIDS czar**. No one even knows what kind of AIDS czar they want. Far **_worse_**, there is **NO HEAD OF AIDS RESEARCH**. Stupid **Ted Kennedy** has pushed an **appallingly dumb plan** through Congress that establishes *another* bureaucracy at NIH. When will everyone realize there has **never** been one single major illness cured by NIH? Why do we continue to put all our trust and hope in NIH? NIH is **incapable** of operating in time of crisis, emergency, or plague. But who listens to us— we who understand what's wrong with the AIDS research system and have ideas how to make it work? **Hillary, Bill the Welsher's Wife**, has placed on her Health Panel **NOT ONE SINGLE AIDS EXPERT**. Dr. Anthony Fauci, for better or worse the government's leading AIDS researcher, has, during these past six months, received not one single phone call or summons to a meeting from **Bill the Welsher, Hillary the Welsher's Wife**, Donna Do-Nothing, or any of her lackeys (Patsy, the patsy, Fleming; Kevin, the invisible, Thurm, Dr. Phil, the hatchet-man, Lee). This is **appalling**. Not one single person of importance at the White House or in HHS has cared enough to call Fauci and ask him: how's it going? what do you need? what can we do to help? This comes at a time when *important scientific breakthroughs* are occuring that need to be pursued IMMEDIATELY. **Time is being pissed away!** Just like it was under ReaganBush! *NOTHING IS ANY DIFFERENT!* What kind of inhumanity is this? **THIS IS YET ANOTHER PRESIDENT AND YET ANOTHER HEALTH SECRETARY WHO DO NOT CARE ABOUT AIDS!** *WHY DO YOU NOT SEE THIS?* WHY ARE OUR SO-CALLED "LEADERS" KISSING THIS PRESIDENT'S ASS? HE MAY BE SAYING ALL THE RIGHT THINGS BUT HE ISN'T *DOING* ANYTHING! While we are dying! Dr. Haseltine at Harvard now predicts **ONE BILLION people** will be HIV infected by the new century. How can we sit by so passively and wait so passively for **Bill the Welsher** and Donna Do-Nothing *to DO SOMETHING*? Where are your voices? Where is your anger? Has everyone turned into AIDS whores? (The longer this plague continues the longer you have a job.) THIS NEW PRESIDENT MADE US PROMISES AND HAS DONE NOTHING TO IMPLEMENT THESE PROMISES OR TO EVEN DISCUSS WITH US THE POSSIBILITIES OF IMPLEMENTING THESE PROMISES. WE HAVE BEEN COMPLETELY SHUT OUT FROM ANY DISCUSSIONS WHICH IS BAD ENOUGH UNTIL YOU REALIZE **THERE AREN'T EVEN ANY DISCUSSIONS GOING ON**! *WHY DO PEOPLE NEVER BELIEVE ME UNTIL IT'S TOO LATE?! WE ARE BEING INTENTIONALLY ALLOWED TO DIE!*
OH, MY BROTHERS AND SISTERS, I BEG YOU TO LISTEN TO ME.

Larry Kramer

Distributed to all the guests at a dinner honoring Health and Human Services Secretary Donna Shalala, Washington, April 23, 1993.

by the National Minority AIDS Council, I was joined in my protest by a person of color, a very gutsy and beautiful young woman, Sabrina Greene. Together we passed copies of my flyers to everyone and then stood flanking Shalala as she spoke her meaningless rhetoric, one of us on either side of her, holding up big posters denouncing her inactivity and hypocrisy.

It was a good experience for me, and I wonder now why I don't do things like this more often! You don't need hundreds of people to make a successful demo.

The weekend was a very inspirational one for everyone who was there. I made a speech on the steps of the Capitol to many hundreds. I'd hoped to speak at the march itself, but, once again, it had pointedly been made known by the committee in charge that I was not welcome. A number of people had tried to get me on the program for many months; toward the end I tried to fight for myself when I discovered that one of the people in charge had directed *The Normal Heart* at Brown University. No luck. The night before the march, when Torie Osborn, then head of NGLTF, heard I wasn't speaking, she, together with Urvashi Vaid and comediennes Kate Clinton, who was to be emcee, and Robin Tyler, offered to sneak me in and get me in front of the microphone. So finally I had the great privilege I'd coveted for so long— talking to my people, not only spread out in front of me as far as the eye could see, but also across the country and around the world via cable television. Since I'd had no time to prepare a new speech, I extemporized one based on this flyer.

I've had many compliments about this appearance mainly because there were few men speakers and fewer speakers in any way connected with AIDS, a shocking and evidently quite deliberate insult on the part of the organizers. Needless to say, all hell broke loose when the committee discovered what had happened, resulting in many nasty articles and accusations in the gay press. I couldn't have cared less what those incompetent youngsters thought. I'd got my message out, thanks to four great dykes.

It was an interesting lesson: the younger generation coming along and having so little respect for the hard work put in by their predecessors. I hadn't thought of myself as an old fart before, but now I guess it was time to notice that others did.

(I did get a few letters from Welsh people. I'd offended them by calling Clinton "Bill the Welsher." Life is a daily lesson in learning how and in what way we interact with others.)

I should mention that somewhere along about this time I fell in love again. It has been a very long time since I have been in love. The two "great love"s in my life have been the friend I wrote *The Normal Heart* about and the friend I wrote *Faggots* about. I guess it's no longer a secret that this "new" love is the latter. We came back together, after some fifteen years, during which we never so much as ran into each other, though we live only a dozen or so blocks apart. It's over a year now and this time it seems to be working out.

Evil *Times* — Part One[*]

Just what does it take to make a newspaper morally responsible? How much heartbreak is required? How much suffering? Before I die, I wish I could write something that, *at last*, would break the hearts of the men who run *The New York Times*. And make them *see*.

To this day there has not been one single in-depth investigation of the scandal that is the United States' government AIDS research program in the pages of the most powerful and feared newspaper in the world.

What does it take to make them *get it?* What confidential memo do they have to read? To make them *see*.

When confronted by accusations that the *Times* still has, quite possibly, the worst reporting about AIDS of any media outlet, Managing Editor Joseph Lelyveld,[**] responds: "What aren't we writing about? What do you want us to write about that we're not writing about?" When presented with long lists, he mutters, "I'll look into it."

---

[*]*The Advocate*, Issue 643, November 30, 1993.
[**]Since these two pieces were published, Joseph Lelyveld has become editor-in-chief, replacing Max Frankel, who has retired, and Jeff Schmalz has died.

The man I'm seeing lost his lover last year. He received a phone call from a straight friend he hadn't seen for some time. "How's Michael?" the straight man asked. David told him Michael had died of AIDS. "AIDS? He died from it? I thought it was all taken care of. I don't read about it anymore."

The bottom line is this: I am going to die—as all my friends have died—because the most powerful and feared newspaper in the world refuses to hold our wretched government's feet to the fire, as it has done on a long list of other scandals stretching back to the Pentagon Papers.

Not one single *Times* article in the thirteen years of this plague has in any way investigated NIH, questioned why in thirteen years they've accomplished so little, noticed what a dead end it is for almost every illness, and identified what a complete failure Dr. Anthony Fauci has been. At the *Times*, the NIH is Lourdes—unassailable.

Not one single *Times* article in the thirteen years of this plague has in any way investigated the Department of Health and Human Services, or its long list of incompetent heads, including its present one, Donna Do-Nothing, for all the same reasons.

Presidents come and go and the *Times* criticizes them mercilessly for what they have *not* done, what scandals simmered on their watches. Reagan, Bush, now Clinton are allowed to get away with murder, as far as AIDS is concerned.

(I am not talking about any of those endlessly repellent "bleeding heart" stories *Times* reporters like Mia Navarro and Jane Gross churn out about us poor AIDS victims. What hypocritical shit this is, just so the *Times* can say: "How can you say we're not writing about AIDS?")

There's only one "out" *Times* reporter, Jeffrey Schmalz, now dying of AIDS, to whom Lelyveld assigns AIDS stories, in so doing putting such a strain on Jeff that it's no doubt hastening his death.

Since 1981, *Times* AIDS reporting has been done by: Richard Flaste, Erik Eckholm, Dr. Lawrence Altman, Nicholas Wade, Philip Boffey, Gina Kolata, and Philip Hilts. All of them have reported to the Science Department. AIDS was and continues to be reported as a medical/science story only. It is not reported as a political story (like the Clinton health plan), or a scandal (like drug pricing or Savings and Loan). But AIDS isn't a medical story. It's a political scandal, which science writers aren't capable of writing about. So the *Times* is not telling the world about AIDS, just as the *Times* did not tell the world about the Nazi holocaust until it was too late. To read the *Times* is to enter a never-never land. I do not live in the city or in the country or in the world that the *Times* reports to me.

The New Yorker of October 4 ran a huge exposé of the scandal in France involving the deliberate sale by government officials of tainted blood. This story was suggested (by me) to Nick Wade before it broke in France (in 1991). Wade was uninterested. (Just as he's uninterested in reporting any other ideas I suggest to him.) Wade does not like me. Indeed, Nicholas Wade has a reputation among his very own colleagues for being homophobic. Nick Wade is now the science editor of the *Times*. He decides what is and what is not written about AIDS. A man his own colleagues claim is homophobic is in charge of what small amount of AIDS reporting there is.

During the first nineteen months of AIDS, the *Times* wrote about it seven times. (The Tylenol scare rated fifty-four articles in *three months*.) Richard Flaste, then the science editor, defends this appalling record in all seriousness by saying "there was nothing to write about," as does Altman, who wrote the first article. (Flaste then went on to join the Sunday *Times Book Review*, where, it's interesting to note, any book that dared to criticize the *Times'* wretched AIDS record was panned. I know of no book that reports the *Times'* abysmal record that has been treated fairly by the book review.)

Evil *Times*—Part Two[*]

D r. Lawrence Altman, the only *Times* reporter covering AIDS since the beginning, once worked for the Centers for Disease Control; he's more government apologist than unbiased reporter. He's currently embarked on a campaign to blame AIDS activists for drugs that aren't working, like AZT or ddC. It's the activists' fault for pressuring for their speedier release. Altman is incapable of writing about the great pretender, Dr. Fauci, with anything short of worship. Since Fauci is the source of most stories the *Times* will publish, this is unprofessional behavior of the highest order.

Phil Boffey had the beat for the crucial years when AIDS passed from disease to epidemic to plague. I have gone into great detail earlier in this book, about how ill-informed Boffey was on even the most basic stuff. (Complaints to editor Max Frankel fell on deaf ears. Max is not a listener.) Phil might have been covering measles—nothing embarrassing or shocking (which is just about everything connected to AIDS). The motto of the *Times*

The Advocate, No. 644, December 28, 1993.

419

is "All the News That's Fit to Print" and for your average heterosexual white man (and *Times* editor), Boffey was boffo.

At the *Times*, after you're a lousy reporter they promote you. Boffey, as bad an AIDS reporter as Wade, was made an editorial writer. (He actually writes a good editorial once in a while.)

Then we got Gina Kolata. Gina is, well, sloppy. She made so many gaffes (the ddI story, the "deaths" from Compound Q, quoting "expert" sources who weren't) that even Max noticed. ACT UP stickers all over the country proclaiming, GINA KOLATA OF *THE NEW YORK TIMES* IS THE WORST AIDS REPORTER IN THE WORLD also did not please. Gina has pretty much been taken off the AIDS beat.

The current incumbent, the only person who reports on AIDS on a regular basis for the most important paper in the world, is Philip J. Hilts. I cannot say enough unkind words about Philip J. Hilts. He is utterly, completely, horrendously, explosively—tragically—useless. There is not an AIDS story out of Washington that he bothers to write about. Important conferences, appointments, discoveries, scandals all come and go unnoticed, unrecorded anywhere in the pages of the *Times*.

Why are such historic omissions allowed in this famous newspaper of record? Why have an AIDS reporter and allow him to remain silent? Is Phil Hilts *not* writing about AIDS because his editors don't want AIDS written about? Is it an intentional act?

The wife of Joseph Lelyveld, the managing editor of *The New York Times*, the number-two man on the editorial side after Max Frankel, runs an AIDS clinic in Harlem. She knows how truly awful this plague is. She knows how truly wretched the NIH is, and every other government agency that pretends to deal with AIDS. When I asked Joe Lelyveld why this very fact—that his own wife works in AIDS—does not spur him on to see his paper do a better job reporting this plague, he answered me with one of the most tragic responses it has ever been my misfortune to hear. He said *because* his wife worked in AIDS was the very reason he had to be careful what he ran in the *Times* about AIDS, lest he be accused of favoring this illness over others.

Joe, does it ever occur to you that you are probably more

responsible than any person in the world for the deaths of your wife's clients?

Joe, at which point does your newspaper pass beyond bad reporting and into evil?

Joe, I think your behavior is evil.

Why does no one at the *Times* listen when so many cry out that AIDS is a national scandal of tragic proportions? Why does no one at the *Times* notice AIDS cases are rising from an original forty-one to one billion? How can a columnist like Walter Goodman, another apparent homophobe, get away with dumping on an NBC report on the danger of contracting AIDS through blood transfusions, telling *Times* readers that several hundred cases is nothing to worry about? Why will the *Times* identify Ted Danson as Whoopi Goldberg's "lover" and refuse to use the same word for any gay man, either in text or obituaries?

It all boils down to the same thing: It's still okay for faggots and niggers and spics to die.

I'm told that the new publisher, Mr. Sulzberger, Jr., is not homophobic and, indeed, gives handsome donations to Broadway Cares. I don't want his blood money. Just as I don't want any more repulsive Navarro-Gross "victim" stories. All these hypocritical tokens to appease liberal consciences make me vomit.

No, they make me die.

The New York Times, in its refusal to report responsibly the scandal that is our government's response to AIDS, is an evil newspaper, run by evil men, performing evil acts. As much as Hitler did, these men are murdering human beings.

Anybody wants to call me crazy, off the wall, round the bend, finally demented, go ahead.

History will bear me out.

T hese were two of my monthly columns for *The Advocate*. They were part of a series on evil, on trying to understand and define it. (They were finalists for a national magazine association award—it's interesting that my anger with the *Times* is so widely shared.) I don't know why I never thought much about evil before—whether I even believed in it or not. Perhaps I just had a certain innocence, a belief learned at my mother's knee that all people were decent. But after so many years of screaming about the horrors gay people and people with AIDS endure, it finally hit me smack in the face that I wasn't writing about the one thing that was probably most behind our ostracism. These *Advocate* pieces were just a beginning of trying to understand evil, and my Yale speech that follows was a continuation of my investigations. The novel on which I've been working for so long, *The American People*, will now focus a lot more on it.

What prompted me to write these attacks was my continuing horror over how the *Times* gets away with doing such an irresponsible job covering the AIDS plague. Despite constant pressure. Despite constant criticism. Shit, even their own reporters know how terribly they report AIDS. It's no secret even there, in their own newsroom!

Several years ago I was on Charlie Rose with Frank Rich (then the *Times'* drama critic). After the program Frank and I found ourselves walking out together and talking. He asked me what I thought of the *Times'* AIDS coverage and I let loose. He listened attentively and offered to see if Joseph Lelyveld, the managing editor, would meet with me. Sure enough, I was invited to lunch with Joe. It was a very pleasant lunch—Joe is a nice man—and I listed many specific suggestions for stories, a few of which he noted down.

To this day, none of these suggestions has metamorphosed into a story in the *Times*. I've written to Joe a number of times, and with increasing severity, to point this out, and he always answers me, now quite defensively. A recent response asked me why I couldn't make my requests nicely, and I wrote back pointing out when

I asked nicely it obviously didn't get done. (Not that it gets done when I ask not-nicely.)

Joe is one of those guys like Clinton: He says the right things, and everybody who knows him thinks the world of him. So it's hard to criticize him and make anyone believe you. People think I'm crazy when I criticize Joe.

Things took a bizarre turn when Jeffrey Schmalz died. Jeff was one of the *Times'* top reporters, not particularly openly gay and certainly not writing about AIDS or gay issues, who discovered he had AIDS only when he collapsed in the newsroom and was rushed to the hospital with PCP. From then on, he was a man possessed, writing with fire and passion about being a gay man on the *Times* and, by the end, with great anger, about AIDS and this country's lack of response to it. That he was sick for his several remaining years circumscribed the number of articles he could actually write, which were unfortunately few and the only really good AIDS stuff ever written in that paper. His last article, for *The New York Times Magazine*, was entitled "Whatever Happened to AIDS?" and it was a very damning indictment indeed of how he felt he'd been abandoned by his country.

We'd become close by the time he died. I asked his sister if I could speak at his memorial service and was told I could. But then someone must have realized what I might say and who might be in the audience for me to say it to, and I was—literally—disinvited by Adam Nigorney, the openly gay *USA Today* reporter in charge of the service. Mr. Nigorney and I did not have a pleasant conversation. A week or so later I got a call from David Dunlop, who told me there would now be *two* memorial services, one "for family and friends" and the other open to the public, and I could speak at the latter. Okay. Didn't mean to cause you *that* much trouble . . .

I found myself at this second service introduced by Nigorney as an activist who had threatened to have both services picketed by ACT UP if I hadn't been allowed to speak. I was livid at his accusation, which was not true.

Afterwards I went over to Dudley Clendinen, with whom Nigorney is writing a book on the history of the gay movement since Stonewall—Dudley had been interviewing me—and told him I did not wish to appear in their book, was ashamed of Adam, and wondered how someone who acted like this could write a history of the gay movement with anything resembling understanding. (I expected more of Dudley, too—an old friend who shared his coming out with me. One loses friends quite often when one is an activist.)

My speech follows. (Imagine the first few rows beneath my podium filled with the top echelon of the *Times*.) I have no idea how it reads or if, as they say, you had to be there. As at Vito's memorial, there was that unearthly silence, as if I was the only person in a sealed box. Because it was so quiet, I could speak softly. The Dalton School auditorium (chosen because Jeff had been filmed for television with these students) was pitch black; I couldn't see the faces of all the hierarchy of the *Times*, whom I hoped were not asleep. I'd worked very hard on the text. I actually thought it quite restrained. (They should only have seen the earlier versions.) This was an opportunity that would not come to me again. I didn't want them to think I'd gone completely nuts.

I have no idea what any of them thought. There was the expected applause from the activists sitting in the rear. When I asked various *Times* people later, I was told they got my point.

Then why hasn't anything there improved? Even Lelyveld's promise to replace Jeff with another strong AIDS reporter has not been kept.

I received a most nasty letter from Jeffrey's sister. In return, I sent her a copy of this book.

No, my relations with the *Times* don't get any better. And after sending everyone there copies of these *Advocate* articles, and after making this speech at Jeff's memorial, I don't expect they will. (I shudder to think what they will print about me when I die.)

I wonder if AIDS will *ever* be covered well, anywhere—with compassion, insight, justice, fairness, depth? Just as I wonder if there will ever be a cure. And just as I wonder if all my criticisms of mediocrity everywhere will *ever* improve things. For all my dunning, when someone second-rate's replaced, the replacement's invariably third-rate.

Who Killed Jeff?*

T here is not a day that goes by when some friend is not dying from AIDS. People like Jeff do not come very often into this world. Most of those who die were not like him. That makes remembering him more painful. What we have lost! I try not to remember people. There are too many to remember and I get confused. Confused that all their faces are fading. Confused there are so many of them. I can no longer hold on to all their names. Confused why there should be so many of them. Confused that so many have been allowed to die. I know now that AIDS is intentional genocide. How could I believe otherwise? Jeff was allowed to die. He knew this, of course. That's what his last article was all about.

I've been going to services like this for twelve years. I have no more tears left. I wanted to make a speech that would make you cry, but I can't make myself cry. I'm empty inside. I'm not certain I can even feel anything anymore. All the Jeffs in my life are dead. All the bright, capable, talented hopes and dreams for our future have died. I live in a wilderness of not knowing where

---

*Delivered at a memorial service for Jeffrey Schmalz, The Dalton School, December 7, 1993.

to turn. One by one, the anchors that have held my reason in place are pulled away. Jeff. If Jeff could get through all this, and write about it with such insight and brilliance and clarity, then I can too.

But Jeff hasn't got through all this. Jeff is dead.

In all these years of attending services like this, one thing always hits me. Why can't the people who come to mourn make the connection between the death of the loved one and *why* he died?

Jeff died asking, "Whatever happened to AIDS?"

He died asking you why he died.

Have you asked yourself why he died?

Does anyone who ever attends these endless memorials ever ask, Why did this person die? I mean, *why?* Not what from, though that too, but WHY?

Have you asked yourself "whatever happened to AIDS" and put that together with "why did Jeff die"?

And then, when you have asked yourself why, have you asked yourself the next big question: What did I do to help save Jeff's life?

You loved Jeff. You came here to mourn Jeff. Jeff died from a plague. What have you done to stop this plague? This plague that killed Jeff, Jeff whom you came here to mourn.

You probably didn't do very much, because the plague is still raging and out of control. And Jeff died.

So I guess you didn't do very much to help save his life. The life of the Jeff you say you loved and have come here to mourn.

Why didn't you do anything? *Why?*

What are you going to do now? Are you going to do anything now in honor of Jeff's memory? In honor of the man you say you loved and have come here to mourn?

Why aren't we all trying to do what Jeff did? That's really what he was asking in his article. Why isn't everyone fighting to stop this plague? He was telling us that our new President is as bad as his two predecessors and that, despite all kinds of public statements, the research for a cure just isn't being done.

That's why I say AIDS is intentional genocide. From now on I am going to say it over and over wherever I go and wherever they will put my face and allow my voice to be heard. I am going to scream it as loudly as I can so that perhaps even Jeff will hear me and know that what he realized at the end is being screamed out loud by his friend and fellow fighter. AIDS IS INTENTIONAL GENOCIDE! It is being allowed by our goverment and sanctioned by the third President in a row. Jeff was allowed to die.

And at the end of his life, Jeff knew all this. That's what his last article is all about.

Genocide is a crime an entire society commits. Presidents and congresspersons and bureaucrats don't get away with murder when enough people won't let them. Jeff may have worked for *The New York Times*, but he was a member of one of the most oppressed minorities. AIDS is an evil act perpetrated on minorities.

The New York Times could have saved Jeff. But it didn't. Since this plague began, in 1981, it has chosen not to. Jeff was probably infected about that time.

You came here to mourn him. If you cared about Jeff, then you are hypocrites if you continue to do nothing and continue to allow so little to be done and continue to allow the Jeffs of this world to die. A great many people in this room have enormous power. The parents of many of you in this room have enormous power. Have you learned to ask your parents how they use their power? Is making money all they do? And have you learned how to read your daily newspaper and notice what is *not* written in its pages? The newspaper that Jeff worked for has enormous power. What has that newspaper chosen to do with its power? Certainly not to fight to save the life of Jeff Schmalz, whom they claim to have loved.

I thought it was the moral responsibility of all of us to use what we are given to fight for the good of mankind. That's what every religion and philosophy commands. Did you? Did you do anything to save Jeff's life?

No, you didn't. Not really.

I know that many of you do not welcome me here. I long ago became accustomed to being unwelcome. I do not think it untoward or a projection of any kind on my part to say that the Jeff I knew would welcome me here and welcome these words.

Please. In Jeff's name, use your power. So that he will not have died in vain. Silence does indeed equal death, and action equal life.

I am going to have distributed among you some articles I've published about the history of AIDS coverage in *The New York Times*. I hope you will read them and believe them and make known your desires for a much improved state to this newspaper's management.

Surely the most noble gesture this paper could make to honor Jeff's memory would be to finally begin responsibly reporting this plague of AIDS.

Good-bye, Jeff. You will be missed. Perhaps it will take your death to make your employers into responsible human beings.

Part Four

Some Thoughts About Evil*

*For as I detest the doorways of Death, I
detest that man who
hides one thing in the depths of his heart,
and speaks forth another.*

Homer, The *Iliad*

I believe in evil.

I believe evil exists. Visibly, tangibly, and recognizably.

My dictionary defines evil in the most benign of fashions: the quality of being morally bad.

I believe evil is more than this. I believe evil is an act, intentional or not, of inflicting undeserved harm on others.

I'm sure this definition is not precise or inclusive enough.

I must tell you that this is *my* definition of evil. It's been difficult for me to find one that defines it this way, which is the way I believe it should be defined. I find it very peculiar that I can find so little that *specifically* tells us what evil is.

---

*This speech was delivered at Yale University on December 2, 1993, where I was the first speaker invited by the Research Fund for Lesbian and Gay Studies at Yale.

I've entitled this talk "Some Thoughts About Evil." I've read many books about evil since I agreed to make this speech and since something made me say to myself, "I'm going to talk about evil. Because something evil is going on. Why haven't I ever addressed what's going on in *that* context?" I've read all these books and still I can't tell you what the world really thinks about evil or how the world defines evil.

Not only is there little consensus on what evil is, as I think there should be—and as there is for, say, war, aggression, holocaust, even sin—but during my investigations I began to realize that evil isn't even thought about much anymore, by the liberals and by the intellectuals (or whatever you want to call the opposite of the bigots and the religious right), the people I once thought of as on "my side."

As I say, it's very difficult to research evil, to find in books the stuff from which one can make sense out of whatever it is. Dictionaries and encyclopedias, indeed all the books I consulted, give only the vaguest and, at the same time, broadest, definitions of it. Even Freud wrote very little about it, and mostly under the concept of sin, or coupled with God, which is not the kind of evil I want to explore. "Something bad," which one finds as part of evil's definition elsewhere, is not nearly a good enough description.

No, no writer, philosopher, or theologian, in any of my research, has been able to define evil for me* in a way that makes

---

*After this speech was delivered, I came upon a remarkable book, *People of the Lie*, by M. Scott Peck, which has indeed been extremely useful to me in defining evil. I wish I'd read it in time to include Dr. Peck's ideas and definitions in these remarks. He has certainly given me intellectual ammunition to support my contention that those in charge of AIDS, be they in Washington or in our own AIDS organizations, are partners in perpetuating this evil. It's interesting to note that when I said this in one of my *Advocate* columns, that magazine received a record amount of mail, all of it condemning me. Dr. Peck defines evil "most simply as the use of political power to destroy others for the purpose of preserving the integrity of one's sick self.... We are far more likely to kill that which is different from us than that which resembles us." "Evil has to do with killing," he says; "I do not mean to restrict myself to corporeal murder. Evil is also that which kills spirit." He talks a great deal about "group evil"—how "human groups tend to behave in much the same way as human individuals—except at a level that is more primitive and immature than one might expect." "Group immaturity," he calls it. The most salient discussion in his book, for me, deals with group responsibility. "I am thoroughly convinced that much of the evil of our times is related to specialization ... how the specialized individual is in a position to pass the moral buck to some other specialized any more sense to me than any of my earlier investigations into trying to make sense of why people don't fight back—particularly gay people, particularly people confronting AIDS, even when, especially when, they're facing extermination.

Yale is my alma mater, and I was taught, as I presume you are being taught, to attack my deliberations and determinations in the most rigorous fashion possible, to state my thesis and marshall evidence so conclusively that the ipso facto can be nothing but. That is the way to be an intellectual.

But then intellectuals tend to intellectualize when they set themselves a problem to make sense of. And perhaps there are times when intellectualization simply does not present a decent enough case for or against the argument. Thinking about it isn't the same thing as living with it. And it seems to me that the people I've read had only the vaguest personal notion of evil and very little, if any, experience with evil, at least the kind of evil I am talking about. These people are philosophers or teachers or theologians who contemplate the issue intellectually, as a concept, at most as a witnessed and not a lived ordeal, and as a concept that, for them, when fully explored, might yield some insight into why God—their God—allows anything awful to exist in the world.

God does seem wrapped up in almost everybody's discussion of evil.

Even if they have endured or been personally exposed to evil, these investigators are looking for a way not only to make sense out of what happened to them, or what they witnessed, but also to find it in their hearts somehow to forgive those who have trespassed against them.

As I grow older I have become increasingly amazed at the willingness of human beings to seek and offer forgiveness, particularly when they have been most sinned against, most trespassed against. I am told that this is the Christian way, or the

---

cog or on to the machine itself. . . . Specialization contributes to the immaturity of groups and their potential for evil through several different mechanisms. One such mechanism is the fragmentation of conscience. 'You've come to the wrong department . . . That's down the hall . . . The problems you're talking about are beyond our purview. . . .' " Dr. Peck's thoughts intersect remarkably well, though he's certainly coming from a different place, with those of Professor Zygmunt Bauman, whose book *Modernity and the Holocaust* I discuss in "AIDS: The War Is Lost" (see page 334).

humanist way, or that indeed, for many so trespassed against, this is the only or best way to regain or retain sanity. That God is love and love is forgiveness.

The problem with any and all of this, for me at any rate, is what do you do when you don't believe in God?

Or when you don't believe that all men are equal.

Or when you don't feel that the human spirit redeems all, or is, across the board, redemptive.

Most of the investigations of evil seem, for some reason, to have been written by theologians. I guess if you're going to believe in God and you're also going to be a theologian, the problem of evil, particularly in relationship to good, and to God, is high up there on the list of matters you're going to have to deal with, intellectually at any rate. I mean, if you're going to talk yourself into believing in God, then you certainly have to come up with some sort of rationale for why there is so much that is UnGodly going on in the world.

I don't mean to be flip about any of this, but it does seem to me that most of the pulpits of this world are inhabited by people who are just a few feet higher off the ground than the rest of us and hence are, to be kind about it, out of touch.

However, this is not what I want to talk about, beyond saying I do not believe in God and I do not care about God and thus all the endless dissertations dissecting the traditional Christian view that God is all powerful and all central to all and everything are beside the point to me. God is God and evil is evil and if ever the twain shall meet they will meet in a more God-fearing person than I.

And I am not interested in defining evil only as a concept that can be compared with good, as in good and evil. This is more germane a statement than you might think. Evil has no separate listing of its own in the *Readers' Guide to Periodical Literature*, nor in the *Encyclopaedia Brittanica*. In the former it is listed under the pairing "Good and Evil." And the *Columbia Encyclopedia* defines evil solely as "the antithesis of good."

Why can't anyone define evil in and of itself? Why can't it be thought of as something in and of itself? Why does every book and dictionary and encyclopedia and intellectual consider evil only in the context of a question—such as this one in the *Columbia Encyclopedia*'s definition: "Why does evil exist in the world?" Death and disease and sin are definable in unquestioned ways. Why isn't evil? In the secular world, I mean. For you and for me. Without any God stirred in. Even the Catholic Church, that most questionable of enterprises, over many centuries has developed elaborate codifications of evil that are unquestioningly definitive. Sins That Cry to Heaven for Vengeance, Sins Against the Holy Spirit, sins mortal and venal. Yes, the Catholics can tell you what evil is. Though, of course, only in reference to their God.

I am interested in trying to make you think of evil precisely, as an entity, a noun, on its own, as a tangible act and deed, part of the daily miserable occurrences in our vocabularies of life, and I am interested in asking you to ponder as well why this word or concept is not much in use anymore, particularly when it's such a useful concept, such a useful, if you will, weapon, one that is certainly used against us often enough by our enemies, those who constantly tell us that gay people are the evil ones, that our "lifestyle"—and how I have come to hate *that* expression (talk about concepts that are indefinable)—is evil and the sex we have is evil and our desire to marry is evil and our expressions of affection are evil and our determination for equal rights is evil and our expectation of protection under the law is evil and our art is evil. And of course AIDS is evil—not because it has been allowed to grow so unattended but because *we* have it. If our enemies have such a certainty of what evil is and that we are the embodiment of it, why don't we—you and I—know what evil is and that *they* are the embodiment of it? Evil is certainly no longer a concept that anyone I know bothers to consider, not even when we confront bigotry and hate, at the most extreme, or just plain lassitude, ass-dragging, stupidity, intolerance, ignorance, and invisibility—intentional or otherwise.

Have we simply given evil away? Are we too superior to acknowledge it, believing that our enemies, in their bigotry, are of lesser intellectual vigor or rigor than we are, and that if they are going to play in such mud, we, at least, proud and of clean hands, will be bigger than they are? I do believe it is something like this. I do believe that we, who are condemned as evil by others, have discarded the concept as somehow beneath us to respond to.

And, in so doing, we have carelessly tossed out a most valuable weapon for our own exceedingly depleted arsenal of defensive ammunition.

Once upon a time, the concept of evil was different. This country was founded on the conviction that evil lived in the land—everywhere—and this fact was breathed into every heart and soul from every pulpit and around every dining table and in every classroom. To the Puritan mind there was nothing else to be so frightened of as evil's lure, evil's call, evil's victory.

But that was yesterday's evil. Not today's evil. That evil was the evil of God the stern father, God the controller general. That evil was the only way they knew to keep the troops in line.

One can only wonder if somewhere along the way, since then, as more and more of the troops refused to stay in line, the very concept of evil disappeared, its parameters and pertinencies blurred and then eradicated, so that, by now, it is absent from the modern world.

Has evil somehow become disdainfully old-fashioned, and on another level, too Stephen King?

■ ■ ■

Here are some of the things I wrote down from my readings in those books I told you about, by those who have written about evil:

This is from Ernest Becker, a professor who wrote *Denial of Death*, a book I very much admired in my younger days and which won a Pulitzer Prize. His last work before he died was entitled *Escape from Evil:* "In this book I attempt to show that man's natural and inevitable urge to deny mortality and achieve a heroic self-image are the root causes of human evil. . . . Men fashion unfreedom as a bribe for self-perpetuation." He goes on to explain how he has come to the realization that man needs material goods and economic equality and that not achieving these is beyond man's endurance:

No wonder economic equality is beyond the endurance of modern democratic man: the house, the car, the bank balance are his immortality symbols. Or, put another way, if a black man moves next door, it is not merely that your house diminishes in real estate value, but that *you* diminish in fullness on the level of visible immortality—and so you *die*. The ideology of modern commercialism has unleashed a life of invidious comparison unprecedented in modern history. Modern man cannot endure economic equality because he has no faith in self-transcendent, other-wordly immortality symbols. Visible physical worth is the only thing he has to give him eternal life.

I was surprised how many other non-theologically-centered books came to more or less the same conclusion. Evil came about because people couldn't bear to be poor and needed concrete symbols that they weren't, if they were going to have their place in the sun. If they didn't have these symbols for all to see, evil was likely to be the result. Then wars and murders and the taking of tangibly valuable things away by one from another could happen.

"We have no sense of sin," Becker goes on, "because sin means literally separation from the powers and protection of the gods. . . . Since we have become completely secular we no longer have any problem with sin, since there is nothing to be separated from: everything is *here*, in one's possession, in his body. If there is no sense of sin, then evil can, ipso facto, flourish with ease."

So he is saying that evil can come about if we lose our sense of sin, which can only be possessed if we believe in some higher power. So I find myself right back where I started and where I don't want to be.

Becker quotes a good deal from Otto Rank, the psychoanalyst who had much to say to those involved in the creative process:

"All our human problems," Rank said, "with their intolerable sufferings, arise from man's ceaseless attempts to make this material world into a man-made reality . . . aiming to achieve on earth a 'perfection' which is only to be found in the beyond . . . thereby hopelessly confusing the values of both spheres."

Then Becker says:

> The thing that makes man the most devastating animal that
> ever stuck his head up into the sky is that he wants a stature
> and a destiny that is impossible for an animal; he wants an
> earth that is not an earth but a heaven, and the price for
> this kind of fantastic ambition is to make the earth an even
> more eager graveyard than it naturally is.

I do not find any of this—Becker or Rank—helpful in my
search. There is something in it that says to me: We're not living
in the same world.

These nontheologians want a heaven, too. I am beginning to
wonder if this search for God, for heaven, for a greater good and a
higher power, is nothing but an exceptionally grand cop-out. If
you can't figure out what's going wrong in the here and now, lay it
all off on the hereafter. Again, I don't wish to be flip, but I'm simply not getting any answers. I believe in evil. I know what I think
evil is. Then why is it so difficult to find acknowledgment that evil
exists at this moment in the twentieth century? Yes, I think blam-
ing it on God is an evasion of, if you will, the highest order.

Perhaps this is a good place to state why this quest for a
definition of evil is so important to me and why I feel a necessity
to impress on you that it is not a Stephen King novel I am talking
about but something that has become an integral part of my life.

Many people don't believe me when I say that AIDS is genocide
being intentionally inflicted upon gay people and other minorities
and marginalized populations. We are being *allowed* to die. Genocide—the deliberate and systematic extermination of an entire national, racial, political, or ethnic group—need not be intentional to
qualify as genocide. Genocide can also be achieved in more sly and
less obvious ways. Every moral code in the Judeo-Christian tradition, as well as in everything from the most ancient Buddhist
monks to New Age humanism, talks about sins of omission and
commission. All prophets make it very clear that either is a griev-
ous sin. He who looks the other way is just as guilty as he who kills
his brother. Responsibility for our brothers is, for any and all of
these moral codes, foremost, imperative, and unquestionable.

If I and many others are being allowed to die, isn't this evil
on a truly grand scale—I would say unprecedented but we have

all too many examples, recent and otherwise, of the extermination of other groups. And if it is evil, so what? What does a word
mean—and what's more a word that isn't used much anymore,
except as a weapon against us, by the very bigots who are happy
we are dying? And we, the attacked, what do we volley back
with? Well, certainly not with countercharges of a bigger evil.
No, the very concept of evil seems to have become so passé, so
retro, that in my crowd the word is used as a joke. "You're evil,"
we say. "She's an evil bitch."

Becker wrote: "If there is one thing that the tragic wars of
our time have taught us, it is that the enemy has a ritual role to
play, by means of which evil is redeemed. All wars are conducted
as holy wars, a testing of divine favor, and as a means of purging
evil from the world at the same time. Since everyone feels dis-
satisfied with himself (dirty), victimage is a universal human
need. And the highest heroism is the stamping out of those who
are tainted. The logic is terrifying."

Hitler's rise to power was based on his understanding of what
people wanted and needed most of all, and so he promised them,
above everything else, *heroic victory over evil;* and he gave them
the living possibility of not only accomplishing this but, at the
same time and thereafter, forever, ridding themselves of guilt.
It was okay. It was okay to slaughter us. And many, many, many
people believed him. And followed him.

From 1930 to 1941, Hitler murdered fifty thousand Germans
in an attempt to cleanse the German people of the "mentally ill"
and the retarded. Jews and gays and gypsies were not his only
targets. And of course there have been, before and since, many
other holocausts. World War I. The Turkish massacre of one
million Armenians. Stalin's purge of 8 million during the 1930s.
The dropping of the atomic bomb on Hiroshima and Nagasaki.
The allied bombings of Dresden and Leipzig. The extermination
of a large part of Cambodia by the Pol Pot regime in the 1970s.
The Ibos in northern Nigeria. The massacre at MyLai. Among
many others.*

Becker says that evil rests on the passionate personal motive
to perpetuate oneself, and for each individual this is literally a

---

*Recent events in Somalia, Rwanda, and quite possibly Haiti can now be added to this list.

life and death matter for which no sacrifice is too great, provided that the leader and the group approve of it. He says that it is a paradox that *evil comes from man's urge to heroic victory over evil.*

Whatever side of heroism we look at, one thing is certain: It is an all-consuming activity to make the world conform to our desires. And as far as means are concerned, we are all equally insignificant and impotent animals trying to coerce the universe, trying to make the world over to our own urges.

In other words, it is evil for someone to want to kill me and just as evil for me to defend myself, because I can only defend myself by destroying someone or something else.

Perhaps this is why evil is a concept no one talks about much anymore. It's a no-win situation, for either side.

So all any humanist or theologian or academic can possibly advise in conclusion is: Put your trust in God.

And so our enemies, the bigots who claim I am sick because I am homosexual and in so claiming—through their control of the political and hence medical agendas of this country and this world—have actually and in fact contributed to making me sick.

As Kant said, "From the crooked wood of which man is made, nothing quite straight can be built."

■ ■ ■

I recently reread all my written AIDS rhetoric, all the shit I've written and delivered since the beginning, and I noted sadly, as I knew I would, that everything I wrote and delivered in 1981 and 1982 and 1983 and 1984 and 1985 and 1986 and 1987 and 1988 and 1989 and 1990 and 1991 and 1992 and 1993 would be just as suitable for me to deliver today. And I wonder why I keep getting invited to make more speeches. I have no more brilliant ideas. I only had one idea anyway: Fight Back.

Well, people don't fight back. Over the years I've written endless analyses and investigations into why it might be so, that people don't fight back. I was trying to understand it, you see. Just like I'm trying to understand what evil really is and why no one except me thinks evil is going on in the here and now. I gave up trying to make sense of why people don't fight back. I couldn't, I can't, and I never will make sense of it. So it's no longer relevant to me why they don't. They just don't. People, even dying people, even threatened people, even people walking straight into gas chambers seem to be comfortable and content to be lambs or pigs or whichever sacrificial animal metaphor you choose.

Academics—the historians and theologians and sociologists and psychiatrists and epidemiologists—have investigated and probed and researched and posited any number of reasons why people don't fight back and why evil exists in the world and have even come up with a few reasons that are convincing. But then— so what? After I understand, then what? What's changed? No- body listens. Nobody changes anything. No new insight stops the situation from happening. The boy kills, either himself or another, because (1) he hates his mother, (2) he hates his father, (3) he hates his mother and father, (4) he hates himself, (5) he hates society, (6) he hates the white man, (7) he hates the black man, (8) he is economically disadvantaged, (9) he cannot read, (10) he is hungry (11) he is in some way genetically deficient. So what? The *thing* still exists. He or his brother will kill again. We are smarter for all our knowledge and we are braver for trying to get others to listen or understand, but the *thing* still exists and progress doesn't get made—in fact matters get worse—and more deaths of whomever or whatever still continue, so isn't one simply forced to say, So what has theorizing gained us?

That's a little how I feel. I don't want to analyze any longer why people don't fight back. Why people don't fight back against evil. Why people don't fight back against evil which they won't define as evil because we can't find a definition of evil anymore that includes anything that is happening to us but which we all know is evil. They don't and I am ashamed of them and of this fact.

So what?

I have lived through twelve years of horror and death. We all have. But have we all *thought* about it? Most of us live through it and have learned to accept it, without thinking about it. This is the way of the world, we seem to say. It happens.

It does not just happen!

Evil has brought us here. The evil of centuries, the evil of angry gods, the evil of devils, the evil of inattentiveness and disdain, the evil of passivity and cowardice.

But these, too, are only words, condemnations thrown against a howling wind that only blows and cannot listen.

So what?

How can I not sound crazy to you? How can I make my arguments in ways acceptable to the rigorous rules that govern the institution that owns the stage on which I stand?

By the time of his last piano sonata, the 32nd, Beethoven, they say, was deaf. If I tell you Beethoven could hear, what proof have I? Only the music. The piercing overlay of soprano notes that cut through the earth of bass. Yes, Beethoven made himself hear.

He made himself hear!

We have made so many excuses for why we do the things we do. Why we are sinned against. Why we are murdered and abused and insulted by others. But no matter what the excuse, and there are many, and these many are filled with truths— excuses have an annoying characteristic of often being truthful— I do not wish to die because of the psychologizing by the latest exponent of some this-must-let-them-off-the-hook theory. If I am going to be murdered, I want my murderer identified, excoriated, publicized, and punished by one or another, if only by exposure.

I certainly do not want my murderer excused, pardoned, forgiven, redeemed, or—as is now the status quo—ignored— not even named.

If we have no concept of evil, then my murderer is excused, pardoned, forgiven, ignored, overlooked, or—as is certainly true in the case of homophobia and the ignoring of the AIDS plague (and you will forgive me for combining them)—able to get away with it scot-free and unreported upon.

No, I insist that it is imperative to have the concept of evil returned into currency. Even if we must print the money ourselves. I insist on naming the evildoers, and if you read my writing or have heard me speak you will see that I have done just that.

■ ■ ■

As with syphilis, the AIDS war, from the very beginning, has not been waged between science and disease, but between those who seek to preserve AIDS as a scourge on sinners and those who seek its cure. Never before, not even with syphilis, have medicine and moralizing been so closely entwined. And this entwining comes, ironically and peculiarly enough, at a time, historically, of great *moral indifference*. Scandals in politics, business, government occur with such remarkable and continuing rapidity, going for the most part unpunished or unchastized—indeed most likely being rewarded by lionizing media coverage—that the citizenry, already filled with disillusionment that their elected officials can bring them little in the way of progress or relief from their various social and economic and very real miseries, is a silent citizenry. The sense that "there is nothing I can do" is ripe and rife in the land. Abdication of what once was considered genuine responsibility is endemic and epidemic.

We must never forget that, as Hannah Arendt has warned us—and because this analogy is so overworked, I believe it is easily forgotten—the Nazi holocaust could not have happened without the complicity of countless others who did not care or did not know what was being done to the Jews. In his remarkable book, *How Holocausts Happen*, published by Temple University Press, Professor Douglas V. Porpora points dramatically to

> a similar moral indifference to the suffering of others on the part of contemporary Americans. . . . When the citizens of a democracy fail to hold their government to account, they become complicit in whatever crimes that government commits and share in its guilt. If . . . the prinicipal lesson of the Holocaust is that we must assume responsibility for the behavior of the governments that rule us, it follows that we must necessarily also assume *responsibility for being informed* about the behavior of those governments, the validity of the justifications those governments provide for their behavior. This responsibility is a never-ending task.
>
> Intellectual reflection holds little interest for the majority of United States citizens, who tend to accept uncritically whatever beliefs have been handed to them. . . . People have a very difficult time challenging authority. . . . In fact, we tend to believe that it is actually illegitimate for us to disobey authority.

For genocide to occur, more is needed than just government bureaucrats willing to obey any order. A genocidal government must have the compliance of its public as well, for if the public outcry is sufficient, the government will be unable to carry on. . . . Genocide is a crime an entire society commits.

There will be no public outcry if the public either approves of what its government is doing or is terrorized into silence. But the disturbing fact is that neither of these conditions is necessary for the public outcry against genocide to be absent. It is sufficient that the public be indifferent about what is happening. And that is true all too often.

When a government is involved in genocide, its actions will usually be ambiguous to most of its citizens. . . . When the victims are remote, the citizens can generally have no first-hand knowledge about their fate. The citizens then become largely reliant on secondary sources of information such as the media, which may well present a biased picture. The further away the victims are, the less of an obligation they present. The citizenry is less apt to care about them as real people. Instead of being perceived as real human suffering, the victimization of remote people takes on the character of abstract statistics. There is little that can be done to counteract the stereotypes the government presents. The religious admonition to love one's neighbor applies only to one's primary group. . . . A state of pluralistic ignorance tends to prevail. People look around and see that their fellow citizens are not reacting to what is happening. This reinforces their conviction that there is nothing to be concerned about. Their own consequent lack of reaction in turn reinforces the same conviction in everyone else.

I have said all this before, ad nauseum, in my own words. I thought that because this is a university, I would use the words of an academic—that perhaps these would prove more rigorous and hence more acceptable to you than my own.

■ ■ ■

For those of you who have heard me speak before, or read my books, or seen my plays, I think you will agree that—save for raising the level of my pitch to respond to evil—I have said nothing new to you tonight. I have made versions of this speech and voiced companions to these thoughts over and over and over again until I am blue in the face and parched in the mouth. I have nothing new to say to you because there is nothing new to say, to you or anyone else, and you—or those who sat in your seat before you—have heard me say these words and voice these thoughts. And I can only wonder, If you or they had listened to me, would I have to be making this speech again tonight?

I'd always hoped my words would make a difference, that anybody who was telling the truth would and could make a difference. I've learned otherwise. I've learned that people can be left to die, quite intentionally, in this country of ours. Many different kinds of people. I've learned that democracy does not protect one and all. I have learned that democracy is a sham. I have learned that democracy protects only the straight white man with the money and the power to demand that he be protected. I have learned that everybody else is pretty much left to die.

But then you must know all this. Do you know all this? In your heart and soul, do you know all this? I mean—you do know all this, don't you? If you do not, then this university of yours, my alma mater, is not doing a very good job.

How comfortable we all have become with mass death, with the concept of holocausts and genocide.

I am not going to conclude these remarks with a recital of all the latest figures and case numbers and infections per second and deaths per moment. I always used to include all that, to truly underline the extent of the evil that is being successfully accomplished—facts, figures, how many infected, dying, dead. No more. I'm also no longer going to give you specific chapter and verse on what this lily-livered President and his hard-as-nails wife and their administration filled with all shadow and no substance are not doing. I did all that—again ad nauseum—in all my other speeches about two other Presidents who were also phenomenal cowards married to bitches on wheels. Nobody listened to them anyway. I gave those speeches and I guess a lot of people heard them, but nobody listened. You didn't listen to them. But then you're younger and perhaps you just weren't around.

I only say one thing in my speeches now. I say it over and over and over wherever I can and to whomever will listen or interview me or put my loud unpleasant presence on TV, and after I die I hope some historian will write a book and say: Somebody said it, when it had to be said, Larry said it. Even if nobody listens to me, I'll rest easier knowing that I said it over and over and over again, and even if everybody else in the entire world is a stupid dumb fuck asshole, I'll know I wasn't.

This is what I say. AIDS is intentional genocide. It is intentional. It is intentional. It is intentional genocide and I know with all my heart and soul that it is intentional and I am not going to spend any more time giving you chapter and verse on the whys and the wherefores. Read my book, and while you're at it ask yourself how come you are in the auditorium of one of the world's greatest universities in the THIRTEENTH YEAR of a **PLAGUE** and how is it that this creep Kramer can make exactly the same speech now as I could make thirteen years ago because nothing has changed except the inexorable toll of infection and death, and the third asshole President in a row is **sanctioning** intentional genocide.

AIDS is intentional genocide. AIDS is intentional genocide. AIDS is intentional genocide. AIDS is intentional genocide. AIDS is intentional genocide. AIDS is intentional genocide and I know with all my heart and soul that it is intentional and I am going to say it over and over and over until I die and I may go to my death with all of you thinking I am crazy but I am going to go to my death knowing that I spoke the truth and I spoke it every single day of this plague and I spoke it over and over and over again.

Another thing. What is going on and around and won't stop, this thing that is going around called AIDS that won't stop, is a **PLAGUE!** When is everyone going to get that through their thick stupid unaccepting brains? Why do you call it an epidemic? An epidemic is three or four cases of something that wasn't there last week. Maybe a couple hundred at the most. After that, it's a **PLAGUE.** Why is this essential truth denied? Why do you have to sugar coat? *WHY CAN'T YOU FACE THE TRUTH!*

***WHY DO YOU HAVE TO FUDGE THE FACTS?* Why can't you call a plague a plague?**

ONE BILLION PEOPLE ARE GOING TO DIE FROM AIDS. The figure is not mine but Harvard's.* Everyone believes everything else that comes out of Harvard. Since the beginning of education, everyone in the world has always believed Harvard as if she were Mary, the Mother of God. So why doesn't everyone believe this? Why doesn't that wrectched wimp in the White House believe this? **ONE BILLION PEOPLE ARE GOING TO DIE FROM AIDS.**

Why don't you believe me when I tell you that intentional genocide is going on and why don't you believe Harvard when they say one billion people are going to die from AIDS and why don't you believe me when I say that the research for a cure is not being done? I don't care what you read in the wretched *New York Times* or what you see on homogenized CNN or the vapid "MacNeil-Lehrer" or what two-faced government liars who say they are doctors tell you, **the research to find a cure for AIDS is not being done.**

For genocide to happen, you need more than just *government* bureaucrats willing to obey any order. A genocidal government must have the compliance of the public as well, for if the public outcry is loud enough, the government wouldn't be able to carry on.

Genocide is a crime an entire society commits. Genocide is a crime an entire society commits. Genocide is a crime an entire society commits. Genocide is a crime an entire society commits.

AIDS is the most evil act perpetrated on minorities by the straight white man since the introduction of slavery into our country.

How long are you going to let your President get away with murder? He's a worse murderer than you are, but the difference between his kind of murder and yours is that his is deliberate and conscious. He knows what he's doing. And he knows you are good little boys and girls who are afraid of him or are too busy

---

*As I've mentioned this figure was put forth by Dr. William Haseltine in a piece he wrote for *The New York Times* op-ed page. Dr. Haseltine was then at Harvard; he is now in Washington, as one of the heads of the National Genome Project.

elsewhere to be bothered to get the facts, so, in the end, you do and believe what you're told. That is how the white master subjugates his slaves!

How many people have to be buried before a society can feel a *responsibility* for ending a plague? How many people have to die before you can feel **responsibility** for ending this plague? How many? Give me a number! **ONE BILLION PEOPLE ARE GOING TO DIE FROM AIDS.** Do you, as a member of a community of liberal and caring and thinking people, accept that a plague can be going on and you are doing nothing to stop it?

I have come here on the useless mission of trying to make you understand that something evil is going on. I have come here to try to define what evil is and what evil is around us and what evil you are participating in and colluding with. I have also come here to say something that has been growing inside of me for years, gnawing at me because I haven't had the guts to say it out loud. I have come to hate almost everyone I know. People who think they're so fucking okay they're at Yale or they're on the right career track or they've got their future taped or they're white and the world is white, and though they would never say this out loud they think it, boy do they think it. And people like your parents, most of whom are in my generation. No, hate is not too strong a word. I condemn all of you for your hypocrisy and your silence. If you are gay, you know better than anybody in the world how awful this plague is and that everything I am saying is true and that an evil of terrifying proportions is consuming your past and your future. If you are straight, you know as well as anybody in the world how awful this plague is and that everything I am saying is true and that one of these days this evil of terrifying proportions is—one way or another—going to gobble up you and yours, too. Yes, I hate all of you for what you don't do and see.

Where, among you, are the equivalent of the Gentiles who risked their lives in Nazi-occupied Germany and Holland and Denmark and Sweden to save the lives of Jews, not to bury them?

Where, among you, are the students of Tienanmen Square?

Where, among you, are our *heroes*?

Where, among you, are those who are willing to fight fights when you don't want to fight fights?

Who, among you, are those who will force yourself to hear?

I used to wind up my speeches by giving long lists of suggestions. What to do. How to do it. I'm not going to do that anymore. Figure it out for yourself. Take some responsibility and figure it out for yourself.

And if I hate you for these things, think how much I hate myself even more because in thirteen years I have not changed one goddamned thing.

When I finished speaking, I found myself running quickly out a side door. Yes, they were clapping wildly, giving me a standing ovation; I didn't want to ask them why they were doing that—how could they be doing that?—and I didn't want them to see my tears of despair. In Albany only days before, I'd delivered an even angrier and more confrontational harangue, to a conference of AIDS health-care providers, screaming at them that all they were doing was helping people die and when were they going to start fighting to help people live. This was followed by that *Advocate* column, "After Seeing *Schindler's List*," in which I unequivocally compared GMHC to Dachau and APLA to Auschwitz.

The fury and the anger are erupting into a pretty constant stream of molten rage these days. And more and more, I find myself refocusing my discussions and arguments and thoughts in terms of "evil." I am certain that what is being perpetrated upon us is true genocide, but beyond that—if there can be a beyond that—is the hand of genuine and palpable evil.

In all my life, I never thought about evil. Now I can't stop thinking about it.

As I've said more than once, it's been exceedingly depressing assembling these additions for this new edition, rereading all I've said for so long. It's actually made me physically ill to my stomach. I want to throw up or fart or shit or something *physical* to void my insides of all this bile that gets spewed in order to keep my sanity in a world run by people far crazier than I. This task, of re-reading and selecting and editing and writing these connecting passages, has taken far longer than it should have. I can't bring myself to the computer each day without depression and this physical discomfort. "And here's *another* one that didn't work."

I realize it's been a pretty depressing journey from the hopeful fury at the beginning of this book to the hopeless despondency at its end. It's hard to see where any successes were achieved, where there were any causes for celebration. This is a pretty grim note to end on.

I spend a lot of time reflecting on these past years. Asking myself questions like: What did I do wrong? Why didn't we get further? Why weren't we more united? What made the two organizations into which I poured so much of myself go sour—neither in any significant way changing the horrific and tragic course of this plague? Should I start another organization? How many times can I write/deliver the same speech/article/diatribe? What do I do next? Where do we go from here?

As far as AIDS is concerned, we have another asshole in the White House. The NIH is, more than ever, an $11-billion-a-year cesspool. And all the bureaucrats may have new faces, but their pollsters have brainwashed them with the same message: AIDS is not a high agenda item.

It's hard not to face the fact that I failed as an AIDS activist.

I am compelled to say I don't know where to go.

Maybe that's the wretched message I should leave you with.

My body is now beginning to give me the signs. Falling T-cells, of course. Skin eruptions. An endless cough no one can find the reason for. Something called ITP, wherein my platelets fall so low I haven't enough of them to clot my blood. I'm on the demon AZT.

So my personal roller coaster ride appears to be commencing. The one I've witnessed happening to so many of my friends. What's coming next? Depending what time of the day or night it is, I'm often frightened. I don't want to die. I still have too much work to do. Too much yet to write.

More than anything, I now have David. Now that I have a friend in my life again and we're happy, I don't want to leave him. We're even remodeling an old barn in the country, overlooking a lake—the dream house I've always longed for, to share with someone I care about. Will I be around long enough to witness some exciting new discovery that will save my life and the lives of so many others? Every day I hear bits and pieces of information from around the globe. Will a few of these coalesce into a cure? Or at least a treatment that will keep us going until another treatment . . . ? The perennial question we all ask—How much time do I have left?—is now joined by new questions: How much time free from the mess and pain that is AIDS do I have left? Do I dare stop screaming? If I don't continue the fight every single second, does that mean death will come? Am I on the verge of finding out?

Have I lost all faith in political activism, either grass roots, organized, or individual? If I were younger and healthier, would I try again?

Could *anything* have worked out and made matters any different?

To quote Hannah Arendt on the Jewish Holocaust: *"This ought not to have happened."* I shall go to my grave convinced this plague of AIDS need not have happened, and that once it started it could have been quickly ended.

But perhaps the satisfaction of a plague-less land is never meant to exist on this earth, for anyone. And perhaps it is part of everyone's journey to try to reach—however unsuccessfully—a promised land. The journey, not the arrival, matters, as has been said since the beginning of philosophy, and I cannot deny that my journey—however far from my goals I still remain—has left me feeling most well-used by the events my times have pressed upon me. Arendt talks about "the venture into the public realm," by which she means "that [in this arena] in every action the person is expressed as in no other human activity. . . . We start something. We weave our strand into a network of relations. What comes of it we never know . . . because one *cannot* know."

So perhaps these many reports from the holocaust will not turn out to be as worthless as I often feel they are. Perhaps they will have started something—somewhere, at some time, of which I may never know.

I've discovered something interesting as I speak at schools around the country. I've discovered I'm often invited to speak, not because I'm gay or talk about AIDS, but *because I am angry.* Kids today—particularly kids of color—seem almost desperate to know how I do what I do, how I turn my anger into something productive, how I can even make a living from it. At a few of the schools I've gone to, I've been so grilled for details about how I write, how I choose my arguments and my targets, how I fashion all this into a speech, that sometimes I never even get to give the speech I was invited there to make. It's exciting to see this, when it happens. It's exciting for me to discover that this book itself is used as a text in many schools, as are my plays. I think this pleases me more than anything. To be used as a text in schools!

As a kid, my father always called me a "sissy." I've learned these past years many times over that I'm not. But as a kid, you believe fights are fought to be won. I guess the last lesson I've learned as an AIDS activist, and the hardest one to learn, is that fights are never won. They just go on and on. They *are.* And yet they must be fought. They must, still, continually, and forever, be fought. Over and over and over, they must be fought.

Of course I'm not stopping my AIDS activism. It may have taught me that I no longer believe in my country, or my President, or my government, or in democracy itself. But it's taught me to believe in myself. And perhaps, in the end, that's what activism, and life, can only be about, its essence and its core.

I'll think of ways to continue to raise hell.